Art Therapy Education

Art Therapy Education:

Teaching, Training, and Research

Edited by

Tami Yaguri and Dalia Merari

Cambridge Scholars Publishing

Art Therapy Education: Teaching, Training, and Research

Edited by Tami Yaguri and Dalia Merari

This book first published 2021

Cambridge Scholars Publishing

Lady Stephenson Library, Newcastle upon Tyne, NE6 2PA, UK

British Library Cataloguing in Publication Data
A catalogue record for this book is available from the British Library

ISBN (10): 1-5275-7500-4
ISBN (13): 978-1-5275-7500-4

CONTENTS

Part II: Training

Part III: Research

INTRODUCTION

DALIA MERARI AND TAMI YAGURI

Faculty members of the Academic College of Society and the Arts in Israel wrote this book. In recent years, teachers from three programs – Visual Art Therapy, Dance/Movement Therapy, and Psychodrama Therapy – met on a monthly basis to discuss teaching and research-related issues. This volume is a result of the belief that it would be a good idea to put on paper the knowledge and insights discussed in these meetings, sharing them with a broader audience.

The faculty members at the College combine clinical work with academic teaching. The chapters of this volume reflect their extensive experience and vast knowledge. Each one of the writers has developed teaching methods and models that constitute the cornerstones of the College's curriculum. Similar to other clinical professions, art therapy as a profession began in the clinic rather than in the halls of academia, and slowly established itself as an academic field. The founding scholars – notably Margaret Naumburg, Edith Kramer, Elinor Ulman, Harriet Wadeson, in the United States and Adrian Hill, Edward Adamson and Rita Simon in the United Kingdome – started publishing their clinical experiences and organized them in theoretical frameworks. This formed the basis for art therapy as an academic discipline.

Art therapy is a young discipline. The first art therapy graduate programs in the U.S. were launched in the late 1960s – early 1970s. Only in 1973 did the American Art Therapy Association issue the first guidelines for art therapy training programs (Junge, 2010; Leigh, 2021). All clinical and academic disciplines are constantly changing and developing. However, as a young discipline, still in its formative years, this endless process is more conspicuous in art therapy than in older professions.

In a recently published editorial in a special issue on education of *Art Therapy*, a journal of the American Art Therapy Association, Editor in Chief, Jordan Potash, wrote:

> In the 20 plus years since I first stepped into an art therapy classroom as a student, much has changed. Programs require many more credits, educational requirements are more uniform, and classes that were once electives are now mandatory – such as social and cultural diversity. (2021, p. 3).

In Israel, as in the U.S. and U.K., academic teaching of art therapy started in the 1970s. Initially, our College, the Academic College of Society and Arts, which started as an extension of Lesley College of Cambridge, MA., was the only institution that offered a formal academic Master's degree in art therapy in Israel. In recent years, the number of academic institutions offering study programs in art therapy has markedly grown.

The curriculum of academic instruction in art therapy in Israel is dictated by the Council for Higher Education, which – as with any other field of science – places emphasis on the acquisition and organization of knowledge. The range of courses offered in academic studies shows that most focus on the transmission of information, be these professions pertaining to behavior and the human environment (such as psychology and sociology) or the cluster of courses related to art therapy. All these emphasize information as a necessary basis for the acquisition of the profession. Information is conveyed through frontal lectures, which require from the student to become a vessel for absorbing information and memorizing it – the ultimate goal being the emission of the same information during the examination, so that the better the student's ability to reproduce the material, the higher the score.

Although it is unquestionable that the formal information component is necessary for the making of art therapists, the informal component of clinical field experience is no less significant. Not only in terms of the effectiveness of teaching, but also since the lecturers constitute a model of the approach to the profession, which they instill in the students, thus developing their professional identity. This experiential component of the curriculum is of critical importance in art therapy education. Moreover, as suggested by Leigh, the unique requirements of art therapy teaching have prompted the development of discipline-specific teaching methods, so as to "teach students how to think, practice, and develop the ethics and values of the art therapy profession." (2021, p. 5).

This book is made up of three parts: Teaching, training and research. The first part focuses on teaching methods and central topics of the curriculum. This part demonstrates the changes that teaching methods in art therapy are undergoing, especially in integrating theoretical information with experiential methods. Studio exercises accompany theoretical courses, and even in the theoretical courses themselves the topics are presented through visual images as much as possible. The second part deals with training, relating to the practicum, workshops and internship periods in art therapy education. Hands-on training accompanies the student throughout the art therapy program of study and later, as a starting therapist. Teachers at the College have developed unique training methods. Training in the campus is done in a group setting, combined with art making.

The third part deals with research related to art therapy teaching. For a long time, the scarcity of research in art therapy has been a source of concern for leaders in the field. More than two decades ago, the American Art Therapy Association (AATA) formed an Art Therapy Research Initiative, in an effort to promote research in the field (Deaver, 2002). The progress that has been made over the years still leaves much to be desired. More recently, Kapitan (2012) and Leigh (2021) have pointed out that little research has been conducted on art therapy education. A survey of the literature conducted by Leigh (2021) showed that between 1980 and 2016 only 48 articles on art therapy education were published in peer-reviewed journals.

Moon and Hoffman (2014) suggested that the unique characteristics of art therapy education call for a different type of research than the form customary in social sciences. These characteristics are demonstrated in this book as a whole. Similarly to the global trend, in Israel the process of academization has boosted the recognition of the importance of research in art therapy, which has been expressed in an increase in academic publications in professional journals in recent years. This development has been prompted by the formal academic requirements of writing theses as part of the master and doctoral programs and the concomitant research-related courses that have become an integral part of the teaching curriculum.

*

The authors of the following essays share their professional experience in three areas: teaching, training and research. The first part contains seven chapters on *teaching* art therapy in multicultural classes. This includes introducing future therapists to a digital world; using visually centered method with cognitive theory; introducing life-story into art-therapy; teaching around sickness and death of classmates; theoretical polyphony and psychodrama training; integration of Dionysian and Apollonian modes by dance movement therapy students.

Hilla Haelyon and **Rachel Hillel-Avraham** use body-identity-emotion model in art therapy multicultural classes. Israeli academies become multicultural. In such a learning environment, teachers and facilitators face unique challenges, enhanced against the background of the Jewish-Arab conflict. Creative teaching methods that combine an original model contribute to a positive learning atmosphere, imparting values and attaining academic goals.

Daphna Liber focuses on art therapy in a digital world, where realities in the hybrid clinic are mixed. Her hybrid approach considers the integration of digital dimensions with the aspects of art therapy methods. The world of expressive art therapy faces the challenges of a digital age. For this hybrid combination art therapists must be aware of distinctions between "Digital Natives" and "Digital Immigrants." The uniqueness of the current generation gap influences a concept of identity and their attitudes towards digital ecology. A tool is presented for identifying the personal position of each therapist in relation to the digital world entry into the art therapy room.

Janice Shapiro and **Elana Lakh** present a method of teaching art therapy theory that integrates the creative imagery with the cognitive aspect of theory. The method is based on dual coding mode and on experiential learning which are integral to art therapy teaching. Active art making by the participants in response to the theory, forms an inherent part of their lecture structure, in a way that contributes to internalization of the material taught. Didactic curation of response imagery is demonstrated.

Amia Lieblich presents an original use of 'life story' in workshops for art-therapists. The workshop includes three elements: theory of narratives of life stories, experience in writing and interviews as a means for obtaining life stories, and the expression of these stories in various art modalities.

Michal Lev, **Aya Kats** and **Gili Navoth** ask how creative-oriented teaching meets with sickness and death in art-therapy graduate studies. Their art-based pedagogy proposes a creative space within mental health graduate programs for personal processing and group resonance as sources of knowledge.

Tsiky Cohen focuses on the importance of theoretical polyphony in training psychodrama therapists. He explores humanistic-existentialist philosophy in the field of psychodrama, and demonstrates how this philosophy alerts psychodramatists to psychic content. He suggests that apart from the typical contribution of Moreno's theory to psychodramatic work, it is important that psychodrama therapists hold a position of theoretical polyphony in their work. This enables them to remain sensitive to various emotional textures and hues moving parallel to one another, without needing to set up a hierarchy among them.

Hilda Wengrower implements Nietzsche's terms of the Apollonian and the Dionysian in the worlds of the performing arts and in science. She introduces these terms in order to look at the training of arts therapists and especially the dance movement therapists. The Apollonian and the Dionysian allow for holistic perception and thinking of the artistic experience and the training process of arts therapists.

The second part of this book contains four chapters on *training.* It discusses the open art therapy studio, a group supervision model that turns therapy and group supervision into a creative experience, an experiential teaching of an art-based training. The training of art therapists is conducted in workshops and internships.

Debra Kalmanowitz and **Janice Shapiro** explore an approach to teaching the open art studio from the perspective of the therapist/teacher. The use of structured, directed reflection following an open art studio process is described with an emphasis on the importance of timing. The significance of the open studio in art therapy trainings is explored. In addition, some broader implications for the advances of the profession and the challenges of academization are considered.

Yonathan Schur and **Lior Schur** formulate and demonstrate a new term: "Mutual Visual Transference." This describes a group supervision model in art therapy. The model's premise is that the patient's artwork seeks to visually "tell a story." Art therapists are invited to an "active reading" through their own work with art materials. Gathering all the artistic responses created in the group reveals a multi-layered picture of the patient.

Reuma Weinberg and **Ronit Amir** present an original term "co ∞ figuration field." It illustrates how the daunting place of not knowing, in therapy and group supervision, may become a creative and inviting experience for both client and therapist. The connections woven between the artwork, the therapist, the client and group supervision, have the potential of being transformed into a dynamic field that facilitates a variety of meanings, realizations, and embodiments of the therapeutic process.

Liat Shamri-Zeevi and **Anat Gilad** describe an innovative ABPT course developed at the Academic College of Society and the Arts. The course is designed to integrate a theoretical-psychotherapeutic body of knowledge and hands-on experience in art-based interventions that can be applied in parental training. The combination of the theoretical and the practical serves to expand the students' therapeutic repertoire, and allows them to make use of the techniques they learn in the course when working with parents in the clinic. This leads to a better, deeper relationship with parents, and by extension with the child they treat in art therapy.

The third part contains five chapters on *research* related to art therapy teaching. It holds research on creativity, intimacy, multiculturalism, 'mushiness,' and applied neuroscience insights to the field of creative arts therapy. Each of the chapters shows unique characteristics of art therapy education that requires unique type of research.

Dalia Merari reviews several theories of creativity and discusses their relevance to teaching art therapy. The second part of the chapter describes a survey, conducted among teachers of art therapy at the Academic College of Society and Arts, designed to examine the lecturers' perceptions of creativity in teaching art therapy, and to assess the concordance of these perceptions with the theoretical notions of creativity. The impact of external stressful constraints, such as those induced by the Covid-19 pandemic, forces the development of creative teaching methods.

Michal Lev explores intrapersonal intimacy through painting, witnessing, and video footage editing. She discusses operational elements of intimacy, the conditions that favor or hinder intimacy, and unique features of artistic media that further intimate experience. Her art-based research process demonstrates six modes of inquiry as interdependent elements: drawing and painting by the co-researchers in three experimental sessions witnessed by the researcher; reflective discussions with co-researchers; artistic responses by the researcher; a private exhibition; editing of video footage and creation of edited videos; and culminating discussions and review with the participant co-researchers.

Noga Ariel-Galor focuses on the experience of teaching a seminar on multicultural art-based research. Guidelines for preparing researchers to engage in such inquiries are discussed, as well as possible sensitivities stemming from the class being multicultural itself. Moreover, considerations regarding teaching art analysis for research are reviewed and applied to a multicultural research context. The learning process and the structure of the class is elaborated, and some final conclusions regarding art analysis from a multicultural perspective are suggested.

Elana Lakh and **Shevy Medzini** introduce the concept of 'mushiness' from clinical experience. 'Mushiness,' the mental quality of shapelessness, liquidity and undifferentiating, affects primal areas of the psyche, and is elicited when working with wet, liquid and slimy materials. Mushiness is based on touch and sensory experience, and is related to the emotional experiences linked to internalized primary object relations. The model distinguishes developmental mushiness, which exists before diffrerentiation is achieved, from traumatic mushiness, which derives from the disintegration of differentiation into a repetitive petrifying experience of loss of meaning.

Sharon Vaisvaser discusses fundamental aspects of brain dynamics and ways to assimilate and apply this knowledge in Creative Arts Therapies (CATs) education. Neuroscience insights are discussed from several angles; an embodied account of brain function; sensory-motor architecture and processing; affectivity and emotion regulation; dynamics of the self and the empathic relationship; aesthetic engagement and creativity; finally converging into the neuroplastic moulding of the brain. The grounding of CATs profession in evidence-based neuroscientific principles may enable deeper and expanded intra- and inter-psychic understanding.

References

Deaver, Sarah (2002) "What Constitutes Art Therapy Research?" *Art Therapy* 19(1), 23-27

Junge, Maxine Borowsky (2010) *The Modern History of Art Therapy in the United States*. Springfield, IL: Charles C Thomas.

Kapitan, Lynn (2012) "Educating the Future Practitioner of Art Therapy" *Art Therapy* 29(4), 148-149.

Leigh, Heather (2021) "Signature Pedagogies for Art Therapy Education: A Delphi Study" *Art Therapy* 38(1), 3-4.

Moon, Bruce and Nadia Hoffman (2014) "Performing Art-Based Research: Innovation in Graduate Art Therapy Education" *Art Therapy* 31(4), 172-178.

Potash, Jordan (2021) "Special Issue on Art Therapy Education" *Art Therapy* 38(1), 5-12.

PART I:

TEACHING

CHAPTER 1

THE CHALLENGE OF MULTICULTURAL CLASSES: INTEGRATING ARTISTIC WORK USING THE BODY-IDENTITY-EMOTION MODEL

HILLA HAELYON
AND RACHEL HILLEL-AVRAHAM

Theoretical review

The academic debate over the past decade has been characterized by an increasing demand to call attention and resources to the study of multicultural learning spaces (Verkuyten & Thijas, 2014). Despite the worldwide acknowledgement that the education system must turn its attention to the handling of multicultural learning spaces, there are still no international guidelines or programs for the world's education system (Verkuyten & Thijas, 2014; Harington & Gelfand, 2015; Flevian, 2017; Kess, 2012). Most of the world's schools implement individual strategies that suit the local educational agenda. Moreover, they define only narrowly the means for handling the issue of multiculturalism.

The State of Israel may be an interesting case study for discussion of multicultural learning spaces. Israel is considered as a Western country sustaining multicultural diversity (Friedman, 2018). This variety has been apparent in recent years in Israeli academic life and in the classroom. The classes constitute a microcosm of the cultural diversity existing in Israeli society. During the past decade, classes contain students from a variety of ethnic backgrounds: Jews, Arabs, Bedouin, Druze, some religious and others secular. Some scholars (Berry, 2016; Haelyon, Rahimi, & Cohen Liverant, 2018) argue that in order for a learning space to be considered multicultural, three conditions must apply. The first one is the presence of varied cultural groups; the second is an appropriate representation of each of the cultures in all areas; and the third is the existence of a social ideology that promotes multiculturalism in society. These three features are a socio-political declaration relating to the structure of society and expressed in all areas of life.

Indeed, during the first decade of the 21st century, many articles have been written about multiculturalism in the Israeli education system (Gladi, 2009; Yogev, 2001; Yonah, 2007; Sever, 2001; Perry, 2007). The central argument accompanying academic study in this area was that Israeli society must recognize the cultural baggage of all the groups and integrate it, or at least parts of it, into its canonical culture. Gladi (2009) claims that the demographic and ethnic reality necessitates the definition of a cultural identity that represents the range of heritages composing the fabric of Israeli society. She argues that multi-culturalism reflects society's true structure, and should not be suppressed but directed to creative channels that will enrich Israeli cultural life – since Israel has to face its demographic and social reality.

The Israeli case aligns with the international globalization processes that impact many areas of life. Studies from around the world indicate that one of the most prominent influences in study spaces is the increase in ethnic and cultural diversity in many parts of the world (Tabory, 2007; Tabory & Sasson, 2010). The buzzwords in the multicultural discourse are: "social climate", providing an appropriate response for minorities (Civitillo et al., 2017; Sam & Phinney, 2012), and "cultural sensitivity" (Cho & De Castro-Ambrosetti, 2005). A study by Haelyon, Rahimi, and Cohen-Liverant (2018) even argues that despite the increasing awareness of issues of ethnic diversity and the need for cultural sensitivity in classrooms, teachers still do not know which situations might arise in the class, and more importantly, how to handle them. Possible situations include: embarrassment, silencing a particular group, opposition and struggle, and so on. According to Haelyon, Rahimi, and Cohen-Liverant (2019), unlike facilitators of conflict groups, who undergo special training for handling complex situations resulting from diversity, such training for teachers is partial, and in Israel completely non-existent.

Multicultural classrooms are an arena for a struggle about definitions, meanings, and interpretations. Frequently, the interpretations and meanings granted to an event have a greater impact than the event itself. Such situations have raised the need for implementing a multicultural policy in schools, and has encouraged researchers to examine the question of the teacher's privilege versus the students. Thus, for example, a study by Cho and DeCastro-Ambrosetti (2005) argued that most of the teachers in the USA are white, belong to the middle class, and have English as their mother tongue. These teachers expressed discomfort and distress from their lack of knowledge about managing challenging situations and handling students coming from different cultures. Streihorn (2010) also classifies multicultural learning spaces as fertile ground for creating cross-cultural misunderstandings, such as: conflict resulting from oversensitivity to one cultural value, while neglecting another value; silencing contents that are important to one culture but opposed in another culture; or culture shock due to behavior acceptable in one culture but condemned in another culture. Also, discussions and conversations about controversial issues in multicultural classrooms can rapidly deteriorate into polarizing arguments related to fixed and essentialist differences between groups, such as "it's genetic and there's nothing we can do", or "that's what it's like with them". This sort of conversation tends to be unfruitful, impolite, and does not promote understanding between participants.

In this study, we shall present a program for applying the body-identity-emotion model in an art education context in multicultural classes at the Ono Campus. The proposed intervention began in 2019-2020 and included three multicultural classes.

Using the material body-identity-emotion model to dismantle otherness in multicultural spaces

This chapter argues that discussion of the political material body is essential for handling multicultural spaces. According to body researchers (Turner, 2012; Hulvey, 2000; Amir-Moazami, 2016; Dolezal, 2015; Criado-Perez, 2019), the material body is the first and central platform for expressing multiculturalism. The body is an active expression, though not usually overt. Thus, for example, skin color, gender, clothing choice (such as a Jewish head covering or a Muslim Hijab), hair styling, and so on, testify to the person's social and cultural location. According to Hillel-Avraham, Haelyon and Rahimi (2020), in Israeli learning spaces, the body expressions appear almost immediately when members of the same sector with their bodily indicators gather into a united group and distinguish themselves from other groups. We have frequently observed classes gathering for the first time, and immediately all the religious female Arab students wearing a Hijab congregate and sit apart from the religious female Jewish students with head coverings. Students of Ethiopian ancestry will usually also gather together and distinguish themselves from other groups in the room. This behavior often lasts an entire semester. In order to handle this dilemma, with awareness of the need to sustain a multicultural learning space, we have created an intervention program based on the body-identity-emotion model (Haelyon, 2007). This model originates in the sociological discourse around the body, connected with the sociological discourse about identity and emotions.

Since the late nineteen-nineties, behavioral science researchers have raised the need to study the body holistically (Grosz, 1994; Gatens, 1996; Shildrick, 1997). The holistic approach aims to replace the concept of the disembodied body with a new term, embodiment. Scholars (Grosz, 1994; Morris, 1993) have argued that the term disembodiment refers to a paralyzed body, a split body, a body discussed by other people, a body shaped and disciplined by social and cultural forces. Many examples, are provided by Turner (2012), from the fields of conventional medicine, anti-ageing medicine, women's health, cosmetic surgery, etc. Elizabeth Grosz's (1994) argued that disembodiment is an expression of a body operated upon by forces from the outside in, and it is merely an obedient receptacle. The need to establish an active internal agency to oppose this external force has encouraged many researchers to seek for the opposite of disembodiment and to propose the "lived body experience model" (Engelsrud, 2005; Wehrle, 2020; Legrand, 2017; Bellerose, 2019; Bullington, 2017; Sheets-Johnstone, 2020).

The lived body is the body that has words, the body that can oppose the disciplining discourse agents. This is a body that creates movement from within itself, makes its own choices, and even refuses to be obedient and subordinate. This new approach proposed replacing the term disembodiment with the term embodiment or embodied body. This discourse was critical to issues relating to women's health and their ability to object to certain medical discourses applied to their bodies, which they did not internalize and obey. The new approach suggested that the feminine inner agency examines the mechanisms of discipline in an enlightened manner of bodily sensations, experiences of pain, embarrassment, and discomfort. The focus on emotions, argued the researchers, is highly relevant and significant in active dialogue with external forces, such as physicians, for example (Haelyon & Gross, 2011; Merari, Shitrit et.al. 1996; Merari, Feldberg et.al 1997).

Haelyon (2007) argues that a truly holistic model must also consider the individual's identity and emotional experience and add this to the bodily experience. The reason for this is the inseparable link between the body and identity. Establishing an individual's identity is also apparent in bodily choices, for example, choosing a religious identity is usually expressed in the body, in choosing particular clothing, hiding or revealing hair, and so on. Similarly, certain bodily choices influence a person's identity. Interestingly, it appears that in the research literature too, scholars of the body and scholars of identity have reached the same conclusion. Scholars of identity have called for the examination of the corporeal self, while scholars of the body have sought to examine embodied subjectivity. It appears that the central drive of these aspects comes from their primacy. The body and the identity are primal elements in the human encounter occurring in the cultural space. Individuals' culture and identity choices are also apparent in their bodily choices, and vice versa. People with a particular skin color or appearance receive a certain social treatment that also later establishes their identity. An important example of this issue is presented in the classical work of Franz Fanon (2008 [1952]) "Black Skin White Masks". When Fanon wrote about the experience of Black people in Western society, he discussed the boundaries of his body in the public space. Similarly, Edward Said (1978) described Lawrence of Arabia referring to the encounter between the body of the desert man and the identity attributed to him.

These works demonstrate what many scholars of the body (Mercedes – Vella, 2015; Nirta, 2015; Strings, 2019) argue, that marginal groups always have bodily presence, while the body of people enjoying social privilege and status is an absent presence.

Another inseparable connection in body-identity relations is the emotional realm. Various emotional states are apparent in the body and influence the person's identity (Lyon, 1997; Haelyon & Gross, 2011; De-Gelder, 2016). Thus, for example, a feeling of embarrassment can be expressed in blushing, or a feeling of great excitement leads to shortness of breath. These relations are also evident in the hurting body, the bodily state of pain, which carries an emotion and constructs the identity of the hurting person. According to Haelyon (2007), holistic body research must include all the three elements, body-identity-emotion, together, due to their primacy and immediate presence in any social space.

We decided to apply the holistic body-identity-emotion model in our work as lecturers in multicultural classes. The assumption was that precisely raising silenced contents that reverberate under the surface would help make the other familiar and enable contact between participants from different groups. Since these contents are not spoken, whether for reasons of political correctness, wishing to avoid falling into the trap of stigma, discomfort in talking about appearance, or other reasons, we found that artistic tools could serve us in bringing these contents into the class space and helping to create contact.

The ethical value of aesthetic education: Art and creativity in the learning space

In (1995), Prof. Yuli (Yael) Tamir, then Israel's Minister of Education, published an anthology including many studies proposing making more active use of artistic tools in teacher training in Israel, and particularly refining the field of art in schools. She argued that in Israel there is a clear distinction between core subjects and accompanying subjects, especially in the preceding decade. This policy almost marginalizes art education. Art education is considered a field of tertiary importance. Primary importance is attributed to core studies, defining the central subjects without which the educational purpose cannot be achieved. Secondary importance is attributed to learning-supporting subjects that help students succeed in the core subjects. Mere tertiary importance is attributed to enrichment studies, including art.

The application of art in schools suffers from several obvious limitations: the shortage of time devoted to art within enrichment studies; low quality art teaching due to employing art teachers as external contractors; and finally, even if there is an "art cluster", as recommended by the Ministry of Education, it only receives two weekly hours per year. These two hours need to include: music, plastic art, theatre, dance, media, cinema, and television. It is clearly impossible to put on a play, to experience a deep creative process, to get to know creative techniques, in just two weekly hours per year. Thus, schools have to choose just one field, as if there is no difference between studying music and studying drama or dance. Any attempt to include more than one field turns the study of art into a sort of empty time slot. The reduced importance attributed to the field leads to the outsourcing and privatization of art studies occurs. Since art studies are not part of the core curriculum, teachers suffer from a loss of employment continuity, which could harm the quality of their teaching. This situation could create a social gap between parents who continue to nurture their children's music studies beyond school hours and others who cannot afford this.

As part of the Israeli effort to put art studies onto the social and educational agenda, several scholars published studies about the ethical value of aesthetic education, both in teacher training and in school implementation. Thus, for example, Frogel (2012) argued that education is supposed to enable people to think while experiencing pleasure achieved through art and creativity. He claimed that aesthetic education enables people to be free of the world of personal experiences in which their existence is measured only by their own focus of pleasure, toward a freer existence where they can express their thoughts. This aesthetic freedom permits learners to think reflectively about reality, honest criticism, and complete human realization. He claims that when we expose young children to art, this exposure can develop their independent comprehension of values, morality, and critical thinking. Finally, Frogel (2012) argues that art contains an interdisciplinary view and therefore we can currently see even high-tech companies investing in creating the product's aesthetic artistic aspect.

Like Frogel, Michaeli (2012) also claims that training learners in art can contribute to empowering their critical judgment and correcting the world. This is because appropriate social protest should include art as a force of observation to create imagination and critical thinking. Education through art trains individuals in society to become more critical and more creative, and to become significant powers to create social change and contact between different groups. Finally, Michaeli argues that the media and digital experiences that surround us lead to powerful attraction to arenas of shallow culture and art, based on the principle of immediate gratification, and our duty as lecturers and educators is to present quality artistic alternatives to the younger generation. We have to expose them to the best works of art in all the variety of their expressions, and to accompany their consumption and nurture their artistic creativity and artistic skills. As he says: "The activity of exposure and creation should not be managed as activity pushed to the bottom of the school food chain… Art education should be part of the fundamental and ongoing core of the education system" (Michaeli 2012: 192). Interestingly, all the advantages of using art listed by the researchers align with the value of "cultural sensitivity," which is so significant in working with multicultural classes.

In the context of these ideas, in 2018, the Ono Academic College opened unique course for teachers using artistic tools. As part of these programs, we worked as lecturers who teach in the program and at the same time we researched the interventions we performed in the field. This project connected the College's educational agenda to that of the Ono Art Company Netanya. This study is based on observations conducted in multicultural classrooms where the body-identity-emotion model was applied using arts. The study's aims were to examine how the body-identity-emotion model, combined with artistic tools, could increase the emotional sensitivity of teaching students and behavioral science students who participated in the courses. And to understand how using the body-identity-emotion model could enable contact between participants from different sectors.

Methodology and research process

This study is an art-based action research. It started in 2018, in teaching multicultural classes that included students from different sectors, genders, ethnic, and religious groups. The courses the students attended were entitled "Education for diversity and multiculturalism" and "Art as an educational tool".

According to Jokela and Huhmarniemi (2019), art-based action research was developed at the University of Lapland's Faculty of Arts, primarily in development projects, where the challenges of peripheral villages, such as population ageing, the isolation of young people, and undeveloped creative-industries and cultural services have been in the background (Hiltunen, 2009; Jokela, Hiltunen & Härkönen, 2015a, 2015b In Jokela & Huhmarniemi, 2019). Long term art-based action research projects are also being conducted on winter art in collaboration with cold climate engineering and tourism (Jokela, 2014) and on cultural sustainability (Härkönen, Huhmarniemi, & Jokela, 2018). Art-based research, is a research strategy that guides the progress of research in the cycles of action research and uses art as a catalyst for development work.

Leavy (2018) suggests that in the background of art-based research, there is a need and objective to develop research to the extent that it produces practical change as well as valid and justified knowledge and understanding related to the production of this change. Leavy (2009) has suggested that while qualitative research is based on verbal expression, art-based research is described with images, sounds, drama, etc. According to Leavy, quantitative research aims for the freedom of values, while qualitative research is based, in principle, on values, and art-based research is political and promotes freedom. Leavy's description is also suitable as the description of art-based action research, where it is typical for this research to be associated with social or environmental politics – more strongly than qualitative research traditionally is. Anttila (2007) describes this paradigm as an interpretation-experiential paradigm, in which objectivity and subjectivity are linked together. Action research-based design research is a cyclical research process based on planned interventions, which aims to solve practical problems and to develop functional theory (Heikkinen, Konttinen, & Häkkinen, 2006). Artist-designers aim to solve the problems of communities and environments by means of communal and interactive methods (Jokela, Hiltunen, & Härkönen, 2015a, 2015b).

Art-based action research usually starts with a place and a community mapping, where the researcher-artist familiarizes with the operating environment and various different methods. The dimensions of the place can be defined as the physical dimensions, subjective experiences, shared narratives, and so forth. The aim of the research is identified and defined on the basis of such multi-level familiarization of the place. An initial research plan can be drafted in interaction with the stakeholder group of the research. Thereafter, the actual research activities begin either on a practice-led basis or with a literature survey. In a literature survey, the researcher familiarizes with what is previously known about the research topic, that is, how other researchers and artists have processed the topics and what knowledge they have gained in similar situations or environments. One of the literature survey's key objectives is to identify the needs of knowledge. In a manner typical of action research, the research questions are reoriented and further specified after each research cycle. Research may also involve side paths and missteps, which are normal in artistic work too. The process is partly intuitive, confusing, and based on experience and tacit knowledge.

In artistic work, the objective and chosen method are usually not very clear at the beginning of the process (Jokela, 2008; Jokela, Hiltunen, & Härkönen, 2015a). Artistic research proceeds intuitively, through trial and error, and leads to unexpected results and surprising insights. The research topic and questions become clearer as the research progresses (Borgdorf, 2009; 2011). It is typical for researchers of artistic and art-based research to even end up in chaos during the research process. Artist-researchers experience a need for space and freedom in order to find their own methods. This may be due to the nature of artistic knowledge and the research questions typical of artistic research (McNiff, 2013). In art-based action research, the artist-researcher does not wander alone, but instead development work is usually carried out in some kind of team or community

In this chapter, we demonstrate how the integration of body-identity-emotion work with artistic tools helped us handle the complexities arising from multicultural learning spaces. Through three cases studies, we demonstrate how we used Art in Action type research and made decisions about using art in real time. We shall also detail the products of the intervention in learning on the micro and macro level. The three cases chosen for analysis are moments we defined as formative learning moments for the class and also for us as lecturers. We should also note that the two lecturers are Jewish, one a religious woman with religious appearance, and the other a secular woman.

Findings

The study's findings are displayed using themes, based on the field work. The themes include the description of events in real time, the choice of artistic intervention, and the conclusions we drew as lecturers. The themes were organized as follows: the first two themes indicate the existence of multiculturalism even within a seemingly homogeneous religious framework. The third theme describes multiculturalism in the encounter that takes place between different religions.

"Permitted and forbidden in the integration of religion and gender": On gender conflict in a Muslim class

The event took place in a class studying education through artistic tools. The lesson's topic was racism, and the lecturer chose sitting in a circle as the setting for learning. The participants included men and women from the Muslim sector, some secular and some religious. Prior to the start of the meeting, the circle was set up in the room, including seats for the number of participants in the group. When the students entered the class, they understood that they should sit down together in the circle. A drawing pad and various types of paints were placed in the center of the room. The meeting started with the lecturer providing instructions, when suddenly a Muslim student broke into the classroom. It was apparent from his clothing that he was a devout religious man. He stood in the center of the circle facing the lecturer and the class, and started shouting at the participants that they shouldn't cooperate with the lecturer and shouldn't agree to sit in the circle. His argument was that a circle including men and women together is a class structure that disrespects religion, and asked the circle to be rearranged into rows, with the women sitting on the left and the men on the right. In face of his shouting, the class fell silent. The first moment was of great embarrassment. It should be noted that the lecturer in this meeting was herself a religious Jewish woman, while the student was a religious Muslim man. In light of familiarity with religious discourse, the need arose to consider a different setting, which had not been planned in advance and was not suitable for the artistic instruction provided earlier. Silence was replaced by chaos, with some of the women in the class, religious and secular Muslims, started opposing the student. In this opposition, two women were central: one was a religious Muslim woman and the other a secular Muslim woman. The secular student turned to the angry student and told him: “If you don’t feel comfortable here, you can leave. This is not the Muslim religion. You took something small from religion and you want to make chaos. People like you are destroying our religion”. The student didn’t hesitate, looked at her, and said: “Look what you look like [referring to her secular clothing], a woman like you doesn’t know what religion is at all”. The woman seemed offended, and then another woman participant, with a religious appearance, her face covered in a Hijab, wearing long clothing, came to her defense. This student turned to the complaining student and told him: “I’m not looking in your eyes [a religious custom commanding that men and women refrain from making eye contact], because I respect you, but I want to tell you that you really can’t address a secular woman in this way and offend her like this. This is not our religion”. The angry student stormed out of the classroom. The secular student started crying, and told everyone: “I come from a religious family. He can’t claim that I’m not religious because of my clothing”. The class was in uproar, and nobody dared speak out. Everyone left the two students alone in the field. The lecturer asked the student to remain with us so we could create a multicultural debate around the event, but he chose to storm out of the class. A few students turned to the lecturer angrily, saying: “Why didn’t you silence him? Why didn’t you throw him out?”

The lecturer explained that even though she did not accept his behavior and his words, it’s important to create dialogue in multicultural contexts. The lecturer tried to examine with him what was inappropriate about the seating, and what was inappropriate about secular clothing, and he chose to be silent and leave the class. It was clear to the lecturer that the central issue at that moment was to discuss the event and not silence it. Also, the immediate purpose was to change the class agenda and the intervention. It was important to start a discussion about gender, gender discrimination, and religion. The issue of racism was abandoned during that meeting. It was clear that it was a foundational moment that required immediate decisions to leverage the event for learning purposes. Situations of multicultural conflict create a powerful reflexive experience for teachers. Decisions have to be made quickly, and the fear is that the class would be unable to contain a wrong intervention that might cause unrest. This is a significant moment in the life of teachers participating in multicultural groups, and there is usually no clear guidance on how exactly to respond. The lecturer decided to calm down quickly from the uproar and not to be upset by the conflict. On the one hand, this was an upsetting moment, but on the other hand a wonderful learning opportunity.

The lecturer decided to reflect her decision to the class, and asked the students to sit in whatever way was comfortable for them, so that each individual could decide. Those who wanted to remain in the circle stayed in this formation, and those who chose to create gender separation could sit outside the circle separately. Most of the participants remained in the circle and two men chose to sit outside, but expressed great interest and involvement. At this stage, the instructions were to choose to use the various paints and drawing sheets that were on the floor. The participants were asked to answer two questions: 1. How do you understand gender? 2. How do you understand gender discrimination. The exercise was allocated 60 minutes, and afterwards there was a complex class discussion, which continued in the following two meetings. The products of the event included the participants' works. Some were paintings depicting Muslim women and Muslim men. Some of the body expressions were women wearing the Hijab and men wearing traditional religious clothing. Other paintings portrayed women and men in secular clothing. These possibilities, as spread out over the floor, demonstrated visually that the issue of the connection between gender and religion can exist on a continuum: in other words, you can be a believing woman and still choose to dress in a manner considered "secular". Other questions that arose included: How much power does clothing have to determine a person's level of religiosity? Who decides what is considered religious and what isn't? And how can spiritual dialogue be conducted when people appear different?

One of the participants, the religious woman who had dared confront the student, chose to show in the class, in the following meeting, a musical piece entitled "Mom went to the doctor", a famous Arabic children's song. After all the class sang the song a few times, and the lecturer was told that any Arabic-speaking child knows this song, the student asked everyone in the class to examine the gender biases in the song. The class observation of the song was conducted critically. Then, the student continued the analysis applying Foucault's understanding of discourse, arguing that from an early age, songs are used to instill gender expectations that continue into the classroom and the way women and men behave in society.

As lecturers, we drew three main conclusions from the event: 1. Conflict events can serve as an excellent opportunity for a journey of intercultural inquiry. 2. The material platform (external appearance, sitting in a circle, clothing) includes significant variables that convey important messages that should be taken into consideration when planning a multicultural creative meeting. 3. The artistic medium contributes to channeling the conflict. The option of connecting with art helps distance direct and focused conflict, which is not always pleasant and easy to discuss, in favor of individual connections adapted to each individual's own expressions. Finally, the experience of sharing in creation enables a dialogue characterized by continuity rather than being one-dimensional.

"Possibility of different religiosity": Accepting the other in the Orthodox Jewish sector

The Jewish religious space is multidimensional and branching. While religious Jewish people may appear identical to others, a deeper inquiry into the religious world reveals many variations. In Israel, there exist over 100 different Hassidic and other religious denominations. Each denomination has its own Rabbis and various religious behaviors. One of the projects we were asked to instruct was a course on diversity for religious and Orthodox women students. The group included over 40 women students from various denominations: Habbad Hassidic, Gur Hassidic, National Religious, Lithuanian Orthodox, and others. Obviously, each participant believed in the way she was brought up. Each denomination has its own Rabbis, synagogues, typical clothing, lifestyle, and leadership. Sometimes, the multicultural campus is the first opportunity in the lives of these women to make contact with Jewish women who conduct a different religious lifestyle to their own. In this type of class, conflicts of a religious nature often arise. Such spaces also test the loyalty of the religious lecturer. The class inquires, over a long period, indirectly, which denomination the lecturer belongs to, or in other words, where does the lecturer's loyalty lie? This issue is often discussed between the lecturers, and they decided to "make the other familiar'. This need resulted from a discussion in the class around head coverings. Married religious Jewish women are commanded to cover their heads. In certain denominations the head covering is a headscarf, in others a hat, and in a few, a wig. Some women wear both a wig and a hat. During one of the social gatherings, the issue of modern Orthodox women arose as part of the course contents. The phenomenon of modern Orthodox women is a feature of the twenty-first century. Such women wear a long wig, emulating natural hair; they wear colorful clothing, which was unheard of in the Orthodox world previously; wear Western brands (Nike, Adidas, etc.); use make-up; and are employed in the secular space. These women engage in a completely modern lifestyle and acquire higher academic education, but at the same time they observe the Jewish *Halakha* (commandments), both minor and major.

In one of the class meetings, an intense discussion arose about what women are permitted and forbidden within the *Halakha* rules. The discussion revolved around head coverings. In order to establish their arguments regarding head coverings, each student used quotations from the greatest Rabbis of her denomination. The class started to argue about what was and wasn't considered *Halakhic* in the context of bodily appearance and behavior. This argument appeared to be a dead end, since each participant claimed that her way was the only *Halakhic* way.

After the meeting, the lecturers met to think about an artistic intervention that would enable the women to get to know and accept approaches different from their own. This intervention included several stages: First, each participant was asked to choose a sector other than her own (for example, a woman from the Gur Hassidic denomination would choose the Breslau Hassidism; a Lithuanian would choose Habbad, and so on). In order to conduct this intervention, which would be considered radical in the Orthodox world that seeks to distinguish denominations from each other deliberately, the lecturers approached the campus Rabbi for permission for this sort of intervention. Even after receiving the Rabbi's permission, at first it was difficult for the students to step outside their sectorial loyalty for a moment. The lecturers decided not to compromise and not to allow the students to stay in their sectorial comfort zone, despite many requests to study their own denomination. After the students consented, with some concern, to choose another sector for study, they were asked to go out and photograph typical clothing and rituals of the sector they had chosen. These were photographs of ceremonies: weddings, circumcisions, Bar Mitzvahs, and of clothing in general. They were also encouraged to photograph the cultural symbols of each denomination and any cultural indication different from those familiar to them.

During the next stage, the students were asked to tell the story of their chosen denomination in the class, using photographs and presentations. We observed how they presented things, and for a moment it appeared that they were really able to stand in the shoes of the other. The presentations were accompanied by singing, and some of the students asked to demonstrate the ceremony in the class. Some gave out candies and sweets, similar to the ritual in their studied sector. There was no trace of the head covering conflict that had appeared earlier. Now, the conflict was replaced by excitement and joy. In the final stage, the students were asked to create a shared exhibition of all the body representations and appearances from the ceremonies they had documented. The presentation day was a sort of celebration. All the students arrived on time and started hanging their works on the walls. They seemed excited when they presented the denomination that wasn't their own, explained and defended it, using photographs and video clips. The students were asked to curate the exhibition themselves, with complete cooperation between them. The exhibition was hanging in the corridors of the Orthodox campus and received great attention. All the appearances of Jewishness, with their variations and mutations, were displayed on the walls.

This intervention led to several conclusions: 1. The best way is to allow people to wander in the world of the other using their senses. Participation in rituals, with the whole array of senses it creates, colors, sights, and flavors, helps people reduce their judgement of others. 2. Photography as an artistic tool sharpens the importance of the Gaze Theory. The use of the camera applied the idea of "observing the other", and this contributed to removing stigmas and prejudices. 3. The exhibition, spread over the campus walls, demonstrated the possible continuum in people's religious choices, as apparent in identity and body relations.

On sculpture and melody: Working in a multicultural group of Jews, Arabs, and Druze

The group included 16 participants, mostly women, from various sectors of Israeli society. There were five Arab Muslim women, three of them religious and two secular. Eight participants were Jewish women, three of them religious and five secular. The other 3 participants were from the Druze sector. For a whole semester, the students learned training skills and were prepared for activist field work, as facilitators with at-risk youth, women's shelters, groups of Israel Defense Forces (IDF) widows, and so on. At each meeting, the students shared dilemmas that arose in their field work, and the other participants gave them advice and shared similar experiences from their own work.

The instructors sensed that this group was creating volatile contents. For example, how can facilitators working with IDF widows share with Arab women and ask them for advice? At the same time, the contents referring to multiculturalism, conflict, and complexity never rose to the surface. The group operated calmly, everyone respected each other and treated each other politely. This experience was exceptional. The lecturers didn't understand it, but followed the group spirit. It transpired that despite the harmony on the surface, underneath things were stormier.

During the course's final assignment, the participants were asked to create an artistic installation to describe their experiences as group participants. They were required to decide for themselves what sort of artistic installation would best describe their learning process. The lecturers decided to observe from the sidelines. After a discussion, in which each participant was well-represented, the women decided to create three dimensional dolls seated in a circle, representing the process they had experienced as students in the group. The students made life-size figures and seated them on chairs. The figures they created had white, circular faces without any features. They were all identical, without any identifying features to distinguish one from the others. The instructors wondered why the students had chosen to erase completely any features of difference. Why, for example, had they not chosen to clothe the dolls, to give them features of religiosity and ethnicity? They understood that this artistic choice reflected the group unconscious, which throughout the year had refused to recognize difference.

In the last two lessons of the semester, the students decided to include music in their installation. They split into groups, with each choosing music to play. The end of the semester approached, and in the final lesson before the installation, each pair played the music they had chosen. The Arab and Druze students chose melodies without words. The Jewish students chose a very political song, whose lyrics are: "I have no other country, even if my land is burning, just a Hebrew word…" This is a nationalist Israeli song that argues that Israel belongs to the Jewish people. The students played their choices in class, and when the Hebrew song was played, there was an outcry. It seemed that the conflict and complexity that had been suppressed throughout the year arose even more strongly at the last moment. The Arab students claimed that the song didn't represent their being part of the group, and that they were unable to connect to such a song as representing the process they had undergone. The Jewish students responded that this was an Israeli song, and if they (the Arab students) were studying in an Israeli college and identifying as Israeli, they should also accept this song. The Muslim students replied that they had deliberately avoided playing songs with lyrics, because they knew that the Arabic language didn't represent all the participants. They said this was why they had chosen tunes without lyrics, and that the Jewish students should do the same.

As part of the facilitation, it was necessary to decide how to express diversity on the one hand and avoid offending others on the other hand. This was a complex dilemma, and the experience itself came as a surprise. The element of surprise, along with the tight schedule for setting up the installation, was a difficult experience. After consultation, the lecturers decided to return the dilemma to the group, even if several more meetings would be required before the end of the semester. These meetings were accompanied by active dialogue around everything that had remained unsaid until now. The meetings included questions about external appearance and head coverings. The Jewish students asked, for the first time, why religious Muslim women cover their heads even when they are not married, while only married women are required to do so in Judaism. Questions about identity appeared for the first time, and thus the Jewish student who worked with IDF widows addressed the Arab students and asked them how they had felt throughout the semester when she had shared stories of women whose partners had fallen in battle. The dialogue became dynamic, authentic, and genuine. For the first time, the lecturers felt that real contact was made in the group. As the date of the installation approached, the students decided unanimously to play a melody they all agreed on, without lyrics. At the same time, they decorated their dolls each with the features of her own religion and sector.

The conclusions we drew from these meetings: 1. Artistic tools can encourage dialogue and open up silenced contents. They can serve as a platform around which people argue when they don't feel secure enough to confront complex political contents. In other words: the struggle was not just about the music, but about the politics of language and positioning relations between Jews and Arabs in the social space. 2. Also, work and study groups in multicultural settings may display shows of politeness, emotional work, and blurring of the diversity. Teachers/ lecturers have to be alert and ready for the appearance of possible conflict. Even if the conflict doesn't appear overtly, its energy might be present under the surface. 3. In situations where the conflict catches the instructor unprepared, it's better to echo the conflict back to the group, trusting the group forces to reach a solution. Using artistic tools can be a catalyst for a solution.

Summary

This study employed art in action interventions, with an emphasis on multicultural issues and the triangle of relations body-identity-emotion as a holistic experience in multicultural understanding. The study's findings show that as teachers, we have to adopt cultural sensitivity and accept that body appearance, clothing choice, and even where people sit in class are important elements for displaying the participants' identity and social belonging. Insensitivity to these elements can create a negative emotional experience for the participants. In these contexts, artistic and creative expression and the use of artistic tools in work can be very important, because they help the teacher and students create a channel that bypasses conversation and respects the differences and subjectivity of all participants. In other cases, the artistic tool actually brings silenced conflicts to the surface and makes them spoken. Speaking enables acquaintance and replaces "politeness" with real, authentic human contact. Teachers and instructors in multicultural groups have to adopt creative, branching thinking and remember that any problem that may arise from the class's multicultural nature could have several creative solutions. Since there is still no ordered doctrine for working in multicultural spaces, and moreover, there is still no platform for working with art in action methodology, as instructors we have to apply art in action when we work with these fascinating human spaces.

References

Amir-Moazami, S. (2016) "Investigating the Secular Body: The Politics of the Male Circumcision Debate in Germany" *ReOrient*, 1(2),147-170.

Anttila, P. (2007) *Realistic Evaluation and Productive Development Work*. Hamina: Akatiimi.

Ben-Amos A., Tamir Y. (eds.) (1995) *The Teacher between Mission and Profession*. Raanana: Levels.

Bellerose, C. (2019) "On the Lived Imagined Body: A Phenomenological Praxis of a Somatic Architecture" *Phenomenology & Practice*, 12(1), 57-71.

Berry, J. (2016) "Comparative Analysis of Canadian Multiculturalism Policy and the Multiculturalism Policies of other Countries" *Psychology in Russia: State of the Art*, 9(1), 4-23.

Borgdorff, H. (2009) *Artistic Research within the Fields of Science*. Bergen: Bergen National Academy of the Arts.

Borgdorff, H. (2011) "Knowledge in Artistic Research" (pp. 44-63) in M. Biggs, & H. Karlsson (eds.). *The Routledge Companion to Research in the Arts*. London: Routledge.

Bullington, J. (2017) *The Expression of the Psychosomatic Body from a Phenomenological Pperspective*. New York: Springer.

Civitillo, S., Schachner, M., Juang, L., Vijver de van, F.G., Handrick, A., Noack, P. (2017) "Towards a Better Understanding of Cultural Diversity approaches at School: Multi-informant and Mixed-Methods Study." *Learning, Culture and Social Interaction*, 12, 1-14.

Cho, G., DeCastro-Ambrosetti, D., (2005) "Is Ignorance Bliss Pre-service Teachers' attitudes' toward Multicultural Education." *The High School Journal*, 89(2), 24-28.

Criado-Perez, C. (2019) *Invisible Women: Exposing Data Bias in a World Designed for Men*. London: Chatto & Windus.

De-Gelder, B. (2016) *Emotions and the Body*. Oxford: Oxford University Press.

Dolezal, L. (2015) The body and shame: Phenomenology, Feminism, and the Socially Shaped Body. London: Lexington books.

Engelsrud, G. (2005) The lived body as experience and perspective: Methodological challenges. Qualitative research Vol 5(3) 267-284.

Fanon, F. ([1952] 2008) Black skin white masks. New York: Grove press.

Frogel, S., Barkhana-Lorand, D., Levi-Keren, M., Barkai. S. (2012) "On the Importance of Art Education" *Hed A'Chinuch*. April 2012, 5, 46-47 (Hebrew).

Friedman, A. (2018) *Dialogue on Campus: Arabs and Jews in a Common Space*. Tel Aviv: Kav-Adom (Hebrew).

Gatens, M. (1996) *Imaginary bodies Ethics, Power and Corporeality*. London: Routledge.

Grosz, E. (1994) *Volatile Bodies*. London: Routledge.

Haelyon, H., Rahimi, D. I., Cohen liverant, R. (2019) "Practice and Ethics in Teaching in Multicultural Spaces" *Keshet – Journal of the Humanities and Social Sciences*, Ono Academic Campus, 3, 66-75 (Hebrew).

Haelyon, H. and Gross, H. (2011) "The Lived Pain Experience: The Case of Women Undergoing IVF Treatments" *The Indo – Pacific journal of phenomenology*, (11) 1-10.

Haelyon, H. (2007) *A Locked Garden: The Experiences of Body, Identity and Emotions of Women Undergoing Fertility Treatments in Israel*. Haifa: Pardes (Hebrew).

Härkönen E., Huhmarniemi, M., Jokela, T. (2018) "Crafting Sustainability: Handcraft in Contemporary Art and Cultural Sustainability in Lapland" *Sustainability*, 10(6).

Heikkinen, H. L. T., Konttinen, T., Häkkinen, P. (2006) "Trends in Action Research" (pp. 39-76) in H. L.T. Heikkinen, E. Rovio, L. Syrjälä (eds.) *From Operations to Information: Action Research Methods and Approaches*. Helsinki: Kansanvalistusseura.

Hillel-Avraham, R., Haelyon H., Rahimi, D. I. (forthcoming) "Silence Multicultural Educational Spheres" *Keshet – Journal of the Humanities and Social Sciences*. Ono Academic Campus (Hebrew).

Hiltunen, M. (2009) *Community Art Education: Performatively in the Sociocultural Environments of the North*. Acta Universitatis

Lapponiensis A160. (Doctoral dissertation). Rovaniemi: Lapland University Press.

Hulvey, S. Y. (2000) "Myths and Monsters: The Female Body as the Site for Political Agendas" (pp. 71-88) in D. Walker King (ed.). *Body Politics and the Fictional Double*. Bloomington & Indianapolis: Indiana University press.

Jokela, T., Huhmarniemi, M., Hiltunen, M. (2019) "Art-Based Action Research: Participatory Art Education Research for the North" (pp. 45-56) in A. Sinner, Rita L. Irwin, Adams J. (eds.). *Provoking the Field. International Perspectives on Visual Arts PhDs in Education*. Bristol: Intellect.

Jokela, T., Hiltunen, M., Härkönen, E. (2015a) "Art Based Action Research – Participatory Art for the North" *International Journal of Education through Art*, 11(3), 433-448.

Jokela, T., Hiltunen, M., Härkönen, E. (2015b) "Contemporary Art Education Meets the International North" (pp. 260-279) in M. Kallio-Tavin, J. Pellinen (eds.) *Conversations on Finnish Art Education*. Helsinki: Aalto ARTS Books.

Jokela, T., Härkönen, E., Yliharju, A. J. (eds.) (2014) *Snow Design in Lapland – Initiating Cooperation*. Rovaniemi: University of Lapland.

Jokela, T. (2008) "A wanderer in the landscape" (pp. 217-240) in G. Coutts, T. Jokela (eds.). *Art, Community and Environment: Educational Perspectives*. Bristol: Intellect.

Mulvey, L. (1989) *Visual and other Pleasures*. Hampshire: Macmillan

Leavy, P. (2018) *Handbook of Arts-Based Research*. New York: Guilford Press.

Leavy, P. (2009) *Method Meets Art: Arts-Based Research Practice*. New York: Guilford Press.

Legrand, D. (2017) "The Living Body and the Lived Body in the Clinical Encounter: How does Body Shape Ethical Practice" (pp. 463-486) in Schramme T., Edwards S., *Handbook of the Philosophy of Medicine*. New York: Springer.

Lyon, M. L. (1997) "The Material Body, Social Processes and Emotion: Techniques of the Body Revisited" *Body & Society* 3(1), 83-101.

McNiff, S. (2013) "A Critical Focus on Art-Based Research" (pp. 109-116) in S. McNiff (ed.). *Art as Research, Opportunities and Challenges*. Bristol: Intellect.

Merari, D., Shitrit, A., Feldberg, D., Elizur, A., Modan, B. (1996) "Psychosocial Characteristics of Women Undergoing In Vitro Fertilization: A Study of Treatment Outcome" *Israel Journal of Obstetrics and Gynecology*, 7(2), 65-72.

Merari, D., Feldberg, D., Modan, B. (1997) "Psychosocial Characteristics of Male Spouses Undergoing In Vitro Fertilization: A Study of Treatment Outcome" *Israel Journal of Obstetrics and Gynecology*, 8(3), 178-183.

Mercedes-Vella, M. (2015) *Boy Image Experiences of Racial/Ethnic Minority Heterosexual Males living with HIV/AIDS: An Interpretative Phenomenological Analysis*. Pennsylvania: Lehigh University.

Michaeli, N. (2012) "Education for Utopia – Educational Ideology of Social Transformation" (pp. 185-195) in Tadmor Y., Freiman, A. (eds.). *Education: Essence and Spirit*. Raanana: Mofet Institute.

Morris, D. (1993) *The Culture of Pain*. California: California University Press.

Nirta, C. (2018) *Marginal Bodies, Trans Utopias*. London: Routledge.

Said, E. W. (1978) O*rientalism*. New York: Random house.

Sasson T., Tabory, E. (2010) "Converging Political Cultures: How Globalization is Shaping the Discourses of American Israeli Jews" *Nationalism and Ethnic Politics*, 16, 22-41.

Sheets-Johnstone, M. (2020) The lived body. The humanistic psychologist 48(1) 28-53.

Shildrick, M. (1997) *Leaky Bodies and Boundaries: Feminism, Postmodernism and (Bio)ethics*. London: Routledge.

Tabory, E. (2007) "Stop The World I Want to Make Peace" (pp. 245-251) in R. J. Eidelson, J. Laske & L. Cherfas (eds.). *Peacemaker 101: Careers Confronting Conflict*. Philadelphia: University of Pennsylvania.

Turner, B. S. (2012) *The Routledge Handbook of Body Studies*. New York: Routledge.

Turner, B. (2005) "Introduction – Bodily Performance: On Aura Reproducibilit" *Body & Society*, 11(4), 1-17.

Strings, S. (2019) *Fearing the Black Body: The Racial Origins of Fat Phobia*. New York: NYU press.

Wehrle, M. (2020) "Being a Body and Having a Body: The Twofold Temporally of Embodied Intentionality" *Phenomenology and the cognitive sciences*. 19, 499-521.

CHAPTER 2

ART THERAPY IN A DIGITAL WORLD: MIXED REALITIES IN THE HYBRID CLINIC

DAPHNA LIBER

Introduction

We are embedded in a digital age, and therefore the world of expressive art therapy faces a challenge. The chapter presents a hybrid combination of digital reality in the field of art therapy. As art therapists must be aware of distinctions between 'Digital Natives' and 'Digital Immigrants.' The uniqueness of the current generation gap influences the concept of identity and their attitudes towards digital ecology. The chapter will present a typology of a therapeutic-digital style. A tool for identifying the personal position of each therapist in relation to the digital entry into the art therapy room. Promoting the Hybrid notion that the combination is a necessary part of the therapist's work.

A hybrid approach will be presented that considers the integration of digital dimensions with the aspects of art therapy methods. The chapter will focus on the digital realms combined in the art therapy room and will conclude with sharing thoughts regarding the role of the teacher in the field of art therapy. The teacher as the agent that combines and promotes the learning, understanding and familiarizing with digital aspects. Those aspects hold a practical element for the teaching of art therapy skills.

Art and art therapy present an opportunity for connecting worlds. An ability to understand what is beyond words through the language of art. The reality around us has changed a lot, and art reflects the time changes and corresponds with them. Art therapy methods, as well as psychotherapy methods, did not go through such extreme changes.

I would like us to draw attention to the reality in which we exist, immersed in a technology embedded world, watch our children and patients grow in a digital ecology. As therapists we meet patients whose digital language is their native language, sometimes even more so than the language of sensory expression in art. We encounter a digital generational gap, but also an exceptional opportunity to enable an integrated learning of the therapeutic field and to connect it with the digital reality in a conscious and clever way.

As art therapists, we should actively address the subject, by understanding our attitudes toward the digital reality, by understanding the ways it enters into the therapy room, by adjusting digital dimensions surrounding us in daily life and in the clinic.

The Covid-19 pandemic stressed the quick and unplanned transition to an all-embracing digital reality, that took place with no appropriate guidance or training. We no longer have the privilege to deal with the question whether art therapy contains digital dimensions or not. Art therapists must examine the ways in which we can train ourselves and our students to integrate the digital reality in the art therapy room.

This chapter will briefly review the unique generation gap of this era, the importance of understanding the attitudes towards the digital reality in the art therapy, as instructors and therapists. Later in this chapter, a typology is presented of different characteristics and their response relating to the digital elements as they are entering the art therapy room. Understanding the stance of the therapist to these attitudes allows future therapists a better self-understanding and beneficial learning. This chapter will relate to understanding the hybrid generation and the need for a training adapted to this reality.

Technology embedded world

The development of technology allows quick communication, and enables overcoming distance, accessibility difficulties and other physical limitations. These technological developments are being used also in psychotherapy. We live in a technology embedded world, influencing us consciously and unconsciously, in an invisible way. The change in technology and the creation of digital ecology made also an intergenerational distinction more intense than the usual generation gap. ‘Digital immigrants’ can be distinguished from ‘Digital natives’ (Prensky, 2001). The digital immigrants were born before the 1980s, they first became familiar with computers as adults. They experience digital dimensions as strange, gradually replacing the forms of communication they were familiar with in their world. The 'Digital natives', born from the 1990s onwards, were born into a cultural setting containing computers, cellular phones etc., a digital ecology constituting a different platform for growth and a different habitat. They are familiar with the computer by default, and the language they acquired in the technological aspect is their 'mother tongue' (Garner, 2017).

Technological means of therapy include psychotherapy via email, therapy text messages and psychotherapy via video conferencing. These types of therapy are possible not only due to the technological capability, but also because their existence is in congruence with the contemporary values, infiltrating the human and therapeutic discourse. Values of availability, immediate response, an all-knowing digital body, seeping into the human consciousness, creating an array of unconscious expectations and fantasies, in relationships, in the therapeutic set-up, and in the learning and training system.

The example that might emphasize this gap is obvious when we look at a classroom, school as an institute that was built during 18th century to provide skills that would be useful for the future of working in a factory (Postman, 1993). During work at the factory the main ability required is to memorize by heart the rules and instructions, where you are graded in every shift on the number of products you manufactured etc. Obviously the 21st century has set different challenges to our students. Sitting in a classroom listening to a teacher standing and talking, only allowed to leave their chair when permitted or when the bell rings, does not resemble their future working place or the skills needed for a meaningful and successful future career.

There is no arguing that our world has changed deeply and dramatically. There is no doubt that art has the quality of meeting a person's deepest needs, in a symbolic language, to the realms where no words are available that allows one's deep strength to be met. Art is dynamic and communicate with the human soul as well as reflecting the Zeitgeist. Therapy, as well as art therapy schools has gone through a minor change, if any. The need to accommodate the environment, tools and skills tends to be slow and minimalistic.

Kamial (2016), describes the importance of further research in the field of learning and education concerning the place of the digital dimension in therapy. In a large-scale study of art therapists, the therapists that reported difficulties and fear regarding integrating digital arts addressed the lack of training in the field and little experience in computerized elements. The respondents related to the digital dimension, giving a sense of lack of touch and a different sensation during the creative process. Despite the long period of time in which we have been experiencing digital abilities, and digital art exhibitions and artworks, there is still lack of adjustment, syllabuses, knowledge and suitable training systems that will allow therapists to use these tools in the best possible way (Kuleba, 2008).

Art materials – App materials

Therapists are ambivalent about technology entering the therapy room and the curriculum. A lot of curiosity is described regarding drawing apps, a variety of documentation and photography options, and the ability to use music from an app. At the same time, there is fear about exposure and violation of privacy, questions regarding the need for "regular" art materials, and questions regarding the issue of boundaries, the 'slippery cellular slope', and lack of professional knowledge on the tech.

The digital aspect of art has a quality that is sometimes experienced as cold, and not liquid or tangible. The art therapist is sometimes worried about lack of contact and sensory experience while using digital art apps or internet, along with its tempting digital ability which allows even those that avoid touching art materials to start a creative process (Garner, 2017, p. 14 ; Malchiodi, 2000, p. 23).

It is possible to identify the limits of our digital view through examining the art materials in the room. Is using colored pencils or marker pens more real than using gouache? Is creating a collage more superficial than working with clay? Is moving or playing more meaningful than dance? Our answer probably depends on the patient and what they bring into the room, and what is difficult for them or what they were deprived of. Providing educational knowledge regarding the digital dimension in therapy will allow the art therapist to examine the issue thoroughly, not just by questions of good or bad, but with more comprehensive therapeutic examination tools. Who is it for, and how? At what stage in therapy and to what extent? Does it represent avoiding the true self, or maybe it alternatively allows experiencing more self-states? An equally important question deals with the therapist, their feelings and views, visible and hidden. Does the therapist experience the integration of the digital dimension as alienating and superficializing? Does the digital dimension confront the therapist with a threatening and unfamiliar place within themself? Does the difficulty originate also from an experience of internal alienation and no connection to the world of the 'Digital natives'? If the answers to some of these questions are yes, then some work is required from the therapist in order to get to know and understand the aspects of the hyperspace and their possible meanings for the 'Digital natives'.

The theoretical writing in psychology does not usually integrate the digital dimension. There is a clear and distinct boundary between the technological writing and writing about the areas of therapy. There is little literature regarding infiltration, and link between these areas, as well as their reciprocal influence. In most studies they are presented as opposite phenomena, contradicting each other, and not necessarily co-existing.

In the postmodern era, it is possible to identify a theoretical transition from monolithic, dichotomous thinking, to broad possibilities of integrating domains in the field of mental health. We witness a theoretical change, identifying the multiplicity of self-component and giving up the attempted unification of the self.

A change in the mental-health definition making a move from a place of unity towards a place of complexity, even at the cost of expressing incoherent self-states (Bromberg, 1996). The ability to exist between changing attitudes and in a constant movement as self-expression as a starting point for healing processes.

In an era characterized by a constant change, art therapists keep the accumulated experience of many years of knowledge and practice. As well as the importance of understanding the flexibility, constant learning and the fear of professional stagnation. Our role as therapists and teachers is to experience the ability to create variation and allow different parts of the self to be expressed. To expand our professional toolbox without fear, as it combines many years of experience, diverse creative tools side by side with digital tools, and an option of expanding the artistic therapeutic tools in a digital ecology. The art presents the option of perspective, ability to experience dimension of distance and proximity, the digital language enables a viewpoint that was not previously possible, of experiencing the near and far at the same time, the past and present alongside as a digital option and an intriguing therapeutic potential. Thus, the mix-up of languages between human and digital can take on a dimension of a new hybrid creation, integrated and exciting (Liber, 2020a).

Mixed realities – the imaginary & the real

The digital reality undermines the usual perception of presence. The imaginary reality is such a tangible imitation, to the extent that the digital objects can be experienced as a true and full reality. Therefore, it might be more accurate to use the term "mixed realities", originating in the field of art, so there is no full separation between the real and the unreal. A virtual representation of a body, human imagination and integrating it in a computer software, are joined together to create an integrated reality, both real and unreal (Lemma, 2017: Brians, 2011). This understanding is in line with the behavior analysis of the 'Digital natives' who are not concerned with the distinction between the digital and the real, and are not busy with the constant attempt to classify and attribute every source of information to the area it came from, but see it as consolidated and continuous information from various sources of information (Palfrey & Gasser, 2008). The digital space is defined as the space created by interpersonal relationships, mediated by technology in such way that the body is not present. In fact, the art therapy experience makes connections and combinations of reality for the benefit of the therapeutic process. Combining art materials and symbols to express a psychological process. Using the spoken language and the artistic language to create a healing intermediate space. Moving from the outside world into the studio and therapeutic work in art, all represent the power of mixed realities, a real dimension and an imaginary dimension, combined into one living space of the therapy room (Lemma, 2017).

In the past, the meaning of the term virtual represented what is not real, therefore imaginary, artificial. As the concept changed, it referred to what is intangible and cannot be touched, and today the term virtual is sometimes used as synonym for the words digital and computerized (Hayles, 1999: Marzi, 2016). The virtual is not an alternative for the real, but rather an addition, another way to express reality, the potential space existing on the border between online and offline events. Recognizing the fullness of the digital picture makes the personal sharing via the digital spaces not to an object, but to an expansion of the interpersonal dimension. By this, the digital reality presents a dimension to which we often refer to in art therapy as the 'potential space', the location between the creation and the creator, the space between the art and the patient, and the digital space between us and the world.

Mixed realities in a hybrid clinic

The classic psychoanalytic approaches suggest that keeping the settings allows the optimal conditions for the development of transference relationship. According to these approaches, the stability of the framework and its unity are used to ensure the patient's sense of security. The relational approaches, focusing on mutual recognition, see a significant therapeutic potential in the tension that exists in the therapeutic encounter between the ritual base and the spontaneous elements. The dimension of digital availability allows further expansion of the settings; therefore it requires awareness and attention (Hoffman, 1998). The training of art therapists includes referring to the studio's settings and the presence of the materials. The materials should be considered as having a varying quality and consisting of different art elements that include also digital dimensions, as well as music, video and pictures.

In the field of art therapy there are prominent studies about the ambivalent experience of the therapists, expressing different and contradicting attitudes regarding the place of the digital in the therapy room. There is a double concern among art therapists. The first arising because they are not familiar with digital tools and lack the knowledge of using them as artistic work materials. The other is a concern due to the difficulty to make therapeutic adaptations of the digital dimensions in therapy and adapting them proportionally and appropriately to the patient and the different stages of the therapeutic process (Thong, 2007; Asawa, 2009; Kuleba, 2009).

We deal not only with digital art materials, but also with a digital clinic. The location of the clinic in the digital age is linked with understanding the perception of the studio as a concept of consciousness. A dimension that exists in a space that is not only physical, and therefore can be transformed to digital dimensions. Orbach (2020) writes sensitively about the experience of the studio as a state of consciousness. A state that can be realized as an internal or external space, digital or physical, nourished with metaphors, with human contexts and in an experience of closeness that creates substantiality. The experience of the meeting, the therapy, the co-creation and the art is the beginning of every conscious experience. Moon describes the ability to make a combined use of the digital dimension and the therapeutic artistic product as promoting the integrative ability (2010).

It is important for art therapists to understand that integrating a digital dimension in art therapy has implications for the therapy. It cannot be assumed that this is "more of the same thing". The digital materials are not "just" another type of art materials; they carry meaning and have implications concerning also ethics, confidentiality, and exposure, not just the qualities of materials. In the training process, it is very important to refer to the studio space with its digital aspects as considerations regarding the therapeutic issues that fade or intensify when using and choosing such tools (Kamial, 2016; Kapitan, 2011). The expanding dimension of the studio and the digital tools available to the therapist, with careful and conscious guidance, makes it possible to see the art therapy as mixed reality, a beneficial space, integrating different sources of information, various self-states and expanding the art therapist toolbox.

It is important to formulate an understanding of the digital ecology giving rise to the H generation, 'Hybrid generation'. Hybridity means linking between various social, cultural and scientific phenomena. A combination of sensations creating a hybrid experience. The possibility of a hybrid product is derived not only from the combination of two different components into an integrative composition, but from the understanding that the uncomfortable and strange encounter between the different forces creates a challenging, lively and unique reality. The hybrid contains unease, and alienation that can lead, in the digital age, to new and unique combinations and aggregations. Lévi-Strauss describes the concept 'Bricolage', relating to combining distinct fragments who were removed from their previous framework, to create a new, coherent picture. Details that may look unnecessary, now receive a meaning and a role and shed light on a new view of the components of this combination and the creation of the new and unexpected contexts. A cultural diffusion that creates a new whole, like combining musical styles, combining lingual styles combining computer language, and creation of a new relationship between man and technology. Hybridity carries a source of vitality, a new perspective allowing acceptance of the complexity, and an understanding that one cannot be fully understood without the other.

Understanding hybridity and its qualities and mixed realities is essential for art therapists. Integration allows the experience of complexity, helps with recognition, and not ignoring the feeling of discomfort that arises when facing the digital dimension. Recognizing the complexity makes it possible to map the experience of alienation, but also the ability to connect and create, and to identify the hybrid power (Liber, 2020).

Hybrid therapy

Identifying attitudes

Following the understanding that a major part of the influence of technology and its invasion into our lives as therapists is unaware, it is very important to consciously identify personal attitudes. With the lack of such identification process, the "dormant" influences of the technology, behaviors and expectations will remain unconscious and it will be difficult for us to refer to them as teachers and therapists.

The therapist's role begins with the possibility to make an "intellectual distance" for examining their attitudes. Identifying the attitudes with a clear new view of the difficulties and feelings, will allow a wide and more understandable perspective in the face of, and within, the digital reality.

Three aspects are presented for identifying the various attitudes more comprehensively.

1. **Personal attitude identification regarding technology** – how I use the digital reality as a human-being, as a teacher, as therapist, as parent. Where do I avoid it and what is my attitude toward each use?
2. **In depth familiarity with my attitudes toward professional identity** – examining attitudes regarding the theoretical dimension guiding my work in the clinic. How do my therapeutic attitudes and the digital arena relate to each other? Identifying assumptions regarding the relationship with the patients inside and outside the clinic. Relating to different modes of communication and making contact via digital communication. The therapist's attitude towards dimensions of accessibility, of being exposed to personal information and regarding disclosing and sharing information. This in depth familiarity process stems from the understanding that all of the above have influence on the willingness to accept in the clinic viewpoints from the digital world that is around us and in us.
3. **Digital inquiry in the clinic area** – what is the place of technology in the therapy room? is it used as a therapeutic tool? Does it enter the room through the patients' attitude and the information they bring? Is it on the boundary between the inside and the outside and is it being used for updating and keeping in touch using digital means? Is there an attempt to block it? And how different are the relations when working with 'Digital immigrant' compared with patients that are 'Digital natives'.

"H generation" – "Hybrid Generation"

After an initial identification of our place and position, by understanding our personal style and the therapeutic identity we are developing now and in the future, I chose to characterize four main identities of therapists, located on the matrix.

The ethical issues influenced by each one of these dimensions, should be considered regarding the level of involvement, information leakage, and the question of the boundaries set between the therapeutic, personal and digital. Our role is to identify the professional and ethical challenges we face when encountering the digital reality in and outside the clinic. After identifying the attitude, it is our role to expand the variety of the personal options as therapists, in terms of personal identity, attitudes, self-states as well as attitudes toward hybrid integration in the clinic (Liber, 2020a, 176).

ADHD therapists' styles relating to digital ecology dimensions

Adapter – updated – lacks control
Drifter – carried away, no agenda
Denial – denies – sterile
Hybrid – alchemist – hybrid

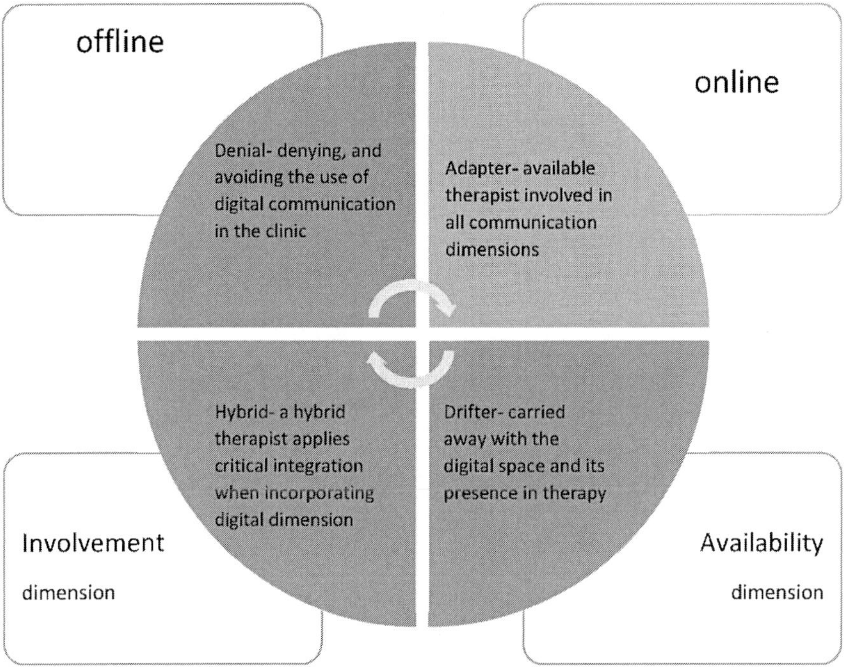

- **Denial** – sterile

The denying therapist is characterized by avoiding the use and integration of the digital dimension in the clinic**.** Believing that it has no place in the clinic, that the digital medium is irrelevant, in an attempt to keep a sterile clinic, ignoring the existence of digital reality, lack of awareness to the digital ecology. Refusal to see the change processes and their relevance to the therapy room. The denying therapist may become angry when the mobile phone is brought into the therapy room and demand to take it out and avoid digital communication between sessions via text messages or emails. The therapist may oppose discourse on the social media, labeling it as inappropriate and shallow, and express a firm view about it as part of "The sickness of our time and decline of the generation."

- **Drifter** carried away, no agenda

The drifting therapist experiences the digital dimension as a natural part of the therapy room. Not as a product of an investigation and learning process, but as an automatic response to the general drift. Taking the digital ecology for granted. The digital enters the clinic while the therapist does not think or consider the materials and issues entering the clinic, but rather as an uncontrolled process, involving digital dimensions inside and outside the clinic, by both the therapist and the patient.

- **Adapter** updated – lacks control

The adapting therapist is available and involved in all communication modes. They adopt the digital changes as means that makes it possible for them to be available for their patients. The therapist is involved with aspects outside the therapy via digital accessibility, and initiates contact if needed. The adapter therapist is usually closer to the digital natives on the timeline. The adoption of a gradual use of the digital media, as well as integrating it in the discourse in the clinic, is more natural for them. Adapting the digital tools is not unaware and uncontrolled, as with the therapist who lacks awareness, but it will not be easy for this therapist to consciously explain and justify their different choices.

- **Hybrid** – an alchemist

The hybrid therapist is characterized by the ability to tolerate the enriching tension between digital ecology and interpersonal psychotherapy. He is aware of the power of being involved, aware of the accessibility and the availability dimensions, aware of the power of art therapy, and has the flexibility dimension for acknowledging the existence of mixed realities in the therapy room and outside it.

Integrating digital dimensions in therapy makes hybrid components available for the therapist

1. Schedule and information updates
2. Referring to online information – psycho-education
3. Update in situations of distress
4. Initiating contact and being contacted by the therapist in special situations.
5. Defining rules for sharing and using social media, like sending a WhatsApp message, sharing videos, and story updates

6. Associating with and relating to the device in therapy as partner, and an analytical third party.
7. Using applications that integrate art and creation
8. Integrating the digital dimensions of the art products in the studio
9. Integrative reference to artistic and digital dimension as expanding the image of the psyche

The hybrid therapist views the dimensions of the change and identifies the importance of what is secure and constant. With the ability of adjusted integration, they can allow the place in which therapy takes place to become a 'sacred place', where a multi-sensory experience exists, and to contain the existence of additional realities challenging and competing for attention as part of our existence in a technology embedded world. The hybrid therapists adopt and practice the ability to create 'joint citizenship' allowing a lively and meaningful place for both digital immigrants and digital natives (Turkle, 2005).

Darwin uses the expression "Survival of the fittest" when referring not to the species that are physically the strongest, but to those who have the ability to adapt when changes occur in their environment. As therapists, we need to adapt to the digital reality without losing the values of our profession. The professional training includes patience, waiting for moments of clarity, and the ability to contain anxiety as opposed to an immediate reaction. The therapeutic field includes the ability to contain complexity, to witness process and not just objects, as well as distinguishing between needs for intimacy and needs for autonomy. The relationships of the patient as well as the therapist's with the digital reality can be a secure base or alternatively a source of distancing and alienation. Art therapy touches the digital dimension with issues of documentation and exposures, using the internet's power for information, sharing, and for emotional support. Being able to internalize a secure base is what allows us to explore the world, to invite new experiences, to become curious and not feel intimidated by change. The new Darwinist term could be "Survival of the digitalist." The therapeutic ability to encounter and cope with the possibilities presented by the digital reality will help us as therapists to meet a wide variety of aspects and viewpoints and make them available as an experience for us, as well as for our patients.

Toolbox for the art therapist

As art therapists we allow our patients to experiment, to get to know the art materials, to meet themselves when facing different experiences with material, symbols and the creative process. Similarly, we should facilitate, offer and invite experiences in the different digital dimensions. Experiencing music chosen by the patient from their cellular phone or private playlist and to accompany a personal creation in digital art. We should dare to experience paintings created on a touchpad, to get to know creative and artistic applications, to become familiar with various materials being expressed digitally. The options of using digital color pallets, being able to make a collage and various effects of artistic origin, before they became an 'Instagram filter'. Our therapeutic and educational purpose is to become acquainted, making it possible to experience the option of mixed realities. In order to allow an accessible therapeutic space, and an integrative full perception of the various elements, in a way that reflects the digital reality as a potential meeting place with our patients.

During an educational process, the art therapists acknowledge the existence of mixed realities and formulate their attitude and accessibility regarding it. The teacher's responsibility for their students is related to their ability to open a door for them to this world and link the digital tools to a wider artistic and therapeutic context. Orr and Malchiodi mention, in different works, the ability of art therapists to adopt the technological changes in a reserved way, at a reasonable rate, same as the general population. The major difficulty emerging from their work is related to the issue of learning and ethical dilemmas. This subject is poorly addressed in the professional educational framework, and this makes it hard to get to know, access, and make an optimized use of the digital tools in the studio (Orr, 2012; Malchiodi, 2018). As therapists we are entrusted with passing on the art therapy profession, we are constantly learning, updating with theoretical innovations, participating in trainings and seminars, dealing with different approaches and innovations in art therapy. As therapists of the future 'digital natives' we must bravely look, experience and even deal with contemporary theoretical approaches as well as with digital accessibility, and to expand our digital toolbox. The digital space allows maintaining professional relationship, become updated with content fields, continuous learning and consulting even from a geographic distance.

Professional organizations offer vast information in the fields of therapy and theory through websites and social networks, and include areas with restricted access, available are only for members of the organization, so discussions and professional and meaningful exchange of information can take place there while keeping confidentiality and according to the rules of ethics. These websites are of great value for the professional field and for personal development, but just as important, by belonging to the professional "family of origin", creating a professional body of teachers and art therapists sharing knowledge and experience and formulating the work tools of integrating the digital into art therapy and teaching it. In the digital learning arena the therapists can choose the level of involvement. One can conduct the amount of intimacy, involvement and affiliation in the professional communities, and trainings as active participants or as viewers and occasional visitors (Cundy, 2015).

As therapists working with 'digital natives' and 'digital immigrants' generation, we must allow ourselves and them to become familiar with the various digital dimensions. Knowing the benefits, risks and the potential will allow them to make an informed choice regarding the technology as a supportive and complementary tool in art therapy. As art therapist in a 'Hybrid generation', We must assist with providing a view that doesn't ignore the existence and impact of digital dimension on the therapy arena, and a possibility to see the hybrid integration as a therapeutic aspect, helping to overcome the anxiety of the technological dimension. Integrating the digital in the art therapy discourse as a creative tool promotes self-understanding and the therapeutic potential on the practical and theoretical levels. An open and hybrid discourse that is not preoccupied with fear of takeover, invasion of privacy and erasing the boundary, but allows to get to know the "digital elephant" in the therapy room (Liber, 2020a).

Integrating the hybrid discourse in the therapy space, whether it is a studio, a clinic, or a digital meeting space, will make it possible to update the therapy perceptions, to link the theory to the Zeitgeist and the work to the digital reality surrounding us, to be willing to undermine the narratives of an external and dangerous digital world. and allow an experience that involves a fresh perspective. A conscious and reasoned use of digital aspect in a way that is not accidental or unconscious but supporting the therapeutic processes, taking place in the room in a conscious and reasoned way.

A word to the teachers

Focusing on art therapist is one dimension, another important angle is held by the art therapy teachers. A different chapter will be dedicated to those dilemmas, but I will point a few important notes on that matter. As teachers we are in charge of transferring professional knowledge, we must allow a conversation tailored for a "Hybrid generation". The mission I see is extending the treatment language taught regarding those digital aspects. The encounter in a digital ecology, between those familiar with digital language and those who experience it with concern, when there is a constant desire to create a collaborative educational and therapeutic discourse.

A reality of distance and a double concern is created. The teachers' fear prevents them from becoming familiar with the digital dimension, in regard to providing work tools, theoretical perceptions and new experiences that integrate artistic and digital dimensions for their students. The practicing therapists are concerned, feeling they lack the tools and knowledge to deal with the digital dimension, and this makes it alienating and maybe even intimidating. In the middle is the patient, to which a whole area of artistic digital expression is unavailable in the art therapy studio.

We are looking for the ability to train a professional therapist, who is art based, and developing inner flexibility for digital experiences adapted for the up-to-date therapy room. This richness of discourse in therapy will be made possible through controlled introduction of the digital dimension to art therapy studies, and will allow the student to formulate a view about digital involvement in art therapy. A therapeutic view that is not grounded in fear of the digital and difficulty to set limits, but an aware therapeutic view. A training that makes the hybrid dimension accessible and a will to integrate the digital with the therapeutic dimension, creating a meaningful space for building a community of art therapists, along with new and meaningful modes of expression in therapy, like photography, digital painting, and digital art expressions (Malchiodi, 2000).

There is room to ask ourselves: do we teach our students about the past and about the materials from which we have learned and developed? Do we teach our students to dare and experience changes? Are they taught to become familiar and deal with new art materials? With new and digital creative skills? Do we really dare and teach them (and maybe teach ourselves first) about the influence the digital reality has on the therapists, patients, and on what takes place in the therapy room? We should ask all those questions as individuals and as art therapy educational institutes.

Conclusion

In the world I grew into there was a home telephone, but the color television was new and exciting, the microwave, walkman and personal computer were all technological innovations in my world. We practice therapy in a world in which the internet is a regular service, available for us at any given moment and everywhere. Our new and excited encounters for the first time with a personal computer and a cellular phone sound to our students and patients like stories from prehistoric times. Our role as those passing on the art therapy knowledge is established, but the knowledge regarding the integration of the digital in the therapy room is partial and fragmented. It is our job and mission, as those leading the way, to be able to mark the professional path for becoming familiar with the theoretical aspect of using the digital aspects in art therapy. It is our duty to develop its integration in the classrooms, in writing and theoretical thinking. Understanding that most of our students, the future therapists, are 'Digital natives' who will treat 'Digital natives' with tools interrelated to this reality, and we must not overlook this blind spot without educationally, therapeutically and theoretically relating to it. We must integrate the vast knowledge accumulated in the past and reach out for the vast knowledge contained in the present for integrating the digital reality in art therapy.

In art therapy studies, there is room to relate to the 'potential digital space'. A place that holds qualities for the psychological well-being, for the artwork and for the therapeutic discourse taking place in it, certainly not as an aspect we can ignore or be blind about. Studying the hybrid understanding of the clinic and art therapy should be encouraged, and understanding that dichotomous division between real and imaginary does not precisely describe the psychological and interpersonal occurrences in a digital reality. Since the digital reality shakes the ordinary perception of presence, and the imaginary reality is such a tangible imitation that virtual objects can be experienced as a full and real reality. It is more accurate to refer to the term 'mixed realities' in relation to the components of the reality and the encounter in the clinic in the digital age (Brians, 2011).

The multidimensional views and the 'ADHD typology' allow the therapist to focus on the different needs and to explore her or his therapeutic attitude and the change of the theoretical language. Understanding one's predisposition can help develop flexibility and an easier adapted movement when facing various self–states, while keeping a hybrid professional and theoretical center. As teachers and therapists, we must enable learning that provides the students with multiple viewpoints, personal and historical narrative, array of cultural attributions and aspects. In order to deal with art therapy in a digital reality we need to train proficient therapists whose viewpoint allows multiplicity and diversity, versatility and hybridity.

Acknowledgments

I would like to express a deep gratitude to the Academic College of Society and the Arts and to the college's leadership, Dalia Ben Shushan, and Prof. Dalia Merari, for the faith and support throughout the research, writing and guidance processes. I also wish to thank Dr. Tami Yaguri for sharing thoughts and editorial guidance.

I would like to deeply thank my mother, Dr. Judith Abrahami-Einat, whose journey is a model and an inspiration to me. She is always there for me, with so much love and confidence. Thank you for sharing my journey.

References

Asawa, P. (2009) "Art Therapists' Emotional Reactions to the Demands of Technology" *Art Therapy: Journal of the American Art Therapy Association,* 26(2), 58-65.

Brians, E. (2011) "The 'Virtual' Body and the Strange Persistence of the Flesh: Deleuze, Cyberspace and the Posthuman" (pp. 116-141) in L. Guillaume & J. Hughes (eds.). *Deleuze and the Body* Edinburgh: Edinburgh University Press.

Bromberg, Philip M. (1996) "Standing in the Spaces: The Multiplicity of Self and the Psychoanalytic Relationship" *Contemporary Psychoanalysis*, 32(4), 509-535.

Cundy, L. (2015) "Surviving as a Psychotherapist in the Twenty-first Century" (pp. 99-123) in L. Cundy (ed.). *Love in the age of the internet: Attachment in the digital era*. London: Karnac Books.

Garner, R. (2017) *Digital Art Therapy: Material, Methods, and Applications*. London: Kingsly Publishing.

Hayles, K. N. (1999) *How we became Posthuman: Virtual Bodies in Cybernetics, Literature and Informatics.* Chicago: University of Chicago Press

Hoffman, I. Z. (1998) *Ritual and Spontaneity in the Psychoanalytic Process: A Dialectical-constructivist View*. Hillsdale: The Analytic Press.

Kaimal, G., Rattigan, M., Miller, G., Haddy, J. (2016) "Implications of National Trends in Digital Media Use for Art Therapy Practice" *Journal of Clinical Art Therapy*, 3(1), retrieved from: http://digitalcommons.lmu.edu/jcat/vol3/iss1/6

Kapitan, L. (2011) "Introduction to the Special Issue on Art Therapy's Response to the Techno-digital Culture" *Art Therapy: Journal of the American Art Therapy Association,* 26(2), 50-51.

Kuleba, B. (2009) *The Integration of Computerized Art-Making as a Medium in Art Therapy Theory and Practice* (Unpublished master's thesis). Philadelphia: Drexel University.

Liber, D. (2020a) "Human Psychotherapy in a Digital Age: Characteristics of the Hybrid Clinic" *Sihot, The Israeli Journal of Psychotherapy*, 34(3), 172-181 (Hebrew).

Liber, D. (2020b) "A Zoom of her Own – The Transition between the Art Therapy Clinic and Digital Therapy" AJCAT, *Academic Journal of Creative Arts Therapies*, 10 (Special Covid-19 edition), 1007-1016 (Hebrew).

Malchiodi, C. A. (2000) *Art Therapy and Computer Technology: A Virtual Studio of Possibilities*. London: Kingsly Publishing.

Malchiodi, C. A. (2018) *The Handbook of Art Therapy and Digital Technology*. London: Kingsly Publishing

Marzi. A, (ed,) (2016) *Psychoanalysis, Identity, and the Internet: Explorations into Cyberspace*. London: Karnac .

Moon, C. H. (2010) *Materials and media in art therapy: Critical understandings in diverse artistic vocabularies.* New York: Routledge.

Orbach, N. (2020) "The Good Enough Studio: Art therapy through the Prism of Space, Matter and Action" *Nona Orbach copyright*.

Orr, P. P. (2006) "Technology Training for Future Art Therapists" *Art Therapy: Journal of the American Art Therapy Association,* 23(4), 191-196.

Orr, P. P. (2012) "Technology Use in Art Therapy Practice: 2004 and 2011 comparison" *The arts in psychotherapy*, 39 (4), 234-238.

Palfrey, G., Gasser, U. (2008) *Born Digital: Understanding the First Generation of Digital Natives*. New York: Basic Books.

Postman, N (1993) *Technopoly: The Surrender of Culture to Technology*. New York: Random House.

Prensky, M. (2001) "Digital natives, digital immigrants" *On the Horizon,* 9(5), 1-6.

Tapscott, D. (2009) *Grown up digital: How the Net Generation is Changing your World*. New York: McGraw Hill.

Thong, S. A. (2007) "Redefining the Tools of Art Therapy" *Art Therapy: Journal of the American Art Therapy Association*, *24*, 52-58.

Turkle, S. (2005) *The Second Self: Computers and the Human Spirit*. Cambridge, MA: MIT Press.

Turkle, S. (2011) *Alone Together: Why we Expect More from Technology and Less from Each Other*. New York: Basic.
Zilberstein, K. (2015) "Technology, relationships and culture: Clinical and theoretical implications" *Clinical Social Work Journal,* 43, 151-158.

CHAPTER 3

THE IMAGERY OF THEORY: A VISUALLY CENTERED METHOD OF TEACHING ART THERAPY THEORY

JANICE SHAPIRO AND ELANA LAKH

Introduction

Visual imagery and sensory experience with tangible materials are the essence of art therapy. Therefore the education of art therapists needs to integrate creative image making with the cognitive aspect of learning. This chapter describes the development of a unique method of teaching art therapy theory and its interactive implementation, using examples.

The method has three main stages. The first is the preparation of the lectures with an emphasis on visual imagery. The second is active response art making to the lectures by the students. The third is our use of didactic curation to integrate the students' response imagery with the theoretical material and present it to the students.

Most of art therapy education uses an experiential visual oriented approach. Response art was traditionally done in studio settings. We have developed a method of integrating the visual aspects of teaching art therapy theory and response art making in a frontal lecture setting. We introduce the concept of "didactic curation" that forms connections between the lessons, elaborates the material, emphasizes key points and creates continuity.

The story of how our approach to teaching art therapy theory creatively evolved is intrinsic to the result. We extend an invitation to the reader to join us in this journey of discovery and for this reason have chosen a narrative style of writing as appropriate. At times we use a poetic tone of phrase to convey the symbolic atmosphere in the course in a style of writing that suits the realm of art therapy. The narrative form aims to share with the reader something of the excitement of discovery that keeps the creative spark alive for our students and for us while teaching and studying theoretical concepts.

The birth of the method

Traditionally art therapy theory has been taught through experiential artwork-based learning models (Honig, 2014) by combining theory and hands-on workshops. Students' art making has been a central part of art therapy education throughout its existence, considered to serve the student's ability to integrate concepts, conceptualize and process clinical work and contribute to professional identity (Deaver, 2012). The role of the arts in facilitating learning has been discussed by many authors.

A comprehensive literature summary was done by Sajnani et al (2020). They summarize the literature discussing the use of the arts in creative therapy student training in all modalities, elaborating on the idea of "aesthetic engagement" – the centrality of arts in art therapists' education. The aesthetic engagement in learning involves social and emotional aspects, as well as higher order thinking skills, creativity, imagination, and is regulated by the learner. Imagination plays an important role in this kind of learning, connecting ideas with experiences and feelings while metaphoric, poetic and symbolic ways of expression influence thinking and learning. We taught this way (McNiff, 2012) when we were adjunct faculty members of Lesley University's extension in Israel and at first continued using the same method when the affiliation with Lesley university came to an end and we became part of the staff of the newly founded Israeli college, The Academic College for Society and Arts. Teaching theory took place in rooms set up for artwork with groups not larger than fifteen, sitting in a circle. Students would express and understand the theoretical concepts we taught through giving expression to their relevant personal associations in artworks.

With the transition to the Israeli Masters of Arts program we were required by the council of higher education to teach theoretical courses to large groups in frontal lectures. The two of us were faced with preparing a series of weekly lectures for a year-long course called "Art therapy: Theory and methods". This paper describes the process we went through in meeting the challenge and the course which was created as the result.

When we began this in 2013 it was the norm for all frontal lectures to be accompanied by power-point presentations usually with the lecturer's spoken text or verbal summaries of its main points displayed on the screen.

We were used to weaving theory into experiential small group classes where for the verbal part of the lesson we sat with our students in a circle. For the part of the lesson devoted to art making the students were scattered around, some sitting at worktables, others standing at easels or working on the floor while we teachers witnessed their creative work in process, moving around the room ourselves. Now we were to change to an auditorium setting where we would stand at a fixed point by the computer in front of a screen, facing a large group of students seated in ordered rows of lecture chairs with armrests for their notebooks or laptops.

Our concern was the fear of losing our art therapist identity by teaching central courses using words only. Aware of Pat Allen's (1992) warnings of being seduced into a dominantly verbal clinical mode, we thought that her qualms were also relevant to the discipline of art therapy becoming increasingly academic. This academization of the profession is clearly an advancement with numerous positive aspects. However, because of the dominance of verbal language in education (Nuzzaci, 2019; Britsch, 2013) we were concerned about getting trapped in the hierarchical concept that words take over other modes of communication during development (Noy, 1999) and the consequent inferiority complex of the art therapy profession itself vis a vis clinicians and academics.

The driving force from the word go was our belief that art therapy theory and art therapy practice are not separate realms and optimally are interwoven. The connecting link is the visual image which gives tangible form to the inner world in practice (Schaverien, 1992) and which expresses theoretical ideas on the screen. Art therapy bridges inner and outer worlds through the image (Case, 2007). We saw visual images as potential bridges between the body of theoretical knowledge existing in the outer world and the evolving inner professional world of the art therapy student.

Our intention was that the images would contain and express the theoretical concepts thus conveying them to the students in the visual language of their profession. We thought this would be appropriate for our audience as people who choose this profession usually have a strong connection to the visual realm. In addition we believed that by emphasizing the visual language we would be role models showing how we use our visual channels to think and process ideas, seeing this as contributing to the empowerment of the students' identity as art therapists.

We identify with the Jungian world view that "image is psyche" (Jung, 1967, para. 75) and that symbolic language cannot be rationally explained or translated into verbal language: "The sign is always less than the concept it represents, while the symbol always stands for something more than its obvious and immediate meaning" (Jung, 1964, p. 41). This unique quality inherent in visual symbols offers infinite possibilities of further understanding of the theoretical concepts thus presented. These concepts are not to be defined and learnt once and for all. On the contrary, they are dynamically alive as described by Jung: "As long as the symbol is a living thing, it is an expression for something that cannot be characterized in any other or better way. A symbol is alive only so long as it is pregnant with meaning" (Jung, 1971, p. 474). Our use of symbolic imagery contributes to the vitality of the relationship between the students and the theories they study.

The central role of vision in learning

We knew intuitively that the use of visual imagery would contribute in many ways to the learning of concepts. This conviction which drew on our own experience has a strong base in existing theory, much researched and discussed.

Gardner (2011) described the strength of the visual-spatial aspect of intelligence. This had been argued earlier by Frances Yates in: The art of memory (1966), who wrote that visual representations guarantee an easier reconstruction of messages than verbal forms and advised translating any verbal message into visual form.

The centrality of vision in learning processes has been described in many texts from various disciplines (Britsch, 2013; Cuevas, 2016; McClanahan & Nottingham, 2019; Nuzzaci, 2019; Kuldas, Ismail, Hashim & Bakar, 2013; Marzal García-Quismondo, Cruz-Palacios & Castros Morales, 2019; Vekiri, 2002 and many others). All these authors agree that visual thinking has an important role in learning. In their wide review of the literature, Shor and Axelrod-Tyer (2014) point out that vision-based learning allows the student to use mediating processes that lead to a transition from primary seeing to looking that organizes the reality perceived. The capacity to see and to look changes as does the possibility of making connections and organizing what is seen. Perception is closely linked with exploration – the discovery of what is seen when looking leads to the building of the student's world, to the creation of new worlds (Roth, 2002). Learning is better when words and images support each other and are connected. This kind of learning also enhances creativity (Nuzzaci, 2019).

Hodes (1998) suggested that images help process information in an efficient way that eases the burden on the working memory because they contain a lot of information in a condensed way. Some of these processes are unconscious: unconscious mental representation can enhance the integration of verbal and visual material in a way that allows students to make meaning (Kuldas et al. 2013). Our use of images appeals to the unconscious as well as the conscious and relies on the collective unconscious as a source of material, in the Jungian tradition. Unconscious aspects of learning involve emotions (ibid), and the response image part of our lesson can give these emotions expression. Hodes (1998) states that illustrations to the text help learning and help turn the abstract information into concrete material. Our use of images goes beyond illustrating the text as we use the images themselves as theory.

According to dual coding theory of cognition, (Paivio, 1975 in Hodes, 1998), learning uses verbal and non-verbal modes at the same time with interconnected but separate information processing systems. Memory of imaged information is stronger, because it is represented in long term memory in two ways: verbal-propositional, and visual-imaginal, that interact and create knowledge.

Before we had encountered the concept of dual coding we embarked on the preparation of a series of lectures based on that theory. The resulting dialogue quickly became fertile. We found ourselves in a field of energy, bouncing ideas off each other. Before long we were dedicating prime time to the project. Seeking, finding and combining images that answered our didactic requirements were exciting and at times even had a numinous quality.

The preparation of the visual dimension of the lectures

We started by thinking about the setting for the lectures as analogous to the definition of the therapy session by physical space and by permanent times of beginning and ending each session (Rubin, 2011). The physical lecture hall and the time frame were set. However, we decided to add a symbolic setting within the lecture itself.

To do this we chose a permanent image template for the opening slide, repeated at the beginning of every lecture. Similarly, every lecture ended with the image we chose as the closing slide. To open we chose the image of a path leading into a green forest, inviting the students to come with us on a walk. To close we chose the image of a wooden bench at the side of the path inviting all of us to stop and rest and reflect on what had been seen and learned. This imagery formed an opening and closing ritual. The function of ritual is one of the key concepts we teach as playing an important role in therapeutic processes and in the setting enabling them (Marcow Speiser, 1997; Bauman, 2014).

Having established the boundaries of our setting we were ready to insert the content. We set out to find images that expressed the concepts delineated in the course syllabus. The image of symbolic "hunting and gathering" came to mind. At times we gathered images from our immediate surroundings – photos of the studio setting, collecting materials in the yards of the industrial zone, pictures from our own libraries of art books, examples of art work from the studio. At times we did not find what we needed nearby and went out hunting, usually in the great hunting ground of the internet, an experience that resonates with the way the English poet Ted Hughes used the metaphors of fishing and hunting to describe the poet's search for the right image, the right words, that exist somewhere but need to be found and captured (Hughes, 1967). As noted by educators of different disciplines, the internet is an educational space with a significant visual component, and a source for many learning experiences (Marzal García-Quismondo, Cruz-Palacios & Castros Morales, 2019). For us, the World Wide Web is a vast and richly populated field full to overflowing with readymade images which can be appropriated to use in our presentations. Hunting demands determination, discipline and focus. It also demands alertness and openness to potential discoveries of finds that we were not consciously looking for. Sometimes we hit on a readymade image that was exactly right while sometimes we created a collage combination to convey our message as in the following example in the lesson on the concept of setting.

Discussing the improvised studio when conditions are far from optimal, we quoted Moon's (2002) vivid description of a home visit where she worked in art therapy with a young boy in the family kitchen. The boot of her parked car was her cupboard of art equipment from which the boy would choose his materials. On the website of a car company we found advertisements showing photos of cars with open boots to display their roominess to potential buyers. In our own studios we photographed rolls of paper, jars of paint, various brushes, a packet of clay, a box of wooden boards and blocks, carpentry tools, a basket of random bits and pieces and more. We "packed" the car boot by copy-pasting these images inside it. This playful and stimulating use of internet imagery combined with photos we took ourselves brought creative energy into our preparations. We made use of found images, similar to the way found objects are used in art therapy (Siano, 2016).

When appropriate we use the power point program to introduce animation allowing an image to make its appearance in stages or to disappear followed by a different image taking its place. For example, when teaching Winnicott's (1969) concept of the positive role of destructiveness in establishing the reality principle, we found an image of an angry boy having a tantrum. Then we chose a photo of a house and positioned the boy as if he was trying to kick down his house. Using the animation function we then removed the house and in its place put a photo of a pile of rubble. After explaining that this was the boy's fantasy of destruction, we removed the rubble and restored the house to its original state. The boy discovered that he was not omnipotent and that his home continued to exist no matter how violently he fantasized its destruction.

We became aware that our creative searching for images expressing the lesson's content caused it to become more our own. This connects to Winnicott's conviction that for theory to stay alive when restated it should be presented in the personal language of whoever is restating it (Grolnick, 1980). For us as art therapists restating theory in our own language means expressing it in the language of visual imagery.

It was an intriguing experience to construct our lectures in this way, restating or interpreting theoretical concepts as images which had to be hunted and gathered and often modified or combined to suit our intentions. When the time came to "deliver" the result to the students we could feel how the creative energy invested by us generated a corresponding experience in the student audience, an atmosphere of active involvement. We hope to generate a similar quality of energy in this chapter. One might see a parallel in the way that when preparing the studio space is experienced as a creative act (Moon, 2002) the creative energy invested is present in that space and influences what happens in there.

Often students ask us to give them our power point presentation. We explain that they would gain far more if they find or create their own images to express their understanding of the theory they are studying as this is a way to make sense of it, digest it and make it their own. This resonates with John Dewey's 1934 suggestion (in Sajnani et al. 2020) that learning happens through experience, while aesthetic experiences enhance reflection and help integrate theory and practice.

Active response art making

At the end of the first course the students' feedback expressed their yearning for making art in relation to the theory studied. We identified with this need. Both of us practice art response as an integral part of our art-based supervision seminars. In this method the art therapist responds in art to the session with a client. The aim is to cultivate therapeutic insight through imagery (Fish, 2019; Brown, Meyerowitz-Katz & Ryde, 2007) especially through making unconscious counter-transferential reactions conscious. Response art making can also serve as an interactive mentalizing process within a therapeutic session (Havsteen-Franklin & Camarena Altamirano, 2015). We liked the idea of inviting response imagery in the different context of studying theory in frontal lectures.

Professor Dalia Merari, the head of our art therapy department, suggested we find a way to include some art making in the course itself. We were responsive to the idea in principle but could not see how art making could be included, given the limitations of time and space.

We have enormous respect for the making of artworks as a potentially numinous experience in a studio that in itself is a stimulating space (Orbach, 2020), with its rich variety of tools and materials and work surfaces. Like therapists who imagine the ideal studio and find it difficult to deal with the less-than-optimal conditions of reality (Moon ,2002) our sacred attitude to the studio space limited us. Locked down into our dichotomous vision of either a frontal theoretical lecture or a creative studio experience, a lecture hall seemed an impossible physical setting for creating artwork.

We are both familiar on a personal level with sketching images as a way to understand and process what we learn, during or after lectures or reading, often in a small notebook using just a pencil or pen as our way of making the material our own, a learning aid. We had not seen this as art making but thought that something like that could work with students. We decided to devote the last fifteen minutes of the lecture to active response image making by the students on their arm sets and provided minimal basic art materials.

The students were curious to see the images created by one another and so were we. Yet time was too short to share the images. We asked them to photograph their images on the spot and email the photos to us.

Didactic curation

The variety of images that soon appeared in our inboxes stimulated us to think of how to develop this intervention further and incorporate it into our teaching structure. This led to the idea of arranging the art responses on slides and showing them at the start of the following week's lecture. We considered how to group them. When several students responded to a particular theoretical concept, we displayed them together. The same concept may have evoked similar images for several students whereas others created completely different ones. The choice of image may reflect a personal or an archetypal association, an emotion evoked by the concept, a link to work in the field or sometimes an unconscious connection. Our creative energy awakened as we played with options for sorting them, actively looking for points in common or points of contrast, relating to various categories such as theme, composition, color or shapes.

As an example, we will describe the art responses to our lesson on resistance. We had discussed its role in therapy in general and art therapy in particular, how to understand it as symbolic communication of emotional states and ways to engage with it on a symbolic level. The images we gathered from the internet for our lecture depicted no entry street signs, gaping holes, closed doors and heroes facing frightening powers. We also showed a photo of an artwork made by a patient, who used nails that he hit into a wooden board to form the words: "I don't want to," expressing his resistance in art materials, rather than by acting out.

Many students responded with personal variations on the traffic sign theme, giving universal signs individual meaning. They created stop signs, slow down signs, danger of flooding signs, danger of rocks falling and others. We grouped these together as warnings that are provided by outer or inner authorities.

Other response images echoed the reluctance to respond at all, like one student who amongst scribbles wrote the words: "I'm tired and I want to go home," communicating resistance tangibly on paper. Two participants sent in empty pages which is very different to not sending anything at all, as act that would be clear acting out. The written objection and empty pages we grouped on one slide.

A less obvious kind of resistance that we had discussed in the lesson was responded to by a student who drew stereotyped flowers in faint pencil as a way of appearing to cooperate yet avoiding any authentic expression of feeling. We paired this with an art response of rows of circles carefully colored in with bright colors which also seemed to us to relate to imagery that is pleasant to the eye but has a defensive function.

We think of this as didactic curatorship. Roya Sachs, curator of the Lever House Art Collection describes a curator as a facilitator who connects people, ideas and creativity (Cohen, 2018). According to a senior editor at Taschen, Julius Weidemann, a curator connects art pieces in a way that creates something new that is greater than the sum of its pieces. "The connection of the art pieces within a context creates a storyline" (Weidemann, 2019). Art educator Claire Robins suggested that: "Stories of art are produced through the curatorial process of selection, juxtaposition and interpretation of art" (2005, p. 150). She stresses that curators' decisions influence what the visitors see, as well as the way they construct meaning and understand what they experience. The curator tells the story of the art, and so do we, emphasizing its meaning in the context of the theory studied. When a curator plans an exhibition and decides how to arrange the works he is guided by a concept that he feels appropriate to the content, the setting and the audience. As facilitators, we are guided by the concept of displaying the works with the aim of enhancing the learning experience of the student audience in the course setting. Arranging the art responses after the lecture, we told the story of the idea that we taught. In our curating decisions we created connections, stressed points, and presented relevant visual and conceptual issues.

We opened the following week's lecture with the curated slides displaying the image responses of the students to the week before. The students pointed out additional connections and contrasts. In the ensuing dialogue we noticed that through the imagery we could emphasize aspects of the previous week's lesson. We could show how each student's choice of image and way of giving it form highlighted a different aspect of the subject taught. We realized that through these slides we were in fact summarizing the key points of the last lesson and elaborating on them.

Discussion

The particular way in which we use visual art as an integral part of our theoretical lecture structure developed organically.

Our extensive use of visual imagery to communicate theoretical ideas in our teaching resonates with the concept of dual coding (Paivio in Hodes, 1998) that is pivotal in learning theories and education research. When the students give form to their own visual images in response to our dual coded powerpoint presentations, they are adding their personal dual coding. This active creation of their individual visual channel amplifies the effectiveness of the visual-verbal duality and fits with the way Hodes (1998) sees imagery as a type of elaboration strategy that serves to integrate new information with existing knowledge. We see a meaningful contribution to this integration in the initiative that each student takes in choosing which aspect of the lesson she wants to elaborate on and how to give it visual expression in her own individual way. This is an active learning mode.

According to Dewey (in Sajnani et al., 2020), the artist actively internalizes elements of the world, relationships and ideas, and then externalizes them in his art, enhancing new understandings and options.

In the field of science education, Britsch (2013) stresses the active part of drawing as means for processing information in learning. Shor and Axelrod-Tyer (2014) claim that sensory relating to the learnt material is required and that learning theory solely through words will hamper internalization of the knowledge. From our experience we know that this is particularly true for the vast majority of art therapy students. Shor and Axelrod-Tyer (ibid) recommend painting as part of processing the material in learning, connecting seeing with conceptual understanding. They state that students develop a unique visual style which they term "fingerprints" (2014, p. 121). We see these fingerprints reflected in the students' response paintings, that show each student's unique artistic language, in the context of the theoretical issues presented.

The students' images responses and our integration of them into the course contribute in several ways to the learning experience. From the feedback we learnt that the way the students listen to, look at and think about the lecture is influenced by their knowing that they will respond by creating an image. Often a mental image will appear spontaneously. Imagining possible image responses along the way makes them more conscious of their feelings vis-à-vis the concepts and issues presented. This state of mind adds to their processing and internalizing the concepts taught even though not all the images envisioned are given tangible form. Being alert to potential visual imagery of their own puts the students into an active mode of learning. When they actually give tangible form to particular images they have seen in their mind's eye this active mode is heightened.

Photographing their works and emailing them to us means that what they have made is going to be seen and thought about by us in itself and in relation to images made by others. They know we will give each and every individual image a place in the opening of the following week's presentation, reflecting it back in the context of its relationship to the images that have emerged from the group as a whole. Knowing that their responses are to be seen adds value to the process, as being attentively seen always does. A playful creativity is communicated by the fact that we have clearly shuffled around all the images we received, arranging them to show our perceived connections and contrasts.

The fact that the students' images comprise the opening of each week's lecture gives their work pride of place. Furthermore, this opening establishes continuity by building a bridge between the previous week's class and the present one, a bridge constructed from the combination of students' individual images and our curation.

This cycle is repeated weekly. We deliver our lecture, the students send us their response art, we curate the responses to form a story with relevant meaning and present this to the students as the opening of the following lecture. This back-and-forth dialogue between the students and teachers adds an interactive dynamic of fertile communication.

Yet another unplanned but welcome result of this weekly ritual is that by the end of the course each student has her own personal series of image responses to the full sequence of lectures as well as her verbal notes and summaries. These images show the evolution of her unique visual fingerprint. They are reminders of the content and development of the course as seen through the personal prism of the aspects that evoked her creative responses.

Conclusion

The teaching method of art therapy theory we present here can be viewed as an aspect of cultivating visual literacy within the students. Visual literacy involves skills of understanding and interpreting visual images, the capacity to communicate them and to use them to elaborate on material and create new meaning (Marzal García-Quismondo, Cruz-Palacios & Castros Morales, 2019).

This method has three main parts, all giving central place to visual language as an integral component. The first part is the preparation of powerpoint presentations that display appropriate visual imagery expressing every concept taught. The second part consists of image responses by the students.

The third part uses didactic curating to integrate the art responses with the theory.

In a narrative style of writing, we have described how all three parts of our method became interwoven, contributing to understanding and internalizing theoretical concepts of art therapy.

When faced with the necessity of changing from experiential teaching of theory in small groups in art studios to frontal lectures to large groups in lecture halls we moved through the stages of seeing it as a challenge, exploring ways of going about it and then embracing the new approach.

With hindsight we have become aware of the shadow side of the reverence for art. We discovered how flexibility in this matter met important and relevant needs in our students. We still believe that art therapy theory is optimally taught in a studio setting which enables in depth artwork as an integral part of understanding the concepts studied. What has changed is seeing this as the only way. We changed our approach, enriching our students and our professional selves by our investment in dual coded presentations. In addition we developed a new variation of response art, building it into the theory course structure and including our didactic curating of the students' images as an integral part of teaching and learning.

Joseph Campbell (2008) writes of the hero who temporarily leaves his home when setting out on a journey, emphasizing that when the hero returns he adds to his original home whatever he brings with him from his time away. Perhaps we might say that we have returned to our studio home and have built on an extension in the shape of a lecture hall. This cultivation of an additional option has enriched our professional space while continuing to deepen our longstanding relationship with our home base.

References

Allen, P. (1992) "Artist in Residence: An Alternative to 'Clinification' for Art Therapists" *Art Therapy*, 9(1), 22-29.

Bauman, A. (2014) "Rites and Games for Creating Sacred Holy Space" (pp. 65-75) in E. Perroni. (ed.) *Play: Psychoanalytic Perspectives, Survival and Human Development*. Routledge: Taylor & Francis.

Britsch, S. (2013) "Visual Language and Science Understanding: A Brief Tutorial for Teachers" *Australian Journal of Language and Literacy,* 36(1), 17-27.

Brown C., Meyerowitz-Katz J., Ryde J. (2007) "Thinking with Image Making: Supervising Student Art Therapists" (pp. 167-181) in J. Schaverien, C. Case (eds.) *Supervision of Art Psychotherapy: A Theoretical and Practical Handbook*. Routledge: Taylor & Francis.

Campbell, J. (2008) *The Hero of a Thousand Faces*. Pantheon: New York

Case, C. (2007) "Imagery in Supervision" (pp. 95-115) in J. Schaverien, C. Case (eds.). *Supervision of Art Psychotherapy: A Theoretical and Practical Handbook*. Routledge: Taylor & Francis.

Cohen, A. (2018) "Everyone's a Curator: That's not (always) a Bad Thing" *Artsy*. Dec. 21, 2018. https://www.artsy.net/article/artsy-editorial-everyones-curator-bad-thing.

Cuevas, J. (2016) "An Analysis of Current Evidence Supporting Two Alternate Learning Models: Learning Styles and Dual Coding" *Journal of Educational Sciences and Psychology*, 6(1), 1-13.

Deaver, S.P. (2012) "Art-Based Learning Strategies in Art Therapy Graduate Education" *Journal of the American Art Therapy Association*, 29(4), 158-165.

Fish, B. (2019) "Response Art in Art Therapy: Historical and Contemporary Overview" *Art Therapy*, 36(3), 122-132.

Gardner, H. (2011) *Frames of Mind: The Theory of Multiple Intelligences*. Hachette.

Grolnick, S.A. (1980) *The Work and Play of Winnicott*. Jason Aronson.

Havsteen-Franklin, D., Camarena Altamirano, J. (2015) "Containing the Uncontainable: Responsive Art Making in Art Therapy as a Method to Facilitate Mentalization" *International Journal of Art Therapy*, 20(2), 54-65.

Hodes, C. L. (1998) "Understanding Visual Literacy through Visual Information Processing" *Journal of Visual Literacy*, 18(2), 131-136.

Honig, O. (2014) *Post-graduate art therapy training in Israel: Personal and professional transformation through dynamic artwork-based experiential transformative courses*. [Doctoral dissertation]. University of Sussex.

Hughes, T. (1967) *Poetry in the Making*. Faber.

Jung, C. G. (1964) Approaching the unconscious (pp. 1-94) in Jung, C. G., Von Franz, M. L., (eds.). *Man and his Symbols.* Dell.

Jung, C.G. (1967) *Alchemical Studies*. R. F. C. Hull (tran.). Bollingen series XX, Princeton University Press. (CW 13) Electronic version. Retrieved November 13, 2020, from: https://www.jungiananalysts.org.uk/wp-content/uploads/2018/07/C.-G.-Jung-Collected-Works-Volume-13_-Alchemical-Studies.pdf

Jung, C. G. (1971) *Psychological Types.* H. G. Baynes, R. F. C. Hull (trans.). London: Routledge & Kegan Paul.

Kuldas, S., Ismail, H. N., Hashim, S., Bakar, Z. A. (2013) "Unconscious learning processes: Mental integration of verbal and pictorial instructional materials" *Springer Plus,* 2(1), 105.

Marcow Speiser, V. (1997) Ritual in expressive therapy. In: A. Robbins (Ed.), *Therapeutic presence* (pp. 204-218). Jessica Kingsley.

Marzal García-Quismondo, M. A., Cruz-Palacios, E., Castros Morales, F. (2019) A didactic innovation project in higher education through a visual and academic literacy competence-based program. *Education for Information,* 35(3), 263-283.

McClanahan, B. J., Nottingham, M. (2019) A suite of strategies for navigating graphic novels: A dual coding approach. *The Reading Teacher,* 73(1), 39-*50.*

McNiff, S. (2012) "Art and Change: A Process of Creative Contagion" (pp. 36-51) in Schwartz, S. Markow Spieser, V., Spieser, P., Kossak, M. (eds.). *Art and Social Change: The Lesley University Experience in Israel*. The arts institute project in Israel Press.

Moon, C.H. (2002) *Studio Art Therapy*. Jessica Kingsley.

Noy, P. (1999) *The psychoanalysis of art and creativity*. Modan (Hebrew).

Nuzzaci, A. (2019) A picture is worth a thousand words: visual thinking between creative thinking and critical thinking in the teaching-learning processes. *img journal,* 1(1), 234-253.

Orbach, N. (2020) *Good enough studio*: *Art therapy through the prism of space, matter and action.* Private author's publishing.

Robins, C. (2005) "Engaging with Curating" *International Journal of Art & Design Education,* 24(2), 149-158.

Roth, W. M. (2002, April) "From Stimulus to Science: The Changing Nature of Visual Perception" *American Educational Research Association Annual Meeting*. New Orleans.

Rubin, J. A. (2011*) The Art of Art Therapy: What Every Art Therapist Needs to Know*. Brunner-Routledge.

Sajnani, N., Mayor, C., Tillberg-Webb, H. (2020) "Aesthetic Presence: The Role of the Arts in the Education of Creative Arts Therapists in the Classroom and Online" *The Arts in Psychotherapy*. Oct., 2020. https://doi.org/10.1016/j.aip.2020.101668

Schur, Y., Tayer-Axelrod N. (2014) "Dynamic Learning – Seeing, Observation, Cognitive Processes and Conceptual Understanding" *Bemaagalei Chinuch,* (4) 96-127 (Hebrew).

Schaverien, J. (1992) *The Revealing Image: Analytical Art Psychotherapy in Theory and Practice*. Routledge.

Siano, J. (2016) *Holy Junk: Lost, Found and Rejected Objects in Art Therapy*. Private publishing.

Wiedemann, J. (2019) "What is an Art Curator?" *Domestika*. Dec., 2019. https://www.domestika.org/en/blog/2543-what-is-an-art-curator.
Winnicott, D. W. (1969) "The Use of an Object" *International Journal of Psycho-Analysis,* 50, 711-716.
Vekiri, I. (2002) "What is the Value of Graphical Displays in Learning?" *Educational Psychology Review,* 14(3), 261-312.
Yates, F. (1966) *The Art of Memory*. Routledge.

CHAPTER 4

THE INTRODUCTION OF LIFE STORY INTO ART THERAPY TRAINING PROGRAMS

AMIA LIEBLICH

Introduction

This paper presents an original attempt to use "life story" as a central concept in the College orientation workshop for art-therapists. Specifically, with the help of my colleagues,[1] I designed this workshop for a special student-group: experienced arts therapists, aged about 30 to 50, some with many years of practice in Israel. Most enrolled in the year-long course of M.A. study because they are graduates of diploma studies programs and the arts therapy regulatory environment has changed to favor holders of a master's degree. Some enrolled to refresh their professional training. This background has naturally influenced the program devised for the group.

Stories, oral and written, are undoubtedly among the oldest and widest spread forms of art. They have their place in academic psychology and psychotherapy. My academic professional expertise is in the field of qualitative psychology and life story studies (see Lieblich, Tuval-Mashiach & Zilber, 1996, Lieblich, McAdams & Josselson, 2004). I ardently believe that one's life story is a major internal vehicle for the construction and reflection of identity and culture (Bruner, 1990), as well as their inter-personal communication. Therefore, when I was invited as a senior to join a group of instructors in planning the forthcoming orientation, I proposed to use life story as the main concept for our three-days opening workshop.

---

[1] My deep gratitude to Tsiky Cohen, Pazit Dushi, Anat Gilad, Elana Lakh, Vivien Marcow Speiser, Samuel Schwartz, Sharon Vaisvaser – Ono Academic College / The Academic College of Society and the Arts, for their creativity and cooperation. (See Schwartz in press).

In addition to my firm conviction concerning the centrality and significance of life stories within the intersection of therapy and the arts, my assumption was that although the students have rich experience in the various modalities of visual, musical, dance or drama art, they are less familiar with the study of life stories and their application. I based this understanding on the fact that narrative approaches and practices have only recently been introduced into the curriculum of art-therapy programs, as well as generally into mental health training, psychology studies etc. Theories and applications of personal narratives and life stories could therefore provide a fresh start to our study year. I expected that focusing on story as art – whether telling, writing or reading – would be beneficial as an orientation for the year- long program with this experienced group of students.

The general plan that will be detailed below was carried out four times in consecutive years in our college. Some of the aspects of the learning workshop that I detail in this paper were not present in the first try, but were added later, with the team's accumulative experience over these repetitions.

In general, the 3-days didactic experience had two interactive elements: Theory and practice of life stories, on the one hand, and the expression of verbal narrative contents that emerged in the variety of art forms, on the other hand. Some of the classes were plenary lectures, while most of them took place in small groups, dedicated to the art modalities of this workshop, namely visual arts, psychodrama and dance-movement. The next two sections of the present paper relate separately to these two elements of the workshop.

Basic theory of life-stories in psychology

This section elaborated the inter-relationship of three areas: life-story, art and therapy.

Some of the stories we all know are literary work, fiction or myth. This paper relates, however, to autobiographical stories that I will name "life stories." They represent events experienced by the narrator, and usually classified as non-fiction. However, life stories do not document reality as such; rather they are the outcome of reality as perceived, remembered and understood, and as the narrator wishes, or is able, to share it with the listener, within a specific context and time.

The way we formulate our stories about experiences, motivations, feelings, values etc., reflects the meaning we give to our lives. Stories abound in our daily lives from early childhood onwards. We constantly tell stories not only to others, as a means of communication, but also to ourselves. Our stories provide a window into our identity and culture (Bruner, 1986). Moreover, there is a reciprocal relationship among these concepts; our autobiographical stories represent our identity and culture while simultaneously constructing them.

Several theories and studies further developed and explored the relationship of life story and identity. McAdams' (1993) classical work proposes that shaping a story about our life is our way of defining our identity. Atkinson (2007) claims that personal narratives reveal how individual identity is constructed and revised by its representation in the form of a story.

Like art, life stories are based on memories and impressions, past and present events, and themes we absorb from our culture. All these elements of our experience, by their nature, are subjective. Neither memories nor present impressions are objectively veridical. Rather, they are selective and deeply influenced by motivation, context and many additional factors. Therefore, in studying life stories, we aim at 'narrative truth'' rather than 'historical truth' (Sarbin, 1986), or, in other words – the subjective, rather than objective experience, is at the focus of life story studies.

Stories, by their nature, are richer in human detail than psychological theories. In an attempt to be systematic, objective and scientific, psychological theory has severely limited itself in the past from working with stories (Gergen, 2001). Daniel Albright clearly described this situation saying, "Literature is a wilderness – psychology is a garden, well-kept, neatly cut, with its divisions and hierarchies." (1994, p. 19).

The manifestation of stories in art is, naturally, a significant contribution to their effect. Storytelling can utilize all of the art forms (Marcow Speiser, 1998). The arts contribute additional or alternative channels of the processes of expression and construction and enable us to 'know the unthought known' (Bollas, 1987).

On the surface, non-verbal expressions, such as painting, movement and dance, may seem quite distant from storytelling. However, current interdisciplinary scholarship conceive of action, expression and narration as mutually influential. This view is supported by several psycho-biological academic fields. Damasio's autobiographical self (2010) or Gallagher's narrative self (2000), as the object of introspection, are composed from the collection of sensory based experiences of the subject interacting with the environment.

Conceptually, there is an inherent connection between life stories and therapy. In fact, therapy can theoretically be constructed as interactive story-making and story-changing (White and Epston, 1990). The client starts her/his process of therapy, whether short- or long-term, with a certain story, which usually includes complaints, conflicts and challenges of different sorts. The therapeutic process can be described as a continuous expression and revision of this original story, thus enabling better understanding of oneself and, hopefully, resulting in improvement (White, 2011). While the therapeutic power of the spoken and written word is undeniable, the visual, dramatic and movement arts give form to experiences located in another layer of the psyche and soul (Schwartz, Speiser & Wikoff, 2013).

The precise meaning of 'a story' or 'a narrative' is ambiguous. For the purpose of our workshop we suggested to use these terms as synonyms and rely mainly on Labov and Waletzky's (1997) classic exposition. According to this widely accepted proposal, a story involves a reported event. It can be constructed as having three stages, focusing on antecedents, change and consequences. In its full exposition, according to this model, a story includes six stages: 1) Abstract – How does it begin? 2) Orientation 3) Complicating Action 4) Resolution 5) Evaluation 6) Coda. This conceptualization was offered to the students as a framework for the experiential section I describe below.

Didactic-experiential methods for life story work

The approximately one hundred students in this introductory orientation for experienced expressive arts therapists participated in this 3-day workshop. Teaching was accompanied by exercises performed in the classrooms. Some modules brought all the students together while other exercises took place in small groups of up to 15 students divided by artistic modality.

The following exercises were devised to familiarize the students with the wealth of personal stories, later to be used for the art expressions in the workshop. They focused on two tasks: composing one's own life story, and obtaining the life story of another. Due to the time-limited nature of the course, the exercises focused on particular memories rather than forming a complete life story.[2] The first section of the course aimed to allow each participant to compose their own life story episode and listen to another's. It involved writing, reading to the group, and listening. The second section provided preliminary experience in interviewing another person for obtaining a life story. Following each of these verbal exercises, the students integrated various art expressions into the storytelling.

a. *Writing and sharing a self- story.*

A1.

Instructions: "Please try to recall a significant event from your early childhood. Write about the event as much as possible following the Labov and Waletzky scheme presented before. Try to be specific: Where and when did it happen, who else was present, how did you feel."

Twenty minutes of quiet time were allotted for the writing.

A2.

When the writing was completed, the students were divided into 3-person groups. The small group participants read their stories aloud to each other. The instructions required listening to the reading without interruption. At the end of the reading, the two listeners offered their reactions. It was clearly counter-indicated to provide interpretations or advice. Rather, I introduced and emphasized "emphatic listening" (Myers, 2000) as the role to be adopted by those who did not read. This section was allocated an additional 20 minutes.

A3.

Immediately after the exercise, the students gathered in the special arts studios, where they expressed and elaborated the stories written or shared, using psychodrama, movement or painting and other visual representations.

b. Conducting a narrative interview

This section was planned for obtaining a life story from the other. It started with a demonstration of a narrative interview, as detailed in B1.

---

[2] One method for obtaining a complete life story, particularly suitable for art-therapies, is included in an Appendix below.

B1.

In the plenary meeting, I asked for a volunteer willing to be interviewed in front of the class. Consequently I demonstrated a short narrative interview in a fishbowl, where all the class attended around us, and a close-up video picture was screened in front. In the beginning I introduced myself briefly to the interviewee, stated the purpose of the interview (collecting stories for an article) and said: "Please try to recall a significant interaction you had with a teacher, within or outside of school, and tell me about it. It can be a memory from childhood or later in your life. What exactly happened, when and where? What started it and how did it end? How did you feel then? How do you feel about it now? Take your time, and start when something comes up."

Following this introduction, I assumed the active listener role. I tried to refrain from questions and attentively follow the narrator, listening. My body language and gestures expressed my interest in the story told. If some periods of silence occurred, I waited without interruption. After a few moments, if needed, I asked: "and what happened then?"' Sometimes, when the account was general, I commented: "Can you tell me more?", "Can you give an example" etc. Towards the end of this demonstration, I asked the volunteer how she felt then and there.

When I felt that the demonstration was not sufficient for representing the method, I sometimes repeated the process with another topic, e.g. "Can you please tell me about your childhood best friend? How did it start, what happened then? How did you feel about her? Does this relationship continue? How did it end?"

B2.

In the plenary, students reflected and discussed the demonstration, focusing on the behavior of the interviewer. I then gave a brief lecture on the principles of the narrative interview (Josselson, 2013) and presented several basic rules for the life story interview. In particular, I emphasized the differences between a clinical intake or a therapy session versus the narrative research interview. In the interview, I explained, the aim is to 'learn' from the narrator, rather than to 'change' or 'cure' her. I talked about ethics, respect, non-judgmental attitude and special rules for opening and closing the interview.

B3.

The students were divided again into groups of three. Each student took her turn in being the interviewer, the interviewee or an observer of the procedure. Each interviewer chose the subject of the interview he/she performed, and the observer took notes on the procedure. Following each round, the three participants shared their experiences in their different roles. This section took at least an hour.

B4.

The students gathered in their art studios to express in art what they have experienced in the interview section. They were asked to focus on one or two of the narrative elements that impressed them and express their impression in art. While in the visual arts studio each student worked on her own in silence, in the movement and psychodrama modalities, the work was frequently carried out in groups.

c. *Closing exhibition and performance.*

The last day of the orientation was dedicated to processing and summarizing the two former days. Each of the modality groups prepared an exhibition or a performance to represent the experience of the workshop. In the afternoon, we held a final plenary festive session where all students shared their work in the presence of the entire team of professors and instructors. Our summary and feedback aimed at the creation, for the participants and the instructors alike, of a meaningful transitional ceremony for entering the year of studies.

Discussion

Life story materialized in the workshop in a multi-faceted manner. Storytelling took place in several phases: *writing*, which transforms personal memory into words, *telling* the story vocally, which emphasizes its inter-personal communicative value, and *obtaining – listening* to the story of another in an interview setting. Following this verbal parts, the participants were engaged in *creating* the story in art materials and *sharing* this complex experience with others in different modalities. All in all this produced a rich academic and personal introduction for the year-long M.A. program that the students were about to begin.

This format has become a successful innovation in our curriculum and was repeated a number of times in our College. At the end of each workshop, every year, the instructors, all of them experienced arts therapists, expressed their appreciation for the impact of the experience. In particular, we all appreciated the joint effect of the life story verbal part with its artistic expressions. Furthermore, the instructors commented about the effect of the new, verbal component on the students' ability and motivation in the different arts.

In writing a joint article about the experience, the different instructors summarized the pedagogic experience from their different academic and artistic perspectives. The following is quoted from that article:

> The group became the "transitional space" (Winnicott 2005) that facilitated and enabled the process, and contained the spoken stories and images that emerged. The participants often expressed that "they are re-living their childhood experiences," with the emotional content attached, through the pictures emerging from the stories. This process shed new light on past experiences. Although the purpose of the course emphasized "pure" non-judgmental, non-interpretative listening to the words and the images, it had therapeutic value for the students, as it enabled processing and assimilating of the emotional psychic content that the art work embodied. This kind of listening is highly valued for every therapist (Schwartz et al, in press).

Similarly, in the separate processing of the stories in the movement-dance group,

> The students were guided to notice their own bodily sensations and movements throughout the process and witness those of their peers, with relation to the unfolding narrative – the written or spoken word and the emotions and feelings evoked. The students took note of and shared their kinesthetic experiences and thus, the continuous input from the body served as a functional anchor of the phenomenal experience (Schwartz et al, in press).

Finally, in the psychodrama group, which is perhaps closest to the field of life stories, the students were asked to think about ways to represent the stories they told or heard in a dramatic and creative language. After each subgroup presented their work to the whole psychodrama class, "all participants assembled into a reflective sharing circle that focused on the transitions that took place between the personal and the social, and between verbal narrative language and the dramatic one" (ibid.). Subsequent to the exercise of the interview as instructed to the entire class, psychodrama students continued the interview, this time "combining it with psychodramatic tools such as doubling, mirroring, concretizing, soliloquy, role reversal, empty chair and more" (ibid.). As we gained experience in this format, the instructors of the modality groups improved their ability to integrate the life story parts of the workshop, both theory and practice, with the variety of art therapy practices and tools. All in all, in our College, this proved to be a productive fresh start for the MA program for experienced art therapists.

Appendix

The complete life story: Optional exercise for future workshops.

If time allows, I suggest an additional exercise, which has two major advantages: It aims to cover the complete life story, and it uses drawing rather than words, therefore it is especially suitable and relevant to expressive arts therapists. Following my colleague Annie Rogers (2006), I have named the task "The River of Life" and have had meaningful experience with this technique in various settings.

Following are the instructions I give to this exercise: "Each of us can envision her life as a river, originating at birth, and going on to the present moment. Please use a blank page and a pencil. If you take the left side of the page to begin drawing your river, reaching the other end of the page for the present moment, how can you draw your river of life? It can be sometimes narrow and sometimes wide, it may go up and down, disappear for a while, join another river or lake, split into several streams and so on. It does not have to be an artistic drawing. Please draw and do not use words!"

People are given 20 minutes of quiet time for the drawing. Following this, the next instructions are: "Now you may use words to clarify the drawing. Put short captions for the various parts of your work."

After about 10 minutes, participants in this exercise are arranged in 3-persons groups to share the rivers of each one, and reflect on the exercise.

References

Albright, D. (1994) "Literary and Psychological Models of the Self" (pp. 19-40) in U. Neisser and R. Fivush (eds.). *The Remembering Self.* Cambridge: Cambridge University Press.

Atkinson, R. (2007) "The Life Story Interview as a Bridge in Narrative Inquiry" (pp. 224-45) in D. J. Clandinin (ed.). *Handbook of Narrative Inquiry: Mapping a Methodology*. Thousand Oaks and London: Sage Publications.

Bollas, C. (1987) *The Shadow of the Object: Psychoanalysis of the Unthought Known.* New York: Columbia University Press.

Bruner, J. (1986) *Actual Minds, Possible Words.* Cambridge: Harvard University Press.

Bruner, J. (1990) *Acts of Meaning*. Cambridge: Harvard University Press.

Damasio, A. (2010) *Self Comes to Mind: Constructing the Conscious Brain.* New York: Pantheon.

Gallagher, S. (2000) "Philosophical Conceptions of the Self: Implications for Cognitive Science" *Trends in Cognitive Sciences*, 4(1), 14-21.

Gergen, K. J. (2001) "Psychological Science in a Postmodern World" *American Psychologist*, 56(10), 803-13.

Josselson, R. (2013) *Interviewing for Qualitative Inquiry: A Relational Approach.* New York and London: The Guilford Press.

Labov, W., Waletzky, J. (1997) "Narrative Analysis: Oral Versions of Personal Experience" *Journal of Narrative and Life History*, 7(1-4), 3-38.

Lieblich, A., Tuval-Mashiach, R., Zilber, T. (1996) *Narrative Research: Reading, Analysis and Interpretation.* Thousand Oaks: Sage

Lieblich, A., D. P. McAdams, R. Josselson (eds.) (2004) *Healing Plots: The Narrative Basis of Psychotherapy.* Washington DC: American Psychological Association

Marcow Speiser, V. (1998) "The Use of Ritual in Expressive Therapy" (pp. 204-218) in A. Robbins (ed.). *Therapeutic Presence: Bridging Expression and Form.* Bristol, PA: Jessica Kingsley.

McAdams, D. P. (1993), *The Stories We Live By: Personal Myths and the Making of the Self*, New York: William Morrow and Co.

Meyers, S. (2000) "Reports on the Experience of Being Heard" *Journal of Humanistic Psychology,* 40, 148-173

Rogers, Annie G. (2006) *The Unsayable: The Hidden Language of Trauma*, New York: Random House

Sarbin, T. R. (1986) *Narrative Psychology: The Storied Nature of Human Conduct*. New York: Praeger.

Schwartz, S., Marcow Speiser, V., Wijkoff, N. (2013) "The Arch of Arts in Health" *Journal of Applied Arts and Health*, 4(3), 237-45.

Schwartz, S., Lieblich, A., Marcow Speiser, V., Lakh, E., Cohen, T., Dushi P., Gilad A. (2020) "Life Story and the Arts: A Didactic Crossroad" *Journal of Applied Art & Health,* 11(3), 315-328.

White, M. K. (2011) *Maps of Narrative Practice*. New York: W.W. Norton.

White, M. K., Epston, D. (1990) *Narrative Means to Therapeutic Ends*. New York: W. W. Norton.

Winnicott, D. W. (2005) *Playing and Reality*. London: Routledge.

CHAPTER 5

IN SICKNESS AND DEATH: AN ART-BASED RESEARCH OF ART-BASED PEDAGOGY

MICHAL LEV, AYA KATS AND GILI NAVOTH

In memory of Michal Aloni and Shulamit Sabag

"Humanity's Resilience
Resigned with diligence"
The politician grinned at the tree
"I demand: Nature-dying and sad!"
But the leaves and the trunk thought-
We'll see.
Alone sat the child,
Under the tree, on the ground
And drew five notes he could sing...

(Michal Lev, 2020)

Introduction

This chapter describes art-based research (ABR) that examined what transpires when sickness and death enter an art-therapy learning group, and how facilitators and students cope with a topic of a taboo nature, which is absent from the syllabus, yet present in the academic classroom.

The chapter begins with a review of literature dealing with facilitation in teaching and therapy, as well as creativity and resilience in coping with illness and death. It then presents the research methodology with its unique qualities, followed by the results, and concludes with the potential contribution of ABR and pedagogy to art-therapy programs. It is written in the first person plural out of respect for the language and properties of ABR.

The art-therapy curriculum is structured as a three-year program that includes theoretical courses in psychotherapy, alongside clinical and experiential exercises, creative/artistic processes, witnessing, and reflective observation within small learning groups (10-15 students). Experiential courses are facilitated by art therapists, experienced in the field of study. The research arose from unfortunate circumstances whereby one student, enrolled in the program while coping with a serious illness, had passed away. Throughout her strenuous, yet striking learning bout she was afforded the space for processing her situation within her assigned learning group, also known as the *core-group*, during the program's first year.

We, the three primary researchers in this study are all intimately familiar with the topic of sickness and loss. Three factors–the creative ways in which we had worked through our own grief, observing our students who had lost their classmate, and their request to process their feelings within the college's framework–led us to inquire which elements in facilitation enable working through sickness and loss, how do these elements encourage the development of resilience, and is all this related to art-based pedagogy?

Therapist-facilitator in the academy

Academics around the world are preparing systems of higher education and teaching to function in a dynamic reality of uncertainty (Amster, 2014) and to implement artistic processes within curricula. It has been amply demonstrated that artmaking, in groups and individually, endows confidence in people's ability, develops abstract thinking and analysis, and instills empathy through experiential learning activities (Greene, 2008).

Alongside the academics, stand therapists. The April 2020 issue of *Sihot* characterizes turning to therapy as a sign of hope and existential vitality (Cohen, 2020). Other contributors write about the therapeutic relationship, which demands from therapists their engagement, authenticity, and trust in themselves and their creativity. This acknowledges that therapists and clients share a similar psychological markup.

In the learning environment, the literature places an emphasis on *modeling*, referring to learning through observation and imitation. Modeling is even more significant in therapy studies, founded on the facilitator-student relationship. Paolo Knill spoke of the group facilitator as a model for therapy clients, and participants as models for one another (1999). Irvin Yalom also describes a participant who faced her approaching death with dignity and courage, serving as a role model for her environment (2008).

Artistic creativity and witnessing in facilitation

Much has been written about art as a holistic realm of knowledge, which develops complex, sensory and experiential observational capacities (Rubesin et al., in press). The roles of facilitators and art as witnesses to students' development has also been comprehensively reviewed (Dewey, 2008; Webster & Wolfe, 2013).

Nisha Sajnani and colleagues demonstrated how facilitators create an aesthetic framework in which students observed themselves – as artists, as artworks, and as witnesses (2020). This way, art connects the individual to the group. In the therapeutic context, to trauma survivors, the therapist as witness enables recognizing a denied or dissociated reality (Ulman, 2019). Artworks as witnesses bestow life outside their relationship with their creators, reverberating memories into the future (Lev, 2019).

Facilitation in art therapy programs adopts therapeutic features of observation and mirroring, with the goal of shaping students' professional identities (Honig, 2014). Alongside the facilitators, art is a robust factor in encouraging group cohesion. Students are expected to dedicate themselves to learning and creative processes that include self-exploration, empathy, listening, mirroring, and confidentiality (McNiff, 1986). When coping with contents such as sickness and death, empathetic and intimate human connection has been effective in reducing anxiety. When facilitators and group members share their thoughts about the finality of life, they lift the taboo around the discussion of this theme (Yalom, 2006). In Amia Lieblich's book *Death café* (2019), group discussions about death were accompanied by moments of fear, anxiety, and shared sorrow, alongside laughter, cohesion, and friendship, which helped lead participants on the path to reconciliation, relief, and resiliency.

Features of resilience

Most definitions of resilience describe physical and emotional health that coexists with vulnerability and/or hardship, as well as competence to cope with/adapt to adversity (Kalish et al., 2017). Resilience can be learned and developed through dynamic processes (Chmitorz et al., 2018), assuming that we possess strengths and resources that can be mobilized under stress (Lahad, 2017).

A panel of expressive therapists convened by the World Health Organization and Create 2030 advocated the relevance of art for expressing instability, uncertainty, confusion, and anxiety, and for reducing their cumulative damages. In an art-based pedagogy research project, immigrant pupils painted their feelings of oppression and rejection on the school walls. The openly displayed images enabled participants to recognize the pain, as a community possession (Garcia, 2015). Experts in pain research also believe that the willingness to be present with, and view pain as integral with life leads to its acceptance and relief of its symptoms (Lynch et al., 2013).

Another feature of resilience is artmaking within a group setting (Ben-Dori Gilboa, 2013). The artistic undertaking by photographer Jean Rene, in which he, together with local volunteers, pasted close-up portraits on buildings around the world, empowered participants with a sense of presence and ownership of their environment (Thompson et al., 2015). Similarly, artist Addam Yekutieli (2020) tattoos slogans on the skins of passersby, thus engaging the margins of society in building resilience. When a group develops cohesion through a shared journey, the group becomes a supportive container for its members in coping with distress and anxiety, revealing participants' resilience.

Faith is another component of resiliency. In the art-based research paradigm, researchers' belief in science, nature, and humanity motivates them for action (McNiff, 2020). The ambiguous space of artistic endeavors builds resilience for those willing to risk failure on the path to developing skill (D'Mello et al., 2014). Additionally, art's materiality emphasizes our ability to create, especially when the creators confront life's finality (Leader, 2008).

Art as mediator for the wound

In one fell swoop, our lives alter when afflicted with a severe illness. Apart from physical and cognitive changes that breed fatigue and anxiety, the approaching death affects our relationships and our identity as a sick person (Bolaki, 2020). Such changes impinge patients' capacity for attachment and communication with their caretakers and hinder their ability to share and process their feelings. For this to occur, a facilitator is needed to act as a conduit between their wounded psyches and their surroundings.

Michal Lev's art-based research (2020a) expanded Vygotsky's instrumental understanding, which proposed the use of an *other* as mediator. In her study, images, artworks, and art tools functioned as mediators of a profound acquaintance with the self. The artistic creations into which the researcher projected feelings and thoughts, created a safe distance for observation, exploration, and for their acceptance as separate *others*. In a different study, Lev referred to her artistic creations as offspring, which became independent entities the world can relate to (Lev, 2020b).

Methodology

The research examined how facilitators and students in a graduate art therapy master's program cope when themes of sickness and loss, normally perceived as taboo, enter the classroom. The research focused on three questions: (1) How does facilitation that integrates creative processes, witnessing, and reflective observation create space for working through sickness and loss in an art-therapy learning group? (2) How do we characterize resilience in the encounter with sickness and death of a member of an art-therapy learning group? And- (3) What creative factors are reflected in a group of art-therapy students in which the process of sickness and loss takes place?

Participants and setting

The research population included 12 participants aged 25-60, differentiated by socio-cultural characteristics, all well-versed in visual arts. Of these, nine third-year students in the graduate art therapy master's program of Ono Academic College, had the role of students-co-researchers, henceforth, "the students." Some of their names have been altered, at their request. Referring to the students as Co-researchers is motivated by their perception as significant collaborators in exploring the research topic, by using their artistic work, and their gained experiences while studying at the program. The students joined us, the Researchers–three art therapists and experienced facilitators, each having a prior acquaintance with one or more of the students through their participation in courses that we facilitated.

Desiring to enhance the generalizability and validity of the research, participants' sociocultural characteristics were diverse in respect to age, gender, ethnicity, socio-economic and marital status. As three secular women artists and art therapists – we, the researchers, are aware of our biases and their potential impact on the research. In addition, we were liable to Ono Academic College as our employer. Notwithstanding, all efforts were made to protect and respect participants' rights, their unique backgrounds, and voices.

The research process

Respectful for the creative way knowledge is produced, the research comprised six phases:

1. Group experimental session

The session took place in June 2020 during the Covid-19 pandemic, in the college building. It lasted three academic hours – the duration of an experimental class session. Art materials were spread out on the worktable, buffet-style. Twelve student-chairs were placed in a circle, and three video cameras were installed to document the meeting.

For 40 minutes, we led a brief round of introductions and an explanation of the session's nature, we read out-loud the research questions, also presented on the board. With background tunes and guided imagery students were lured to reflect on their selves, and then invited to the buffet of art supplies to create freely for an hour, as they contemplated the research questions. While they worked, we witnessed and observed their creative processes, and when asked, assisted them with technical aspects of their work. Our thoughts and feelings were documented in observational journals.

2. Group discussion

The ensuing discussion was held after the artistic process and lasted 90-minutes. The students exhibited their artworks within the space of the circle and returned to their seats. They were invited to observe the works silently, identify their aesthetic features, and share with the group, with a goal of answering the research questions. Attention was given to students' creative processes and to the artworks' materials and attributes. Most of them positioned their works on the floor, close to their seats; one work was hung from the ceiling. The discussion was concluded with a temporary farewell from the students and the promise of a culminating session, to review the research outcomes.

3. Researchers' discussion and art-responses

After the students left, we remained in the classroom, conversed for 60-minutes, and then responded artistically to the meeting, to decipher meaning. The same buffet of art supplies was used, with the student artworks serving as witnesses to their creative processes.

Phases 1-3 were documented in audio, video, and still photographs. The files were saved in chronological order and uploaded to the cloud.

4. Art-making-meaning

This phase was accomplished by each researcher individually, in her own studio. The systematic examination of the research material included listening to the audio-recordings, watching the video footage and transcribing them. In addition, we engaged in artmaking to process the varied information: Gili used collages integrating images and texts; Aya created pottery, drawing and painting; and Michal combined painting, creative writing, editing video footage and creating short videos. Artmaking was used to interpret our experiences from the group session and to examine the findings. We thus enabled access and attention to the many ways of knowing which are not comprehended by linear analysis alone.

Next, each researcher reviewed the information independently with the goal of answering the research questions. The time that had elapsed from the group-session invited an in-depth inquiry of the video files: of participants' body language, their voice-tones and speech-sequences, the facilitation's distribution between the three of us, and our journaling. Inspecting these details engendered new understandings. This phase concluded when each of us distilled findings pertaining to each research question and uploaded them to the shared folder in the cloud.

5. Triangulation of findings

For the sake of interpersonal integrity and the research's validity and transferability, we employed triangulated observation, during three online meetings of 120 minutes each, due to Covid-19 restrictions.

Each meeting- adhering to a unified structure- was devoted to answering one research question, with each of us sharing her distilling process and answer, while the other two responded, in a circular fashion. We discussed the various points of view and concluded with a holistic, empirical, and condensed formulation of answers to the three research questions.

6. Concluding works

The research process was suspended at this point for the sake of drafting a chapter for an academic volume. The culminating session with students-co-researchers was postponed. In the meantime, we critically reviewed existing literature, created a summarizing video titled *In Sickness and Death*, after which the writing of the chapter was completed.

Outcomes

First question: How does facilitation that integrates creative processes, witnessing, and reflective observation creates space for working through sickness and loss in an art-therapy learning group?

Three operative-mutually-influencing factors were identified: (1) acceptance and invitation to create, (2) observant presence, and (3) connection and cohesion.

The influence of the deceased student Shulamit and her creative processes in the shadow of illness raised questions about the place that was given to her and to her classmates in the learning groups of an accredited graduate Master's program. We hoped to illuminate the nature of learning in the college but were concerned that the research's implementation would provoke controversy. However, in late 2019 and early 2020, reality as we knew it, changed. Sickness and death enveloped the globe, affecting and even dictating the course of the research.

Acceptance and invitation to create

The research was conceived in parallel with the global outbreak of the Covid-19 pandemic. Reality required re-conceptualizing the research and its design. The lockdown imposed in Israel and in higher education dictated changes to the research proposal that had been approved by the college's ethics board. We were granted exceptional authorization to hold the group-session in the college building, on condition of compliance with the Health Ministry's directives. This was a manifest expression of accepting reality, as well as of the motivation to action on all stakeholders' parts.

The group session, originally planned for March 2020, was postponed. Its rescheduled date in June 2020 coincided with the participating students' graduation. Holding the session during the pandemic required flexibility, and adaptation to changes reality dictated.

During the group-discussion, we were aware of an intensiveness, which we attributed to the limited time allocated. The time factor was conspicuously felt in the students' hurried pace of speech, lack of pauses, and in the various phrases referring to time, in the transcription. The student Lee, said: "this is a journey of memory into things that she [Shulamit] did, I felt that I had more to do but no time". We drew attention to this issue when mirroring, to the students, Shulamit's temporariness in their lives. The student Shira understood that time demanded a sanctification of life: "when something earth-shattering like death happens, it shakes you up and lifts you out of the usual denial of death." The student Oshrat spoke about experiencing empowerment through her encounter with death, stating that separation from close people bestows their meaning in us.

Observant presence

We created what the students described as a "safe creative space" by witnessing their creative processes, attentive towards them, and their own selves. During the group-discussion, their artworks, positioned one next to another inside the ring of chairs, became witnesses in a second circle of participants. Their subsistence was how the students examined the research questions.

Observant presence was manifested as we mirrored and gave meaning to the ideas that came up in the group. When student Odelia shared her difficulty to examine her mourning within a research project, the researcher Michal addressed her: "I observed you while creating. You were gathered-in on the floor, holding your work in your hand". Michal's observant attention led Odelia to associate holding the artwork in her hand, to holding her friend's death. Odelia then said "I held Shulamit's death alone. Did anyone gather me up? Was anybody there?" Throughout the discussion, students rose from their seats to look closely at their peers' creations, brought up memories of Shulamit, and discovered connections with her artworks.

Connection and cohesion

In the examination of video footage, connection and cohesion emerged as significant factors. In the group-discussion, participants exchanged direct gazes; in artmaking, intimacy was experienced despite social distancing; and throughout, in the respect shown to each other and to the materials.

At times, making connections between the students encouraged them to speak in the circle. For example, Michal encouraged student Keren: "I observed you winding branches with a rope"; she then connected to student Galia, "you created a repetitive kneading motion"; and with the students' gazes fixed on her, she used her hands to demonstrate their work movements, while turning to Odelia and saying: "It was the same with you". Linking participants echoed the *core-group's* coherence in the first and second years, as well as Shulamit's capacities for self-revelation and in-depth processing of her illness.

Cohesion was also apparent during artmaking and the artworks. In *the collage* researcher Gili created, the boughs of trees interlink as their roots interweave. During the triangulated-discussions, we associated the work's aesthetic components with therapeutic elements of the collage – gluing as a metaphor of binding/healing, and a second skin as a symbol of protection. Gili's assorted texts and images were derived from different content worlds on a single surface. The researcher Aya saw this as "an expression of the mutual support/reinforcement of each detail in the work, in which the tree archetype confirms the fear and validates the reality during the time of the research". Michal's artwork *The Gaze,* dealt with her relationship with her advisor Shaun McNiff. She painted his wounded, sensitive eyes with watercolors and placed them in a camouflage and war-like environment, rendered in acrylic. In her work, the background penetrates the theme, and the gaze observes the occurrence.

Cohesion and connection were manifested in students' comments at the end of the group-discussion. Student Uri said: "the timing of this meeting is very critical. Because of the Coronavirus we did not have a graduation ceremony at the college." Shira added: "this is the first time I make art since leaving class…it's hard to separate from this place", and Galia summed up: "This connected us as a group, and connected each of us within herself." Holding the rescheduled meeting on June 2020, afforded the students space for separating from college, and invited participants to observe the parallelism between the research topic and reality.

Second question: How do we characterize resilience in the encounter with sickness and death of a member in an art-therapy learning group?

As noted, there are many definitions to resilience. We approached resilience as the ability to cope flexibly with crisis and loss, and to recover (Lahad, 2017). Three features of resilience were found, manifested throughout the research: beholding pain; faith; composition and support.

Beholding pain

Gili's *core-group* students' requests to hold a session that could help them cope with their friend's death, reflected a need to behold pain.

Additional expressions of this need were seen in the works of students Abeer and Galia. Abeer, a paramedic, painted *a lioness* in watercolors on paper and placed it on fragments of glass, so that one side showed a roaring lioness, and the other side showed a weeping lioness. Abeer recalled that the close encounter with death led her to look squarely at the finitude of life. In Galia's work, *two containers* were placed on a cardboard substrate. One – a ready-made clay container, and the other – made of gypsum-coated clay with gold fragments, which she created. She said:

> I was drawn to the bowl and placed it near me during my work. Only after I photographed the piece did I realize the presence of that bowl… I am dealing with breast cancer. Touching pain is important. I could project onto the material knowing it would absorb everything, mend, and merge it.

Galia recounted how her pain and coping with cancer were afforded a place in Michal's *core-group* during the program's second year, and added that contact with and observation of the pain led her to growth.

Student Lee was able to transform the denial of her friend's death into recognition: "Shulamit brought herself this way, without defenses, and her openness to the topic enabled the group to observe sickness and pain as part of life." Student Uri observed that an adaptive response to an obstacle or stress contributed to the group's resilience: "There is no doubt that Shulamit, with the disease, was constantly present, but at the same time she also gave us a place." The participants' nods of agreement to his statement confirmed that looking directly at the disease, however painful, encourages growth, and builds resilience among the group members.

Faith

A faith that reckons with Force Major was recognized in the group, as well as a trust in the self. Indeed, the choice of all participants to engage in artmaking as allowing the unknown to transpire symbolically, validates a sturdy commitment to trusting the process (McNiff, 1998).

Evidence of a greater existence was apparent in the work of Oshrat *The illuminated shadow*, in which a yellow plasticine human figure stands on a cardboard, in front of a building façade painted in black acrylic on white Bristol. The façade looms taller than the human figure and leans-over diagonally, threatening to fall. The shadow emanating from the building's windows casts a yellow light toward the figure. Oshrat shared:

> I danced between the words *finality* and *meaning*. Like two ends with me in middle. In the work – the shadow is the light. I asked, would life have meaning if not for the presence of the end?

Her words reflected a search for transcendent wisdom and knowledge hoping to balance between the ends. Student Keren told how she prepared for the group-meeting in the morning, and in a symbolic ceremony she devoted time and thought to her friend Shulamit and lit a candle in her memory. Keren came to the meeting without knowing where it would lead, drawing on her faith for strength. She hung her artwork, *Star of David*, as a mobile from the ceiling:

> I dwelled in the space of the candle, the earth, and the sky. I asked, what could symbolize this kind of connection? I created a Star of David as an amulet that has accompanied me this past year, in thought and creation.

Keren explained that she hung her work between heaven and earth and connected them, as a representation of the ability to connect life and death that the late Shulamit demonstrated.

The participants' belief in a greater existence than man and themselves, led the participants to the college building amidst the Covid-19 pandemic, covered with masks, video cameras, and art supplies. At one triangulated-session, Aya said:

> I pottered a series of flat plates after my father's death. Three sessions later Shulamit passed away. The first plates had imprints of plants, as a life that passed and left a mark, like fossils.

In her remarks, Aya emphasized her appeal to the work as holding and balancing.

Composition and support

The student-body was a partner in destiny, and the holding of hope took place simultaneously for the diseased and the circle of support. We recognized the students' difficulty in looking directly at the subject of research amidst the Covid-19 pandemic, and so they used their circles of acquaintance to recruit co-researchers. The students demonstrated resilience to meet themselves and their colleagues in the study with dedication to the process and their support.

Emergent structures were identified in the research information: the research's division into phases, the structure of the group-session. The systematic structure was also retained in the division of labor amongst the three researchers. The triangle–the most stable of geometric structures-was present in the three triangulated sessions for the three research questions. In addition, the researchers' working method was circular.

From an aesthetic point of view, the circular structure stood out throughout the group-session. At the beginning of each experiential-lesson in the curriculum, the circle of chairs is conspicuous; it disperses during artmaking and recomposes while observing the artworks (image 1). At the group-session, student Keren added an empty chair, as Aya had habitually done in their *core-group,* after Shulamit passed away.

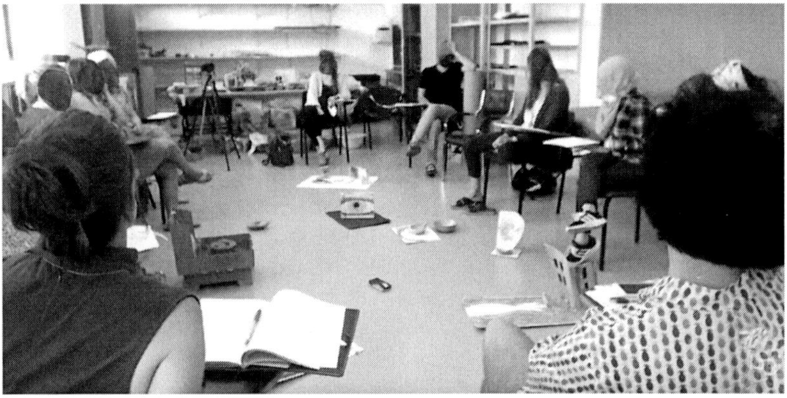

Image 1. Artworks presented in the group session © Michal Lev, Aya Kats, Gili Navoth.

In keeping with the principles of structure, which require foundations and support, the students also supported the materials in their hands until their creations were stable. Eleven of the twelve artworks created in the group-session and in our responses to it, were three-dimensional. We wondered whether the global pandemic urged participants to delimit and to hold? We were required to support one another during the research and to spontaneously create space for three facilitators in one group. Furthermore, we maintained a structure similar to an experiential-lesson in the college, while also focusing on the research objectives to examine what happens when outer reality pervades the group.

The participants' personal connection to the subject underscored their support in the art-based paradigm. Michal, who lost her close friend during the year of research, journaled while editing the video footage:

> Student Shira's words take me back to that night in the hospice with Mikey. We moved from the couch in the great room, to her bed, and back. I felt it was the last night, and I wanted to be with her until the last second.

The study provided a holding framework for the grief and pain she experienced.

Resilience was also reflected in Gili's artworks. The single tree in the center of the first two works was no longer alone. In her *third piece*, she created an environment for that tree, and painted additional trees, "The tree manifests resilience in its ability to nourish itself from the air, the light, and the soil." Her work emphasizes the infinite forces of creation, and the renewal of nature in which coping with pain, sickness, and loss can be supported.

Third question: What creative factors are reflected in a group of art-therapy students in which the process of sickness and loss takes place?

Three elements in coping with disease and loss were found to match the definition of creativity- as the capacity and competency to produce innovation and originality: (1) ex-nihilo, (2) seeing in perspective, and (3) place, between matter and spirit.

Ex-nihilo

In essence, innovation confirms that which pre-exists and relates to it. In the study, the original-new required recognition and respect for the present and absent. Through the modes of inquiry, the abstract was translated into concrete actions and methods of work; observing the taken-for-granted-unknown, factorizing it, and recreating it.

In the group-session, materials such as old pieces of fabric, shreds of paper, strings, leftover wood, and scrap metal were gently handled, and carefully transformed into works of art. This was apparent in student Anietta's delicacy around chicken-wire and cardboard. In student Lee's work, she wetted, and wrapped pieces of linen rags covering on wood scraps, like shrouds that wrap the dead before burial (*In Sickness and Death*, sequence 01:44-02:02).

The group's composition as *new* was discussed in the triangulated sessions. Motivating the group required devotion, self-disclosure, and sharing, which occurred based on prior acquaintances. The silence that prevailed during artmaking in the experiential-session also confirmed the group's newness.

Student Uri shared: “Because of our preoccupation with death and personal loss, we were more cautious and quieter.” Care was also taken in the participants choosing their workspace, art materials, and finding creative solutions to maintain distance guidelines.

Listening to the audiotapes of the session, some ten long pauses in the speech sequence were identified. Sometimes the pauses indicated recognition and agreement, but some silences disturbed the quiet and reflected the void. The content that violated all silence, was a response to the artworks present in the circle. The video footage showed the participants’ eyes extended to the center-to the works on the floor. The art that was at the center filled the circle with content, which was easier to relate to.

Co-researchers’ reflections on their creative processes led to insights. Student Galia understood what she created only when she photographed the completed artwork. Student Abeer was surprised by a watercolor teardrop squeezing out of the lioness’s eye. Student Keren acknowledged moving her work from the floor and hanging it from the ceiling, and student Odelia, who usually works on a substrate discovered that she had created the work *inside her hand.*

Seeing in perspective

As creators, we understand the world through an artistic gaze. Our choice of art-based methodology germinated from our belief in inquiry as creative action.

Creativity requires seeing the familiar in a new way. Accordingly, we were not surprised to find the roots ‘gaze’ and ‘see’ cropping up in the transcripts. Moreover, the aesthetic choices of one participant inspired the work of others in the group. Also, ten of the artworks comprised several materials, and some were a series of works symbolizing their complex feelings. For example, *the collage work* of student Shira was a metaphor of the multifaceted persona of Shulamit.

During artmaking, a search for liminality was identified – betwixt and between. Between light and shadow, control and release, the concrete and the abstract, between life and death. Creativity allowed movement from one zone to the other, while shifting perspectives. In Uri’s work, he drew an eye on both sides of a rectangular cardboard box, and tied it with strings:

> I chose a two-dimensional paper, and wanted the eyes to face each other, and in two-dimensions it wasn't possible. Here, the two eyes are connected but don't see each other, they are positioned back-to-back.

When he said these things aloud, he came to enlightenment, and continued: "I thought to make my eye and her [the late Shulamit's] eye look at each other. And I realized we could not look at each other." Uri spoke about his anger that was replaced by guilt, distance, and once again closeness to Shulamit. As he spoke, his gaze revealed confusion and embarrassment. Perhaps he asked-is his grieving legitimate, despite the kind of relationship they had? The process of creating and sharing in the group allowed Uri a new perspective and served as a mirror for other participants in observing themselves. Uri's reflection emphasized art's use of corporeal materials to symbolize intangible existence.

Place, between matter and spirit

Our holistic standpoint as facilitators and art therapists was also expressed in the research. In the equal value to the earthly and the abstract; in our approach to photographs and the written text; the belief in materials and artistic imagery; for thoughts and feelings, as engendering understanding and creating meaning.

In the group-discussion, student Anietta referred to her mourning rendering:

> I didn't feel I had a place to bring it, to speak it, but only through artmaking. It spilled over and permeated from all direction. I couldn't find words. Precisely here, the work and the group served as a significant container. Now, in this research process.

When the students created, actions of cutting, cleaning, exposing, connecting, sewing, drying, and wetting were witnessed (image 2). Actions reminiscent of medical treatment.

The corporality and tangibility of the materials held the research topic creatively, providing space for reality in the study group, in facilitation, and in reflective processing. During the group-session, the place given to Shulamit was observed. Out of respect to those present and to her absence we decided to forgo exhibiting her works and made do with mentioning her name and creating the research as a container for the memories and experiences with her.

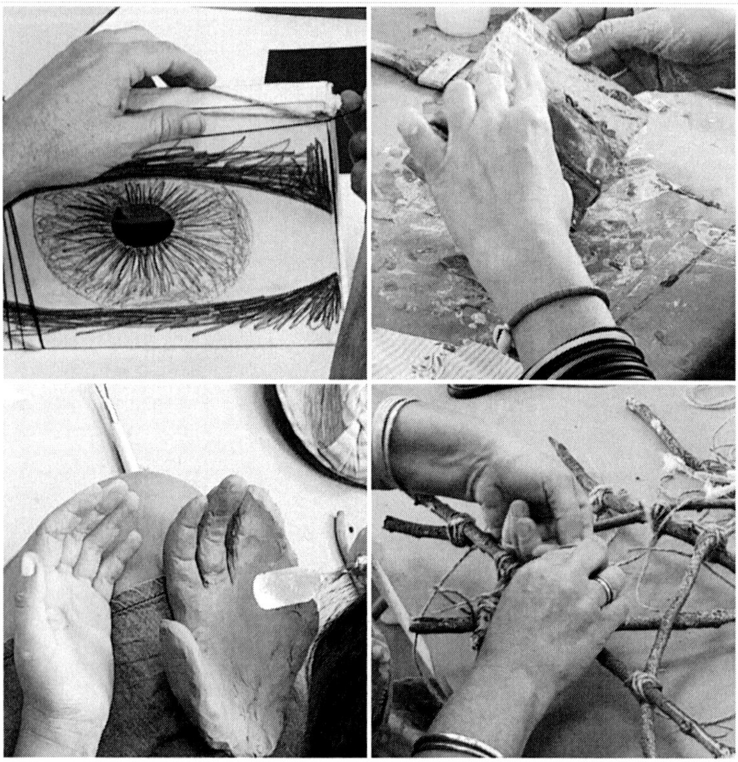

Image 2. Students during the creative process © Michal Lev, Aya Kats, Gili Navoth

When people create, they normally do not set-aside sufficient time to observe the process and its outcomes as done with clients and students. With completion of the work comes release. The time spent observing the research process allowed participants to endow the loss with meaning. Naming the different components, the group holding, and the cohesion, sheltered participants from a reality encompassing madness, pain, and sorrow, and contained these dimensions in a systematic and focused manner in the study.

Discussion and summary

Facilitators in the Art Therapy program are required for personal inquiry, to accompany students on the path to their selves; bound to one another in mind and heart, in sickness and in death.

Choosing an art-based paradigm-in which researchers use art as research tools – best fits the field of research and reflects our position that all research components are equals. Nine student-co-researchers, worked with us, three facilitators-researchers, in exploring three research questions systematically and empirically, through six mutually informing inquiry modes.

The findings identified three components of facilitation that afford space for sickness and loss within a study group: acceptance and invitation to create, observant presence, connection and cohesion. At various stages, we faced professional and personal dilemmas: is the pedagogical approach that accepts sickness and loss as content in a study group, legitimate? Will the students cooperate with the research plan, even when they are not committed to the study framework? Are participants resilient to look at sickness and loss, again, up close? Life's uncertainty required courage and dedication to produce and complete the research project.

The College had never sponsored art-based research involving facilitators and students as primary and co-researchers. The research topic was also ethically and pedagogically controversial. In fact, throughout its phases, the audacity of all research components stands-out, to practice the concept in concrete form. Courage was displayed in participants' choices to be exposed within the creative process, remain in the imaginative realm, play, and explore. Indeed, the research findings revealed three qualities of resilience: beholding pain, faith, composition, and support.

Furthermore, the research demonstrates three components of creativity: "ex-nihilo", "seeing in perspective", and "place, between matter and spirit". Processing grief in creative tools has led, in research, to contain complexity. This idea was manifested in mirroring and gazes within the group, in which participants saw parts of themselves reflected in works and responses of others. The public display of artworks invited an extension of the grieving process from the creator to the participants who observed it. The artworks that germinated, ex-nihilo, emerged omnipotent and eternal, inviting associations and connections from their environment.

The chapter sparks light on a research topic that often remains obscure in pedagogical literature. For us, the research enabled processing of grief, and provided a meaningful anchor within our lived realities. We hope to contribute and enrich the existing knowledge in art therapy curricula, and to offer a creative pedagogical approach to research and facilitation, in which reality functions as study material.

References

Amster, R. (2014) "Teaching to the Test: Climate Change, Militarism, and the Pedagogy of Hopefulness" *Journal of Peace Education*, 11(3), 267-278.

Bolaki, S. (2020) "Introduction: Artists' Books and Medical Humanities" *Journal of Medical Humanities*, 41(1), 1-5.

Ben-Dori Gilboa, R. (2013) "Empoying Art in Group Dynamics: As Means to Develop Resiliency in Professionals Working with Youth at Risk" *Journal of Society and Education*, 24, 34-37.

Chmitorz, A., Kunzler, A., Helmreich, I., Tüscher, O., Kalisch, R., Kubiak, T., Wessa, M., Lieb, K. (2018) "Intervention Studies to Foster Resilience – A Systematic Review and Proposal for a Resilience Framework in Future Intervention Studies" *Clinical Psychology Review*, 59, 78-100.

Cohen, Y. (2020) "Hope During Corona" *Sihot: The Israeli Journal of Psychotherapy*, April, 36-37 (Hebrew).

D'Mello, S., Lehman, B., Pekrun, R., Graesser, A. (2014) "Confusion can be Beneficial for Learning" *Learning and Instruction*, 29, 153-170.

Dewey, J. (2008) *Later Works vol. 10: Art as Experience*. Carbondale: Southern Illinois University Press

Garcia, L. G. (2015) "Empowering Students through Creative Resistance: Art-based Critical Pedagogy in the Immigrant Experience" *Diálogo*, 18(2), 139-149.

Greene, M. (2008) *Towards Pedagogy of Thought & Imagination*. Teachers College, Columbia University. https://www.youtube.com/watch?v=Q1RfuW1WanA&feature=youtu.be

Honig, O. (2014) *Post-graduate Art Therapy Training in Israel: Personal and Professional Transformation through Dynamic Artwork-based Experiential Transformative Courses* [Dissertation, University of Sussex] Sussex.

Kalisch, R., Baker, D. G., Basten, U., Boks, M. P., Bonanno, G. A., Brummelman, E., Chmitorz, A., Fernàndez, G., Fiebach, C. J., Galatzer-Levy, I. (2017) "The Resilience Framework as a Strategy to Combat Stress-Related Disorders" *Nature Human Behaviour*, 1(11), 784-790.

Knill, P. J. (1999) "Soul Nourishment, or the Intermodal Language of Imagination" *Foundations of expressive arts therapy: Theoretical and clinical perspectives*, 37-52.

Lahad, M. (2017) "From Victim to Victor: The Development of the BASIC PH model of Coping and Resiliency" *Traumatology*, 23(1), 27-34.

Leader, D. (2008) *The new black: Mourning, melancholia and depression*. Penguin UK.

Lev, M. (2019) *Painting Intimacy: Art-Based Research of Intimacy* [Dissertation, Lesley University]. Cambridge, MA.

—. (2020a) “Art as a Mediator for Intimacy: Reflections of an Art-Based Research Study” *Journal of Applied Arts and Health*, 11(3), 299-313.

—. (2020b) “Intimacy through Painting” *Academic Journal of Creative Arts Therapies*, 20(1), 1003-1019.

Lieblich, A. (2019) *Death Café*. Kineret, Zmora-Bitan, Dvir (Hebrew).

Lynch, M., Sloane, G., Sinclair, C., Bassett, R. (2013) “Resilience and Art in Chronic Pain” *Arts & Health, 5*(1), 51-67.

McNiff, S. (1986) *Educating The Creative Arts Therapist: A profile of the profession* (1st ed.). Charles C. Thomas.

—. (1998) *Trust the Process: An Artist’s Guide to Letting Go* (1st ed.). Shambhala.

—. (2020) “’Tears on the Flowers’: Worldwide Natural Experiments of Art Healing” *Creative Arts in Education and Therapy (CAET),* 6-12.

Perry, T., Steele, C., Hilliard, A. G. (2003) *Young, Gifted, and Black: Promoting High Achievement among African-American Students*. Beacon Press.

Rubesin, Hillary, Chen, Yu-Ying, Fried, Dina, Lev, M., Teoli, L. (in press). “Building Bridges and Transforming Identities: Reflections on an Art-Based Conference Workshop” in R. Prior, M. Kossak, Fisher T. (eds.) *Applied Arts and Health, Education and Community: Building bridges*. Intellect.

Sajnani, N. (2020a) “Aesthetic Presence: The Role of the Arts in the Education of Creative Arts Therapists in the Classroom and Online” *The Arts in Psychotherapy*, 69 https://doi.org/https://doi.org/10.1016/j.aip.2020.101668

Sajnani, N. (2020b) *WHO Panel Discussion Taster: The Role of Arts & Arts Therapies in the Context of the Pandemic 1m30*, (June 23).

Thompson, N., Remnant, J., Azoulay, M. (2015) *JR: Can Art Change the World?* Phaidon Press.

Ulman, C. (2019) “Witnessing in Psychoanalysis and Philosophy” https://www.youtube.com/watch?v=7y-a7ydXQs8

Webster, R. S., Wolfe, M. (2013) “Incorporating the Aesthetic Dimension into Pedagogy” *Australian Journal of Teacher Education*, 38(10), 21-33.

Yalom, D. I., Leshetz, M. (2006) “The Therapist – Foundamental Actions” *Group Therapy: Theory and Practice*. Kineret, Zmora-Bitan, Dvir (Hebrew).

Yalom, D. I. (2008) *Group Therapy: Theory and Practice*. Kineret, Zmora-Bitan, Dvir (Hebrew).
Yekutieli, A. (2020) "Know Hope" Retrieved Dec., 24 2020, https://thisislimbo.com/truthandmethodproject/

CHAPTER 6

THEORETICAL POLYPHONY AND ITS IMPORTANCE IN TRAINING PSYCHODRAMA THERAPISTS

TSIKY COHEN

Introduction

Polyphony is a concept from the field of music, describing a musical texture that includes several independent voices moving in parallel, side by side. The uniqueness of the polyphonic creation is that it does not feature a definite hierarchy between the voices, so that each voice is rhythmically or melodically independent. It is a work that requires great concentration from the listener, since the latter is required to listen simultaneously to the combined movement of different melodies. In the field of literature, it is customary to use the term "polyphony" to describe texts characterized by a multitude of opposing ideological voices. The uniqueness of the polyphonic text is expressed in its capacity to allow the expression of heterogeneous modes of discourse, without the intermediacy of an editing or judging authority. It enables all the voices in the piece to sound without a particular preference of this or that point of view, thus spanning a poetic, ludic and carnival like space.

In the training process of therapists, in general, and expressive therapists, in particular, a position of theoretical polyphony is required. Such position will train students to become acquainted with various therapeutic approaches and to familiarize themselves with various personality theories such as psychoanalytic theory, object-relations theories, Jung's theory of archetypes, behavioral-cognitive theory etc. (see, for example, Rubin, 2001; Malchiodi, 2005; Elkins & Stovall, 2000). Studies that tried to examine the question of "what makes therapy successful" (Wampold & Imel, 2015) have indicated that the therapist's personality and ability to move flexibly and adapt to the patient without being trapped in a single theoretical approach are the key to a successful therapeutic process.

However, it is precisely among students and psychodrama therapists that there seems to be deep ambivalence and suspicion about the use of personality theories that go beyond the one developed by the father of psychodrama, Jacob Moreno. Many psychodramatists tend to regard psychodramatic therapy as an emotional and cathartic experience whose main goal is to help the person become more spontaneous and creative within the constraints of their personality. Accordingly, many psychodramatists tend to prefer spontaneous action and intuitive interventions over the use of psychological personality theories, analytical investigation and question posing (see, for example: Bustos, 1994; Moreno, 1994; Kellermann, 2006; Telias, 2019).

According to Kellermann (2006), this position of rejecting diagnostics or reliance on a robust personality theory already appears in the writings of Moreno, who did not believe in labels and protested the depiction of human beings as a collection of statistical traits. Although psychodrama was described by him as “a method of diagnosis and treatment” (Moreno, 1946 [1972]), he objected to resorting to the ideology underlying psychiatric and psychological thinking and suggested looking at human suffering based on health rather than pathology.

Indeed, in my experience as a lecturer and supervisor in various institutions for art therapy instruction,[1] one of the things I have noticed is that there are psychic discourses with which psychodrama students may find easier to identify with. However, other discourses, which deal with more archaic and primeval aspects of the human mind, provoked the need to repair, embellish, make them more positive and so on. In psychodramatic work, this phenomenon was particularly noticeable given the unique nature of the tool that relies on the extroversion of the psychic world through the use of dramatic action and role play. The most common scenes to which students turned following an encounter with negative emotional content such as jealousy, envy, or rancor were scenes that purported to create a reparation that rewrites the history of the protagonist. Some examples include an imaginary encounter with the good mother the patient never had; turning a class boycott into a scene where the patient becomes class leader;

[1] Ono Academic College, school of Society and the Arts, Israel; Kibbutzim College of Education, Technology, and the Arts, Israel.

converting a sense of inferiority and futility into feelings of grandiosity and omnipotence, etc.

It is important to clarify that there is no problem, in principle, in using reparation scenes in psychodrama and in treatment generally, and their therapeutic value is clear and important. Nevertheless, in my professional career, I often felt that these scenes were used mechanically and artificially, relying on an unconscious preconception according to which every psychodrama must end with a feeling of acceptance and a happy end (see, for example, Hollander, 1969; Kellermann, 2006). I recall that at the start of my career, I assumed that this was a personal tendency related to the inability of certain students to make contact with certain psychic components. Subsequently, I adopted a systemic perspective whereby this is due to the developmental stages of professional identity and the tendency of young therapists to idealize the therapeutic practice and the therapist's role.

Over the years, however, I have come to the conclusion that there is another variable that contributes to the antagonism and suspicion that characterize psychodrama therapists in relation to the use of personality theories – which is the humanist-existentialist infrastructure of psychodramatic theory and practice. Although scholars and commentators have referred to the interrelationship between the humanist-existentialist school and psychodramatic theory (see, for example: Moreno, 1994; Bustos, 1994; Blatner, 2013; Kellermann, 2006; Telias, 2019; Cohen, 2020), few focused on the resulting implications on the teaching and training processes of psychodrama therapists and of the formation of the psychodrama practitioner's identity.

In this chapter, I would like to focus on the effects of the humanist-existentialist ethics on the formation of the figure of the paradigmatic psychodrama therapist. I will try to show how the humanist-existentialist infrastructure typical of psychodramatic theory functions as an ethical paradigm, which, alongside its encouragement of psychodramatists to be attentive and sensitive to certain psychic contents, also reduces their awareness of alternative emotional discourses. I would like to suggest that alongside the didactic challenges that may arise out of a position of theoretical polyphony, it can help train psychodrama therapists to be attentive and sensitive to emotional textures and hues, moving parallel to one another, without needing to set up a hierarchy among them.

The Infrastructure of psychodrama values – humanist-existentialist ethics

In the professional literature, the discussion of ethics in therapy tends to focus on the level of formal professional ethics that gives the therapist a set of normative values that regulate proper etiquette and reflect the identity of the profession and its practitioners (see, for example: Pope & Vasquez, 2016; Moon & Nolan, 2019). Such ethics generally includes the definition of the profession's identity, its values, and the rules of proper professional conduct. It offers the therapist a set of standards, rules, and norms for work, such as the obligation of confidentiality; the prohibition of sexual relations with the patients; protecting the patients art creations etc.

Occasionally, the discussion of the presence of ethics within therapy focuses on the norms and values that both the therapist and patient believe in, and that may also affect the therapeutic relationship through the processes of transference and countertransference. In psychoanalysis, for example, one of the changes brought about by the postmodern age is an epistemological turn – from a monadic theory of the mind (one-person psychology) to a dyadic and relational theory (two-person psychology). Several contemporary scholars, such as Steven Mitchell (1988), Irvine Hoffman (1983) and Louis Aron (1996), proposed abandoning the traditional characterizations of the therapeutic framework (anonymity, neutrality and abstinence) and acknowledging the mutual effects that exist between therapist and patient.

This transition is to be done with an emphasis on the presence of norms, values, beliefs and worldviews. This has led to the point where many therapists started defining themselves as specializing in therapy that is, among other things, also sensitive to gender, politics, religion, society, culture and so on.

However, there is another level of ethical presence in therapy, on which I would like to focus, and it is the ideational infrastructure derived from the therapeutic theory on which the therapist relies. This ideational infrastructure, consciously and unconsciously, affects the therapist's expectations, interventions, and understanding of the patient. It represents a whole of beliefs and values pertaining to human nature and the meaning of human existence – are we, for example, free and in charge of our own fate or is our behavior circumstantially and deterministically dictated? Do we live primarily in the intra-psychic and subjective world, or are we fashioned by external and objective forces? Is the person's initial motivation homeostasis, set at reducing tension and achieving internal equilibrium, or are we striving towards heterostasis, that is, towards growth, stimuli seeking, and self-realization?

Psychodramatic theory is commonly defined as being inspired by humanist-existentialist philosophy (see, for example, Moreno, 1994; Bustos, 1994; Blatner, 2013; Kellermann, 2006; Telias, 2019; Cohen, 2020). Of course, some psychodrama therapists also work from a psychodynamic perspective, or a cognitive-behavioral one, or combining different therapeutic methods, etc., but from a disciplinary point of view, the field of psychodrama is infused with the ideational mindset of the humanist-existentialist school. This is expressed, among other things, in the tendency of many psychodramatists to emphasize the positive and autonomous human nature; to focus on the phenomenological and non-empirical experience; to think about the human being in a holistic and inclusive manner; and to focus on unique human characteristics that have not been seriously addressed by other therapeutic approaches such as creativity, spontaneity, growth, and self-realization.

Jacob Moreno, the founding father of psychodrama, is considered one of the first thinkers to identify themselves in the therapeutic context with the humanist-existentialist conception (Moreno, 1959; Fonseca, 2015; Telias, 2019). Although he was a psychiatrist by profession, he objected to using the professional jargon widely used in psychiatric and medical thinking, claiming that this jargon objectifies the person and takes the person to be an object of prediction and investigation. Like other existentialist psychiatrists such as Karl Jaspers, Ronald Laing and Thomas Szasz, Moreno maintained that psychiatric disorders are the product of social and cultural forces that hinder people in achieving self-realization and fulfillment (Bustos, 1994; Kellermann, 2006). He assumed that a person who is labeled as having a sick personality, becomes more disturbed and sick because they identify with the social role of the mentally ill, and therefore human suffering has to be examined based on the person's health rather their pathology. The role of psychodrama, accordingly, is to help the person connect to the spiritual and creative dimension within them, while finding meaning in their life.

Moreno developed psychodramatic theory as a practice of group therapy that assumes that a person needs an interpersonal environment that offers love, mutual sharing, and trust. He believed in the healing power of the group, the importance of meeting others, and the assumption that we are social and relational creatures from the outset. In his paper *Spontaneity Theory of Child Development* (Moreno, 1944), Moreno argued that the main problem of classical therapeutic theories is that they tend to elucidate human development from a reductive and pathological perspective: on the one hand, the behaviorist approach, which uses animal studies and applies them to human beings, and on the other hand, psychoanalysis that analyzes the child's development through reliance on the mental model of the neurotic personality. Moreno suggested that instead of looking at the baby as an animal positioned high on the scale of the animal world, or, alternatively, as a young wild savage, we should try to look at it from the highest point that man has ever reached, the one that can embody the lofty achievements of the human race and explicate them.

Moreno believes that in expressions of genius, as reflected in the achievements of human civilization, we are witnessing the creative and generative nature of the human phenomenon that distinguishes it from the rest of the natural beings. He hoped that through psychodrama, humans would be able to connect with the sources of spontaneity and creativity inherent in them. This assumes that spontaneity and creativity are unique human traits that constitute the infrastructure of a person's mental well-being. In psychoanalytic terms, it can be added that Moreno's ideas implicitly link Kohut's idea of the *nuclear self* (Kohut, 1977), or Winnicott's *true self* (Winnicott, 1960), with human capacity for spontaneity and creation. They assume that a connection with the sources of playfulness, spontaneity and creativity encourages mental health and wellbeing, whereas a stagnation of roles and lack of spontaneity indicate a high level of anxiety and the absence of potential space.

Kellerman argues that when one maintains Moreno's humanist-existentialist thinking while performing psychodrama, the concepts of health, normality and pathology in fact become sterile, and therefore the use of various personality theories also becomes irrelevant and unnecessary. Psychodrama is not perceived from this perspective as a mental therapy in the medical sense of the word, but rather it represents an emotional and cathartic experience in which an interpersonal and intrapersonal encounter with personal, social, and spiritual values is brought about.

Indeed, Moreno argued that contrary to Freud's deterministic view that reduces man to such terms such as drive, libido, id, ego, superego, etc., his own theoretical thinking expresses a humanist and spiritual model of the person that is "more than a psychological, or social or biological being. He is a cosmic being" (Moreno, 1964, p. 158). He chose to place at the center of psychodramatic theory the ideas of spontaneity and creativity because he assumed that they reflected the source of vitality of the human phenomenon *qua* a unique being that aspires to authentic self-expression. These ideas instruct the psychodrama therapist to ask *how* a person is acting in a descriptive manner, rather than *why* a person is behaving in a certain way (Kellermann, 2006). They reject the orthodox conception of the therapist as a "physician" or "*tabula rasa*" and substitute it with a therapeutic model that allows group members to meet the therapist as a real and unique subject:

> I do not think an outstanding caregiver or therapist will look or behave like Freud. I imagine the caregiver as a spontaneous, creative therapist, who is in equal relation with the patient, or in the middle of every group (Moreno, 1989, p. 62).

Unique psychodramatic concepts coined by Moreno, such as social atom, encounter, tele, etc. also illustrate the strong humanist-existentialist influences that exist in psychodramatic theory, since they assume that the self can be revealed and evoked only in a social and interpersonal context. The term "tele", for instance (Moreno, 1934; 1954), refers to people's ability to feel, communicate, and understand one other based on each individual's actual and real personality. Unlike projective or phantasmatic psychological phenomena such as transference or empathy, the phenomenon of tele occurs *between* human beings, and not inside them. It represents the human capacity to perceive the other person's personality not only as a whiteboard for projections, but as a real person. A tele encounter rests on the existential reality of the other and involves mutual recognition of the same reality (Moreno, 2000; Kellermann, 2006). It represents an intersubjective dynamic in which two people meet and communicate with one other based on what the existentialist philosopher, Martin Buber, called the "I-thou" affinity (Cohen, 2020).

A thorough discussion of Buber's "I-thou" concept is beyond the scope of this chapter, but succinctly, it means an interpersonal encounter, in which social and cultural constructions collapse, and the two parties meet as two pure subjects or, as Buber described it, as two people sitting on a solitary seat located outside the limits of the world (Buber, 1923). It is important to clarify that the ethos of authenticity often relies on the opposite starting point, according to which a person who seeks to connect with himself and with his inner truth must break away from society and from other fellow men, often referred to as derogatorily as herd, crowd, or mob, and withdraw into himself to discover himself from within. In psychoanalysis, this position is clearly reflected in the intra-psychic emphasis that exists in the theories of Freud and Melanie Klein, but also in the theories of Winnicott and Kohut, which require the therapist to function as an object in the service of the patient's self. In all those cases, an encounter with the subjectivity of the therapist *qua* "otherness" has no place, and therapy is done merely by the therapist's willingness to become an object serving the patient's needs.

In Buber's philosophy, and that of Moreno, one can find an opposite position that assumes that it is the very encounter with the other that represents the central stage on which the self is formed and constituted (Moreno, 1914; Buber, 1923). Only when we succeed in meeting with one another as subjects, not objects, as being that are, on the one hand, similar to us but, on the other hand, different and incongruous, can we succeed in connecting with our own deep subjectivity. The therapeutic power of this encounter stems from its being a unique moment in the "here and now", in which each party evokes for the other party their true self, while also experiencing their own evoked self. The purpose of psychodramatic practice, accordingly, is to establish a liminal space that cancels out the identities and constructions of the group members and regroups them based on universal solidarity and a strong sense of humanity:

> A meeting of two: eye to eye, face to face. And when you are near I will tear your eyes out and place them instead of mine, and you will tear my eyes out and will place them instead of yours, then I will look at you with your eyes and you will look at me with mine (Moreno, 1914, p. 3).

The importance of theoretical polyphony in the training process of psychodrama therapists

At the beginning of this chapter, I suggested that at the foundation of any therapeutic theory, an ethical conception is necessarily reflected, which affects, consciously and unconsciously, the therapist's expectations, interventions, and understanding of the patient. This conception functions, so I claim, as a paradigm of ethical thinking, which, apart from encouraging the therapist to be attentive and sensitive to certain mental contents, it also restricts the therapist's awareness of alternative discourses. The question arises, then, what are the emotional and psychic discourses that psychodramatic theory tends to call fourth or focus on, and which emotional and psychic discourses does it tend to ignore or suppress?

In my experience, the humanistic-existentialist mindset that characterizes psychodramatic theory naturally encourages the engagement with universal human contents, or, as Peter Kellermann justly worded, "engaging in human dilemmas that poets and writers write about" (1997). Many psychodramas tend to focus on actively investigating normative life events or crises and events that are not necessarily unique to a particular person but characterize many people. This could be a psychodrama that focuses on the extasy of love, on the tormenting pain of death, on conflictual family relations, on the question of belonging to a group of peers, on tensions that inhere between the subjective self and the social one, on the experience of existential absurdity, and, of course, on the question of authenticity.

Alongside this, psychodramatic theory, understood as an ethical paradigm of thinking, does not so much call for delving into interpsychic contents belonging to more archaic and primeval strata of the human psyche. The attempt to hold on to a holistic worldview that refuses to reduce the human being into personality particles, complementarily excludes psychodrama's preoccupation with regressive contents, such as sexuality and perversion; envy and greed; homicidal fantasies and psychotic anxieties of disintegration; and so on. This is due to the humanist-existentialist narrative that is less inclined to focus on these themes, and because psychodrama operates in a collective space, thus making it difficult to touch on topics that are more easily discussed in the dyadic space.

The advantage of a pedagogical position that adheres to a conception of theoretical polyphony lies in its seeking to distinguish between theory and practice, thereby allowing psychodrama therapists to adopt a more ludic way of thinking, one that is capable of moving between different theoretical perspectives and containing the paradoxes that exist between them. It does not exclude the humanist-existentialist ideas that characterize psychodramatic theory, but rather suggests that they be taken as one possible tune, inside or alongside which other theoretical melodies and rhythms can be integrated. This position features a pragmatic concept of truth, which assumes that the truth value of a therapeutic theory depends on the effectivity of its implementation.

Pragmatism, in its philosophical sense, deals with the question of the most effective ways to achieve what we want to achieve. On the one hand, it accepts the postmodern argument that knowledge is always context-dependent and contingent on the definitions of value behind it; at the same time, it also assumes that at any given moment, there is a single truth, which is truer than others. Things are always judged through the executive question – does this theory currently help me better understand and adapt to the patient? This is also the thinking that underlies scientific practice – knowledge as an ongoing act of investigation.

Thus, notwithstanding the uniqueness of psychodramatic theory, it is important to recognize that no therapeutic theory, however rich, can capture and describe the full gamut of manifestations of the human phenomenon. Many psychodramatists are integrated into public institutions such as psychiatric hospitals, prisons, child daycare, special education frameworks, etc. The people who receive their therapy from them do not necessarily come because of their identification with humanist-existentialist ideas but because of actual, sometimes acute, distress. Like therapists of other specializations, psychodramatists are required to use the common terms in the framework of mental healthcare as well as to perform diagnostic evaluation processes that can help select appropriate clinical interventions.

The problem is that even when psychodramatists want to inject their work with a theoretical rationale, and to use therefore Moreno's theory, they realize that it is difficult to rely on it as a solid theory of personality from which definitive therapeutic interventions can be derived. Many of the concepts that Moreno coined are described in his writings in an impressionistic and poetic way, presented in a chaotic and non-systematic writing style.

Boria argues (Boria, 1989) that from a meta-psychological perspective, the theory of psychodrama is actually nothing more than a frame or skeleton that still needs to be built. Kellermann, too, claims that one of the reasons that psychodrama has not gained popularity among therapists in other sub-field is that it lacks a well-developed theory of personality (Kellermann, 1997; 2006). Moreno's role theory – which describes human beings according to the variety of roles they play, the flow of spontaneity, their sociometric position, their tele relations, etc. – can explain situations that occur in psychodramatic work, but it struggles to provide therapists with a uniform and coherent theoretical framework for mental development (for further details, see Yablonsky & Enneis, 1956; Polansky & Harkins, 1969; Boria, 1989; Blatner, 2000; Kellermann, 2006).

Holding the pedagogical viewpoint of theoretical polyphony may help train therapists who move with flexibility and integration between different approaches and therapeutic tools. It would enable psychodrama therapists to enjoy the technical and methodical uses of the psychodramatic instrument, without being subjected automatically to Moreno's philosophy and values. According to Kellermann (2006), traces of this idea even appear in Moreno's own thinking, as he believed that psychodrama can be regarded as both a technique and a therapeutic idea. This standpoint allows psychodrama therapists the freedom to choose the theory or set of theories that work best for them and their patient. Accordingly, it makes them more attentive and sensitive to emotional textures and hues moving parallel to one another, without needing to set up a hierarchy among them.

Conclusion

In this chapter, I tried to show how the humanist-existentialist infrastructure of psychodramatic theory functions as an ethical paradigm, which, apart from its encouragement of psychodramatists to be attentive and sensitive to certain psychic contents, it also reduces their awareness of alternative emotional discourses. I suggested that beside the pedagogical and didactic challenges may arise out of a position of theoretical polyphony, its advantage lies in the fact that it is characterized by a pragmatic concept of truth, which assumes that the truth value of a therapeutic theory depends on the effectiveness of its application.

I believe that the fact that there are so many theories and answers, sometimes mutually contradictory, to questions such as what is human nature? and what are mental health and sickness? mainly tells the story of the human phenomenon that, from the dawn of history, exceeds the boundaries of any framework and structure that attempt to capture it, a story that also attests to the meaning of this phenomenon. Perhaps, in our current pluralistic *Zeitgeist*, we must allow psychodrama therapists to choose the theory or set of theories that work best for them, rather than subject them to the philosophy and values that characterize the artistic *modus* in which they specialize.

References

Aron L. (1996) *A Meeting of Minds: Mutuality in Psychoanalysis*. New York: The Analytic Press.

Blatner, A. (2000) *Foundations of Psychodrama: History, Theory, and Practice*. New York: Springer Publishing.

Blatner, A. (2013) "Meta-theoretical Perspectives on Psychodrama" (pp. 5-21) in Baim, C., Burmeister, J., & Maciel, M. (eds.). *Psychodrama: Advances in Theory and Practice*. London & New York: Routledge.

Boria, G. (1989) "Conceptual Clarity in Psychodrama Training" *Journal of Group psychotherapy, Psychodrama & Sociometry*, 42, 166-172.

Buber, M. ([1923] 1970) *I and Thou* (trans. W. Kaufman). New York: Charles Scribner's Sons.

Bustos, D. M. (1994) "Wings and Roots" (pp. 63-76) in P. Holmes, M. Karp & M. Watson (eds.). *Psychodrama since Moreno*. London: Routledge.

Cohen, T. (2020) "Between Tele Relation and I-Thou Meeting: The Therapeutic Value of the Psychodramatic Concept of Tele from a Buberian Approach" *The Arts in Psychotherapy*, (68),101647.

Elkins, D., Stovall, K. (2000) "American Art Therapy Association, Inc.: 1998-1999 Membership Survey Report" *Art therapy*, 17(1), 41-46.

Fonseca, J. (2015) *Contemporary Psychodrama: New Approaches to Theory and Technique*. London and New York: Routledge.

Hoffman, I. Z. (1983) "The Patient as Interpreter of the Analyst's Experience" *Contemporary Psychoanalysis*, 19(3), 389-422.

Hollander, C. (1978) *A Process for Psychodrama Training: The Hollander Psychodrama Curve.* Denver: Evergreen Institute Press.

Kellermann, P. (2006) *Focus on Psychodrama: The Therapeutic Aspects of Psychodrama*. London: Kingsley.

Kellermann, P. F. (1997) "Diagnosis in Psychodrama?" *Journal of the Portuguese Company of Psychodrama*, 5, 25-32.

Kohut, H. (1977) *The restoration of the self.* University of Chicago Press.

Malchiodi, C. (2005) "Expressive Therapies: History, Theory, and Practice" (pp. 1-15) in C. A. Malchiodi (ed.) *Expressive Therapies*. New York and London: The Guilford Press.

Mitchell, S. (1988) *Relational Concepts in Psychoanalysis: An Integration*. Cambridge, MA. and London: Harvard University Press.

Moon, B., Nolan, E. (2019) *Ethical Issues in Art Therapy*. Springfield, IL: Charles C Thomas Publisher.

Moreno, J. D. (1994) "Psychodramatic Moral Philosophy and Ethics" (pp. 69-81) in P. Holmes, M. Karp & M. Watson (eds.). *Psychodrama since Moreno*. London: Routledge.

Moreno, J. L. (1914) *Invitation to an* Encounter. Vienna: Anzengruber Verlag.

Moreno, J. L. (1934) *Who Shall Survive? A New Approach to the Problem of Human Interrelations*. New York: Beacon House.

—. (1959) *Psychodrama, Volume 2*. New York: Beacon House.

—. (1964) "The Third Psychiatric Revolution and the Scope of Psychodrama" *Group Psychotherapy*, (17), 149-171.

—. (1972) *Psychodrama, Volume 1*. New York: Beacon House.

Moreno, J. L., Moreno, F. B. (1944) "Spontaneity Theory of Child Development" *Sociometry*, 7(2), 89-128.

Moreno, J. L. (1989) "Autobiography" *Journal of Group Psychotherapy, Psychodrama & Sociometry*, (42), 1-73.

—. (1959) "Transference, Countertransference and Tele: Their Relation to Group Research and Group Psychotherapy" in Moreno, J. L., *Psychodrama: Second Volume: Foundations of Psychotherapy*. Beaco.

Polansky, N. A., Harkins, E. B. (1969) "Psychodrama as an Element in Hospital Treatment" *Psychiatry*, 32, 74-87.

Pope, K., Vasquez, M. (2016) *Ethics in Psychotherapy and Counseling: A Practical Guide.* Hoboken, New Jersey: John Wiley & Sons.

Rubin, J. A. (ed.) (2016) *Approaches to Art Therapy: Theory and Technique*. New York: Routledge.

Telias, R. (2019) *Moreno's Personality Theory and Its Relationship to Psychodrama: A Philosophical, Developmental and Therapeutic Perspective*. London and New York: Routledge.

Wampold B., Imel Z. (2015) *The Great Psychotherapy Debate: The Evidence for What Makes Psychotherapy Work*. London: Routledge.

Winnicott, D. W. (1987) "Ego Distortion in Terms of True and False Self" (pp. 140-152) in Winnicott, D. W. *The Maturational Processes and the Facilitating Environment*. Madison, CT: International Universities Press.

Yablonsky, L., Enneis, J. M. (1956) "Psychodrama Theory and Practice" (pp. 149-161) in Fromm-Reichmann and J. L. Moreno (eds.). *Progress in Psychotherapy*, Vol 1. New York: Grune & Staton.

CHAPTER 7

INTEGRATING DIONYSIAN AND APOLLONIAN MODES IN THE EDUCATION OF DANCE MOVEMENT THERAPY STUDENTS

HILDA WENGROWER

Introduction

New winds are blowing in the skies of arts therapies: the 'aesthetic turn' (Samaritter, 2018). After decades of the arts serving the health, wellbeing and resilience of clients, and after deepening the knowledge of the disciplines of psychotherapy and allied areas, clinicians, researchers, lecturers and trainers are enquiring about the intrinsic health factors of dance in therapy (Ho, 2021; Koch, 2017; Wengrower, 2021) and of dance movement therapy itself (Lauffenburger, 2020). In the vein of this aesthetic turn, philosophy – especially, but not only when studying aesthetics (Wengrower, 2021) – and anthropology have much to contribute to this new perspective. In this chapter the term aesthetics refers to sensorial perception and its emotional meaning and impact (Wengrower 2021).

This chapter proposes the integration of Nietzsche's terms of the Apollonian and the Dionysian, into the teaching of arts therapies, with a focus on dance movement therapy.[1] In "The Birth of Tragedy," Nietzsche ([1872] 1968) regarded the attributes of the ancient Greek gods Apollo and Dionysus as features of human experience, the arts and aesthetic experience, which are simultaneously opposed and complementary, forming a whole. Following Nietzsche, these attributes have been implemented by theorists of arts to describe characteristics of life, art and characters in plays (Evans, 1986; Jones, 2013) and styles of dance (Jones, 2013; Jovitt, 1998). They have also been used to portray attitudes to science and ways of constructing knowledge.

---

[1] In the following sections, Dance Movement Therapy will sometimes be abbreviated as DMT.

Holton (1974) utilized Szent-Gyorgyi's 1973 proposal to apply Nietzsche's terms to science. The Dionysian aspect represented the element of intuition in enquiry and the logical and rational Apollonian epitomized other approaches to research (Szent-Gyorgyi, 1973 as cited in Holton, 1974). Dancers/choreographers with different agendas, such as Duncan, Wigman, Martin, Schlemmer, manifested their ideas using this terminology (Straus, 2019).

Following Freud's concepts of primary (non-rational, unconscious thought) and secondary process (rational, logical thought) as well as theories of creative process and integrated psychological life, I find an interesting correlation between Nietzsche's and the aforementioned psychoanalytical concepts (Arieti, 1976; Fiorini, 2007; Wengrower, 2016).

In this chapter, the Apollonian and the Dionysian are also considered as:

- Complementary parts of the self
- Aspects of the nature of the arts therapies as professions
- Facets of education that our students have to acquire

All these aspects converge in this present text.

The integration of the Dionysian and Apollonian modes fulfills the requirements the students of arts therapies have to meet in order to amalgamate the intelligence of feelings, i.e., sensibility, intuition and creative characteristics of dance or art in general, with a professional understanding, practice and discourse appropriate to specialists in the twenty-first century.

This chapter presents the written report – a didactic device designed by the author through years of educating and training students in DMT. Colleagues across the world may be using similar techniques, but what might be special here is the conceptualization; the integration of aesthetic (Dionysian and Apollonian modes) and psychoanalytical concepts (primary and secondary processes). Thus, this chapter provides a contribution to the 'aesthetic turn' (Samaritter, 2018) in arts therapies. The Dionysian and the Apollonian are considered aspects of the students' selves and their training. The written report also constitutes a complementary tool for a face-to-face learning methodology and is adequate to respond to factors influencing the institutional education of arts therapists.

The Dionysian and the Apollonian according to Nietzsche

Apollo is the sun god, an ethical deity that demands and implies individuation, self-knowledge and restraint, and heralds balanced beauty and light. Dionysus, the god of vine, incarnates irrationality, intoxication, darkness, transgression of boundaries and chaos, as well as fertility. In a statement very reminiscent of Winnicott's (1971) words about religion as a transitional phenomenon, Nietzsche ([1872] 1968, p. 42) claimed that the ancient Greeks created their gods to help control a willful existence in a harsh environment. They projected themselves into their gods and saw themselves reflected in them.

The following table presents the traits allocated to each *god-mode*:

Table 1. Apollonian and Dionysian traits

APOLLONIAN	**DIONYSIAN**
Thinking	Feeling
Self-controlled	Passionate
Disciplined	Chaotic
Rational, restraint	Irrational, unconscious
Dream facilitating self-awareness	Drunkenness, mystic alienation
Logical ordered	Instinctual
Propositional knowledge, science	Wholeness of existence
Principle of individuation	Loss of boundaries, communal body
Value for human order and culture	Celebration of nature
Celebration of appearance, illusion	Brute realism and absurdity
Plastic and visual arts, especially sculpture	Music and dance

The characteristics of the Dionysian and the Apollonian are entwined in the human self; although with a different terminology, we teach students of arts therapies that both components exist. This is especially true for DMT, which is a time art (Wengrower, 2021) and like music, has Dionysian aspects. Just as Nietzsche thought the Greek classical tragedy was an integration of both god-modes, so too do professionals and trainers need to integrate the Dionysian foundation with the Apollonian in their practice. The author considers this terminology offers an overall way of defining dances not only in societies but also in the clinic of DMT, staying thus close to the language of art.

The chapter will now introduce an analysis of aspects related to the teaching of DMT and the contribution of Nietzsche's concepts to the training of dance movement therapy students and students of the other arts therapies.

Educating students of DMT

Factors influencing the teaching

There are several factors that mould the teaching of DMT, and probably the other arts therapies:

1. The subject matter. DMT is interdisciplinary and multidisciplinary. As a discipline, there is an understanding that its knowledge has been constructed along ages of human life through intuition, feeling, cognition, sensory impressions, art and scholarship (Chaiklin, 2016). DMT is constructed upon the lived experience of a person dancing/moving, and integrates knowledge that stems from dance, body movement, psychology, psychotherapy and anthropology.

2. Professional definitions and requirements. There are several national and international associations of DMT, with a variety of standards and regulations. These, in turn, are influenced by developments in the helping professions, in sciences and in society.

3. Organizational factors. Teaching DMT also depends on the institutional context, i.e., where the training is carried out. There are differences between programs in private institutions, professional associations or at universities or colleges of different sizes. No matter in which country they are located, and aside from cultural differences, universities share common requirements that are almost always related to the theoretical-cognitive fields. This organizational mode is typically Apollonian (Wengrower, 2017). According to Gardner's (1999) taxonomy of different types of intelligence, it is the logical-mathematical and the linguistic intelligences which are stressed. Arts therapies studies involve other intelligences as well as the Dionysian a-rational mode. It may be this that deters universities from potential arts therapies projects under their auspices.

4. Economic factors. Both in the microcosm of the institution imparting the education and in the macrocosm of the society where this institution is situated, the economic factor impacts educational arrangements; although this is rarely openly mentioned or discussed. One of manifestations of these factors is the need to extend students' learning in a way independent of the higher education institution.

5. The Bologna Treaty on Higher Education in Europe. Equally important in influencing teaching and connected to the economic factors, are the effects of technology on teaching and the associated move from face-to-face teaching to work being done by students via the use of new technologies. The European Credits System Transfer (ECTS)[2] is the manifestation of this change. The Bologna Treaty of the European Union recognized—before the Covid-19 pandemic—the usefulness of including distant learning in curricula. It also established that students' work away from the higher education institution has to be evaluated and considered in their learning load. How to respond to this challenge in an educational tradition of close, interpersonal contact between students and trainers has been one of the tasks of DMT educators in Europe.

Most of these factors are in the background when planning a training program or a course teaching DMT or any other arts therapy in today's world. Educating therapists in a university has advantages, challenges and constraints. One of the challenges is to accommodate the learning process of the students to an academic schedule that may conflict with this process. In a class of 16-20 students, as happens frequently in Israel, the sharing of the experience and the reflection about it as well as other stages necessary for training, may take more time than the schedule allows. Due to economic considerations or traditional academic structures, as opposed to longer and more flexible periods of time in experiential workshops, not everybody can verbalize their experience and reflect about it in every particular class. This constraint, however, can prove to be an advantage as shown in the next section.

A personal-written report

This teaching method is one of the devices implemented to integrate the Dionysian and Apollonian, which means accommodating intuition, emotion, drives and chaos with reflective thinking, order and harmony. It also responds to the aforementioned factors influencing teaching.

In dance movement therapy training situations, after the movement/dance experience, students may have time to keep a record of it or reflect in some

---

[2] ECTS User's guide.
https://ec.europa.eu/assets/eac/education/ects/users-guide/index_en.htm

way about it: writing/drawing in their log and many times sharing this talk in the group if they wish. Later, the related subject of study may be introduced verbally.

The dance/movement experience is initiated with one or more of the following specific goals:

- In the first stage in the learning process, dance/movement experiences are introduced to focus on intrinsic aspects of the profession, and later they will be integrated with theoretical/research material.
- Dance/movement are used to learn a therapeutic skill.
- They are also utilized to learn a method in DMT.
- Dance/movement helps to uncover the meaningful complexity implicit in working with images and metaphors, their elaboration and outcome in a process of self-transformation, as it is done in DMT.
- Such experiences broaden the movement repertoire and its embodied meanings.
- Many times, certain dance/movement experiences integrate all of these aspects.

In the educational field, and even in the therapeutic setting, the use of a personal journal is common, and communication and elaboration of embodied experience through a written report is adopted in teaching. These reports should then be sent to the lecturer by e-mail or through a digital platform, which in European countries, meets the requirement of the Bologna Treaty both with regards to distance learning and use of new technologies. Written reports also constitute a method of independent work by students encouraged by the agreement.

The rationale of the written report

The written report is a tool that facilitates the working through of the movement experience in different stages. Although experiential learning has been recognized as promoting holistic learning that touches emotion, thought and behavior, it has been acknowledged that it may provoke anxiety or stress (Hobbs, 1992; Meekums et al., 2010; Wengrower, 2017).

Another important theoretical source for the written report comes from the work of Dr. Pichon Rivière, who created in Argentina a school of thought and practice related to social psychiatry and other connected subjects (Rippa & Rippa, 1989; Tubert-Oklander, 2011). When Pichon Rivière analyzed the learning-teaching process in psychiatry, he determined that there are two kinds of obstacles to apprenticeship when approaching an object of study. One of these he named the "epistemophilic obstacle" (*Diccionario de Psicología Soc.*, 2011), meaning emotional or motivational difficulties, the anxiety that arises when approaching an object of study such as – in his case and in ours – issues related to mental health. Students' anxieties may impede different aspects of the learning process. One of the solutions Pichon Rivière suggests for this is to encourage students to observe their learning attitudes and process. The written reports are intended to be a tool for such self-observation.

Foucault (1990) brought an interesting contribution to these issues when he analyzed the practical meanings of two ancient Greek imperatives: 'Look after yourself' and 'Know yourself.' Foucault said that one of the ways to carry out these moral and psychological duties to oneself is through writing. In many of the reports, expressions such as 'while writing I realized...' are a proof of the power of this undertaking.

In some countries (not in Israel), the core DMT courses are taught in intensive weekends that take place approximately every four to six weeks. The mentors have to stay in touch with the students—and they communicate among themselves—through methods other than the face-to-face modality in order to sustain the caring-teaching relationship and be alert to the students' psychological wellbeing. As noted earlier, the movement experiences may demand more working through and backing than what can be offered in the time allotted to the class in an academic setting. Thus, the reports also allow the monitoring of the students' emotional wellbeing related to the experiences they went through in their learning.

A further aspect taken into consideration for determining the need for written reports is related to the quality of dance-movement as an art of time (Wengrower, 2021). Dance does not leave an external, concrete trace as a work of visual art does; its memory fades and changes with time, part of it remains unconscious and not symbolized. However, the experience is engraved in the body, but for various reasons, the learner may not continue to work through the experience.

Students might stay with their first realizations and not further the process of introspection and reflection. Defenses, such as avoidance, denial, the frenzied pace of life many of them live, studying and working intensively, etc., are common. The Western cultural emphasis of 'doing' over 'being' (Winnicott, [1945] 2018) also has to be taken into consideration as another factor that may hinder reflective working-through of the dance-movement experience. However, pushing students to reflect on their experiential learning should not be the intention of these reports; the purpose behind them is adopted from Pichon Rivière's work mentioned above and from tenets of focal psychodynamic psychotherapy that are considered appropriate to experiential learning as well.

Focal psychodynamic psychotherapy, as created by Balint (1972), focuses on one theme, addresses the client as an adult, does not stimulate regression and avoids the establishment of a strongly charged and dependent relationship without losing closeness. In our case, the focus is on the themes of study. Focal psychodynamic psychotherapy supports the independent discovery of psychological issues of the client or the group and encourages a creative stance. Other sources are Hobbs' (1992) experiential learning, and Yalom and Leazcz (2005) who stated the benefits of a group in therapy. Writing may be a complementary tool to enhance learning from experience, allowing for introspection, self-awareness and taking an observational distance.

Due to the progressive assignments presented to the students, there is a transition from the personal-subjective experience towards integration with theory and clinical implementation. Thus, theoretical knowledge, linked with an embodied experience, is stronger, clearer and more emotionally connected than a learning based exclusively on experience or theory. By resorting to verbal expression and articulating the experience with cognitive knowledge, students improve their communicative skills in the area of the helping professions. In other words, the written reports allow them to go from moving/dancing/playing to developing their inner witness (to exercise an observing ego), and finally becoming professional, integrating all stages without losing their personal significance.

The written report consists of several parts

Section 1. Students are asked to record their lived experience, including their emotions, sensations, associations and thoughts. They are advised not to be selective; it is their personal dairy. However, they are given leeway in how much they want to share in the class-group. The guidelines require a phenomenological description of the body/sensation/movement experience. It is recommended to use "keywords" that may remind them of the experience when they come back to and expand their writing later.

Section 2. The guidelines to this section are intended to allow students to engage in the reflective process. They are invited to answer to questions such as: What was the contribution of this experience for you? Did it give you a new perspective? Did it reaffirm anything for you? Sometimes they may be asked to relate and connect the present experience to a previous one, so they can see the common thread running through the classes.

Section 3. This is an academic segment. It sets out to link the experience with the reading material or with a particular research question. During the first year of studies, the reading is assigned. As the training progresses, students may receive the option to choose their own sources or to add them to the assigned reading.

Section 4. During the second year of studies, they may be asked to consider the clinical applications of the movement experience or their conclusions about it.

The students send the reports to the trainer via the internet; the trainer reads and returns them with written comments a week later.

A written feedback by the instructor

The feedback of the mentor on the students' reports performs the role of a witness (Pallaro, 1999) by acknowledging the students' experiences and reflections, giving sustenance, supporting the process and being attentive to the learners' wellbeing.

The mentor's written comments have other functions as well:

1. They clarify the subject matter or aspects of the students' text/experience.
2. When necessary, they offer a reframing, another meaning of the experience or connect it with a vignette of a clinical situation.
3. The written comments are an extension of the empathetic trainer, involved yet careful not to slide into the role of a therapist. Students' difficulties in learning are first of all treated in relation to the task of acquiring a profession. If a personal issue may be hampering the learning process, the goal of the trainer is to encourage the student to think about it or to seek an adequate framework to deal with it.
4. Sometimes a question is raised by the trainer when some content, experience or thought expressed by the student is unclear. Some queries are intended to promote the reflective process of the trainee. Others do require a concrete answer, such as clarifying an emotion, a criticism, a sensation, a specific concept, etc.

The reports are another resource for the lecturer-trainer, indicating how to proceed with the teaching, what to propose further, what has to be emphasized, etc.

Examples of the written communication between trainee and trainer in the written reports

The following section includes excerpts of the communication between trainees and a trainer taking place through the written report, demonstrating the connection between theory and practice. A brief analysis of these fragments is included. The trainer's comments are preceded by the letter H.

> 1. *When the activity began I felt* [...] *my thoughts were in another place and I wasn't receptive.*
>
> H. *This helps you to know how a patient could feel, many of them might be in a similar state.*

In the student's description we can perceive self-awareness and openness. The answer is receptive, respects the student's privacy and focuses on helping the student learn empathy towards patients, helping to see commonalities with themselves and those they will work with in the future.

> 2. *Now that I write I realize that part of the sadness and anguish which I talked about at the beginning* (of this report) *is connected with* (being aware of) *having introduced into my life a high level of disarray that left almost nothing known from before* [...] *who am I here* (the student came from other country to study in the DMT program), *here I am not a therapist, nor lecturer, nor daughter as I was in* [—...] *now I am a student and a partner* (to a man), *so I am looking for who I am in this place and who I want to be and may be* [...]
>
> H. *Thank you for sharing this with me. I appreciate very much your heartfelt report, it unites introspection and reflection about aspects of the (learning) task. We shall be answering the professional questions along the course.*
>
> *It seems that part of the emotional processes you share here are related to the changes implicit in this temporary move from your country, which has similarities with migration and with the learning of a profession or practice* [...] *They are always challenging questions* [...] *I am available for you if you want to talk.*

The answer expresses empathy, witnessing, clarification and connects the situation to the learning process.

> 3. *I have always felt strong* [...] *physically and mentally* [...] *the movement experience helped me to add other qualities to my strength... The 3rd part* (of the movement experience) *was to improvise* (with strong movements). *It suggested slowness* [...] *I feel different when I move slowly, as if another dimension of me appears* [...].
>
> *Different elements originated that turned into a creative process. Creative: producing out of nothing. I don't know if it is from nothing, because with a thing like a sheet, with a concept such as strength and my bodymind, the result was that we carried out a creative activity.*

This student integrates the theoretical material in her narrative.

> H. *This is learning on the personal level something that will be carried over to your professional life.* [...]

The student continues: [...] *When I analyze it for a second time, I am aware that it kept me safe from unconscious anxieties.*

This excerpt is another example of self-observation and awareness of her embodiment of strength.

> 4. *I realize that the movements* (made by a partner to be empathically reflected) *are comfortable to me when they are known, I could have proposed them by myself or that I would like to perform them. However, I feel uneasy when the movements* (in the group) *come* [...] *not from my repertoire, I also recognize that they arouse my criticism.*
>
> H. *Do you know which emotion comes up with the criticism?*

This student depicts experiences that are not easy to share openly with the group at the beginning of the year but nevertheless, are vital for her process to manifest them and enter into a dialogue about them. She does it in the written report.

5. This is part of the report a student wrote after a workshop with a percussionist that takes place in the last semester of the program. She is from a country that suffered a destructive earthquake two months earlier. Her family was safe; although her mother lost her house. We talked after the workshop and the process continued in the written mode.

At the beginning of the workshop, she enjoyed the presentation of the instruments. When the drums joined in, however,

> *I felt a strange anxiety, directly connected with the earthquake. I tried to deal with it through my breathing, which helped me to calm down.*

H. *Good choice.*

> [....] *I chose the berimbau*[3] *because it has the opposite sound to the drums, with the idea of cleaning myself and releasing the strange anxiety and paralysis. It was good.*[...] *I tried to calm down by walking slowly and breathing deeply* [...] *I tried to be conscious of the drums that I could hear in the distance, incorporating them in a calmer way* [...]

The trainee was surprised to realize how troubled she still was by the damage and pain suffered by her relatives and her country. She took this experience to her personal therapy. Elsewhere she wrote she was satisfied to see how she could handle the stress during the workshop with skills she learned along classes in the training program. To the question of how the experience contributed to her as a future therapist, she answered that she had learned a lot about the effects of vicarious trauma, the unexpected reactions a therapist has to be ready to handle and how to relate to a patient who may be in a similar situation. She recalled, in great detail, how she moved, how she used her breathing and body postures. The trainer's responses gave her support, praised for her way of dealing with the stress, added information and clarified concepts.

Conclusion: The contribution of the written report

The written report is a teaching method suitable for the demands and conditions of learning and teaching in the twenty-first century. Arts therapies—in this case dance movement therapy—were shown, in this chapter, to be an integration of the Dionysian and the Apollonian modes as conceptualized by Nietzsche. The Dionysian is the intuitive, the letting go of rigid control, allowing oneself to enter into the irrational, instinctual, primary process, leaving logical thinking aside, that is part of the creative process (Wengrower, 2016). In the students' experience, the Dionysian aspect manifested in the dance/movement practice throughout the learning process. Some students have to learn to be nearer to this aspect of themselves and of the profession they are discovering. The Apollonian mode allows for psychological balance, organization and elaboration of the dance experience, logical thinking and self-control for practice and research. It is manifested mainly in the secondary process of thought in wakefulness (Wengrower, 2016). For many of our students, it is challenging to acquire some of the traits of this mode; however, all have to integrate both the Dionysian and the Apollonian as, in psychodynamic terms, we have

[3] A Brazilian musical instrument. During this workshop, each student chose an instrument to be played for their movement.

to reach a balance between the primary and secondary process (Arieti, 1976; Fiorini, 2007; Wengrower, 2016).

The method of the written reports furthers reflection on the experience, enhancing introspection, self-awareness and verbal expression, and aims to be a tool that orchestrates these modes. It allows the participant to observe the dance/movement experience in order to work through emotions, sensations and images. It builds transitions between the mover to the inner witness, i.e. to introspection and the embodied theoretical knowledge which are key stances in the development of a dance movement therapist. According to Nietzsche, "The continuous development of art is bound up with the Apollonian and Dionysian duality – just as procreation depends on the duality of the sexes, involving perpetual strife with only periodically intervening reconciliations" ([1872] 1968, p. 33). As Nietzsche saw the integration of these dualities in Greek tragedy, we can aspire to achieve it in our teaching and in our professional practice. In the light of turning to inspect the aesthetic values and contributions of the arts in the arts therapies, learning from philosophers and artists involved in arts making, is crucial since those involved in arts making have an insiders' knowledge.

References

Arieti, S. (1976) *Creativity, the Magic Synthesis.* New York: Basic Books.

Balint, M. (1972) *Focal Psychotherapy*. London: Tavistock.

Chaiklin, S. (2016) "We Dance from the Moment our Feet Touch the Earth" (pp. 3-12) in S. Chaiklin & H. Wengrower (eds.). *The Art and Science of Dance/Movement Therapy. Life is Dance*. New York: Routledge.

Diccionario de Psicología Social (2011) Retrieved Sept., 6, 2011.

Evans, J. (1986) "Death in Venice: The Apollonian/Dionysian conflict" *Opera Quarterly,* 4 (3), 102-115.

Fiorini, H. (2007) *The Creating Psyche. Theory and Practice of Tertiary Process.* Vitoria-Gasteiz, Spain Agruparte.

Foucault, M. (1990) *Tecnologías del yo.* Barcelona: Paidós.

Gardner, H. (1999) *Intelligence Reframed: Multiple Intelligences for the 21st Century*. New York: Basic Books.

Ho, R. (2021) "Back to Basics: The Aesthetic, Poetic, and Contemplative Movements' Attributes that Heal in Dance Movement Therapy" (pp. 25-34) in H. Wengrower, S. Chaiklin (eds.). *Dance and creativity within Dance Movement Therapy. International perspectives*. New York: Routledge.

Hobbs, T. (ed.) (1992) *Experiential Training: Practical guidelines.* London: Tavistock/Routledge.

Holton, G. (1974) "On Being Caught between Dionysians and Apollonians" *Daedalus*, 103(3), 65-81.

Jones, S. (2013) "Nietzsche, Modernism, and Dance: Dionysian or Apollonian?" (pp. 44-70) in *Literature, Modernism and Dance.* Oxford: Oxford University Press.

Jovitt, D. (1998) "Dance: On the Move: Merce Cunningham Dance Company" *The Village Voice*, 43(32), 160.

Koch, S.C. (2017) "Arts and Health: Active Factors and a Theory Framework of Embodied Aesthetics" *The Arts in Psychotherapy,* 54, 85-91.

Lauffenburger, S. K. (2020) "'Something More': The Unique Features of Dance Movement Therapy/Psychotherapy" *American Journal of Dance Therapy*, 1-17.

Meekums, B., Allegranti, B., Bunce, J. (2010) *Developing Constructive Tutor-Student Communication by Becoming More Aware of 'Thinking through the Body'* http://www.health.heacademy.ac.uk/scevents/fol/fol2010/workshops/tutorstudent.ppt

Nietzsche, F. ([1872] 1968) The Birth of Tragedy (pp. 3-146) in *Basic writings of Nietzsche*. New York: The Modern Library.

Pallaro, P. (1999) *Authentic Movement.* London: Jessica Kingsley.

Rippa, B., Rippa B. (1989) "Group Analysis and Pichon Riviere's Grupos Operativos" *Group Analysis*, 22, 397-403.

Samaritter, R. (2018) "The Aesthetic Turn in Mental Health: Reflections on an Explorative Study into Practices in the Arts Therapies" *Behavioral Sciences*, 8(4), 41.

Straus, R. (2019) *Reception and Analysis of Nietzsche's Apollonian and Dionysian Aesthetics in the Writing and Choreographic Practice of six Dance Figures 1900-1948* [Doctoral thesis]. University of Roehampton. https://ethos.bl.uk/OrderDetails.do?uin=uk.bl.ethos.800424

Tubert-Oklander, J. (2011) "Enrique Pichon Rivière: The Social Unconscious in the Latin American Tradition of Group Analysis" (pp. 45-70) in E. Hopper & H. Weinberg (eds.). *Social unconscious in persons, groups and societies*. London: Karnac.

Wengrower, H. (2016) "The Creative-Artistic Process in Dance/Movement Therapy" (pp. 13-32) in S. Chaiklin & H. Wengrower (eds.). *The Art and Science of Dance/Movement Therapy. Life is Dance*. New York: Routledge.

Wengrower, H. (2017) "The wellbeing of students in Dance Movement Therapy Masters Programs" in V. Karkou, S. Oliver & S. Lycouris (eds.). *The Oxford handbook of Dance and Wellbeing.* Oxford: Oxford University Press.

Wengrower, H. (2021) "Dance Comes to the Front Stage in Dance Movement Therapy" (pp. 9-24) in H. Wengrower & S. Chaiklin (eds.). *Dance and Creativity within Dance Movement Therapy. International Perspectives*. New York: Routledge.

Winnicott, D. (1971) *Playing and reality.* New York: Basic Books.

—. (2018) "Primitive Emotional Development" (pp. 145-156) in *Through Paediatrics to Psychoanalysis*: *Collected papers*. New York: Routledge.

Yalom, I., Leazcz, M. (2005) *Theory and Practice of Group Psychotherapy.* New York: Basic Books.

Part II:

Training

CHAPTER 8

TEACHING THE OPEN ART THERAPY STUDIO: DIRECTED REFLECTION ON NON-DIRECTED ART PROCESSES

DEBRA KALMANOWITZ AND JANICE SHAPIRO

Introduction

Art therapy trainings necessarily include a combination of theory, experiential learning and practice. A deep and personal understanding of artistic and creative process is essential for the practice of art therapy. This kind of knowledge is not about reading, but about experiencing. With pressure on the field to become more academic and evidence based, external education bodies are requiring more theoretical courses, sometimes at the expense of the hands – on art experience.

Advances in the profession have many positive aspects to them. Art therapy is found in an increasing variety of frameworks. Research in art therapy has become more prevalent, with arts-based research being explored as a viable option for knowledge creation (Prior 2018; McNiff 1998). However, while the academization of the profession plays a meaningful role in the professional advancement it can also lead to a diminishing role of the arts in the trainings.

This chapter looks at the importance, relevance and significance of the *open studio* to the teaching of art therapy and the capacity of this style of teaching to bridge the divide between academics and the practice of art therapy. The open studio is an approach used in art therapy with art making at its centre. It is non-directive, non-structured individual work within a group setting. We will set out a method for teaching the open studio and show that its inclusion in academic art therapy training does not compromise on the rigor of thinking, rather adds to it.

Theoretical framework of the open art therapy studio

History

Much has been written about the open studio in art therapy including the history of its origins in studios led by practicing artists in psychiatric hospitals in the 1940s (Waller, 1992; Rubin, 1999) establishing the concept of individual art centered work within a group studio setting as healing. Subsequent variations showing different adaptations of the basic model have also been reported (Allen, 2005; Finkel & Bat Or, 2020), Kalmanowitz & Lloyd, 2005; Moon, 2002). In this paper, the development of methods for teaching the open studio is our primary concern. To start let us explore the meaning of each of the two words "open" and "studio".

Open

The word *open* refers first and foremost to the choices made by the participants in the studio regarding their artwork. The approach is non-structured and non-directive. Integral to this approach is the freedom to choose subject, materials and technique. Following the making of the artwork, there is no structured or directed verbal sharing. It occurs if and when the participant chooses to talk. This element of open choice is seen as empowering and central to the creative healing process.

Besides the empowering aspect of freedom of choice there are other compelling reasons for the centrality of this openness in the approach. In a Winnicottian spirit we value his understanding that "The spontaneous gesture is the True Self in action" (2003, p. 148). This refers to an authentic creative act that arises from the self's natural and healthy need to express itself. It does not come about as a response to a suggestion from outside. This means that the teaching includes experiencing and becoming conscious of the therapeutic value of privileging fully free choice over directive approaches.

Studio

The word *studio* evokes a space where art is created. We understand the choice of name for the space in which we work as meaningful. The name reflects the nature of the work done within the space and the professional credo of the therapist carrying out this work. For art therapists the term "open studio" grounds the therapeutic practice in an art-based approach. In the context of teaching this means conveying to the students the centrality of the artmaking itself not only in their clinical work but for themselves.

The studio is a space furnished for art making and the atmosphere stimulates and facilitates immersion in the art making process.

In this context it is interesting that transference often develops to the studio space itself and even on an archetypal level to the world of art encountered there. In psychoanalytic thinking transference refers to the primarily unconscious transferring of feelings for a significant person (parent or caregiver) onto the therapist. Countertransference refers to feelings originating in the therapist's life transferred onto the client. In art therapy theory it is understood that transference and countertransference also occur in relation to the artwork. Art therapist Schaverien (1992) refers to this as "aesthetic countertransference". When the libidinous energy of the participant is deeply invested in the creative artwork, it is less directly involved in the person-to-person transference emotions. In the Jungian (1961) sense, the libido refers to the totality of psychic energy, or *chi* in Eastern tradition. The transpersonal realm belongs to the spiritual aspect of studio art therapy (Allen, 2001).

The role of the art therapist in the open studio

Given that the art is clearly positioned in the center of the therapy, we work towards having the person's libido optimally involved in art making. The nature of the libidinal investment is very much influenced by the way in which the therapist is present. Winnicott wrote of the paradox of the capacity to be "alone in the presence of someone" (2003, p.33), as necessary for experiencing true creativity. The art therapist in the open studio needs to learn to develop the capacity to be that someone in whose presence the individual can be safely alone. This is essential and enables the participants to be immersed in a way that allows for a deep and personal connection to their own creative source and authenticity.

To develop this capacity in the teaching setting requires showing our students how not to act on the inclination to help by suggesting what to do. This is not easy in situations where the participants are anxious because of not finding an idea on which to work or feeling inadequate or unskilled. Rather the nature of our response would be to teach the student therapist to encourage the client to relinquish the need to quickly reach a solution. Instead, we encourage waiting, playing, wandering around the space as healing in itself. To do this, as teachers we ourselves may also need to get out of the way by relinquishing our own need for a solution, challenging our own preconceptions and observing the process of searching with curiosity, compassion, care and patience.

The role of the group

The group in the open studio has several important functions. In the context of teaching this approach, it is important for the student to be aware of these functions in order to understand and make optimal use of them. Firstly, the group can be seen as a container within which the individual's process takes place. The individual in the open studio can be contained by the presence of the therapists, by the group as a whole and by the physical space itself which once inhabited (Kalmanowitz, 2016) has significance beyond the four walls. Secondly, the group generates contagious creative energy as described by McNiff (2015). The collective energy of the group and the evolving images can be infectious, impacting on everyone in the studio space. Thirdly, the group can serve the role of witness. Whether consciously or not, group members are aware of the presence of the other participants and of what they are doing. Fourth, it is not only the individuals in the group who may impact on each other, but the images too. It is our experience that the images play out their own group dynamics, affecting one another and evoking interactions on an aesthetic level. Lastly the open studio group offers the possibility of experiencing a sense of community. Every participant is part of the studio community, by virtue of doing his own personal work within the group. This is particularly meaningful for those who find direct interpersonal communication difficult.

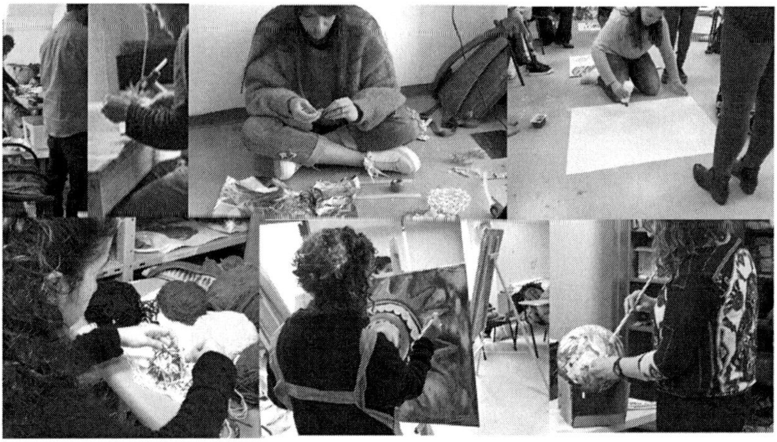

Figure 1. Every participant is part of the studio community. © Debra Kalmanowitz and Janice Shapiro

Teaching the open studio

Experiential learning and teaching as a model

Teaching the studio includes the teaching of curiosity, creativity, critical thinking, problem solving and analytic thinking. It is not about teaching what to think, but rather encouraging conscious awareness of the process and experience in the studio. This can lead to insight on both a personal and professional level, as well as an integrated understanding of theories and practice. Learning about the open studio demands practice, patience, active engagement and structured inquiry. What has emerged over the years is that teaching the open studio in this way allows the student not only to experience and learn this mode of work but serves to bridge the gap between the arts and psychological theory.

Teaching through experiencing is not a new idea. John Dewey ([1934] 1986) and Paolo Friere (2017) have written on this at length as did Confucius, the Chinese philosopher and politician, many years before (551-479 BC). Confucian quotes on education highlight this idea as seen in the following sentences: "I hear and I forget. I see and I remember. I do and I understand" or "By three methods we may learn wisdom: First, by reflection, which is noblest; Second, by imitation, which is easiest; and third by experience, which is the bitterest." (The Free University, 2019). In the open studio the active experience may at times be sweet, exciting or uplifting and at times bitter, upsetting or painful. In keeping with the Confucian understanding, all of these experiences are necessary aspects of learning and the implication is that people understand best through active engagement.

An exploration of the ideas of experiential learning resonates with the teaching of the open studio. This style of teaching is common in art therapy trainings as art cannot be understood through words alone. Two concepts of experiential learning mirrored by the Confucian quotes at the start of this section are *experience* and *reflection.* Through action, experience and reflection, students gain new knowledge about themselves, the art making, creative process and the field of art therapy. Miettinen (2000) suggests "Through its humanistic connection, the concept of experience also has an ideological function: faith in an individual's innate capacity to grow and learn" (p. 54).

The central tenet of experiential learning is that "knowledge is created through the transformation of experience" (Kolb & Kolb, 2005, p.194).

According to Dewey (1938) knowledge is not information passed down to students to recall and catalogue, but instead is an understanding based on past and current experience, used to test previous conceptions and inform new practices (Roberts 2003). For Dewey, "Education must be conceived as a continuing reconstruction of experience… the process and goal of education are one and the same thing" (1986 p.79). Learning is an endless recurring cycle and not a linear process - an exchange between our internal understanding and external environment. In this way we are both receivers and creators of information (Kolb & Kolb, 2005), taking in and putting out, impression and expression. Everyday experience is steeped in the interpretations of past generations as well as our own personal past. It is significant however, that experiences that defy our expectations activate our learning (Kolb 2019).

We need both concrete experience and abstract thought to make sense of the world. Freire (2017) stressed the importance of praxis, the transformative dialectic between reflection and action. He believed that where either action or reflection is out of balance, learning becomes difficult. "Dogmatic beliefs can close us off to new experiences, while total immersion can cloud clear thought" (Dewey (1986) in Kolb 2019 4:57). A new experience can lead to reconsideration of an entrenched belief. Both directions can enhance learning and understanding – acting on reflection and reflecting on action (Kolb, 2019).

This balance is indeed vital to teaching the open studio. After enough time for experience and experimentation, our students are able to begin to reflect and conceptualize. This model of teaching suggests that while it is essential for the students to have time to experiment freely, a structured reflection helps them to pull out the lessons learned with great accuracy. The structure we give is a list of questions to stimulate thinking, reflection and understanding.

Time and timing: Chronos and Kairos

In teaching the open studio this cycle that moves between immersion in experience and the conscious extrapolation of learning from that experience is connected to another cycle that balances different attitudes to time.

The ancient Greeks had two words for time – *Chronos and Kairos*. Chronos is the quantitative aspect of measurable time with a sequence as measured by the clock and calendar. *Kairos* refers to the quality of time, in particular the right moment to say or do a particular thing, identifying that moment and acting on it (Kalmanowitz, 2013).

The open studio setting is contained within the bounds of Chronos time. The session begins and ends at a particular time. Within these Chronos boundaries the participants are invited to totally immerse themselves in their studio experience. Kairos is in the air, inviting the participants to be intuitively aware of what feels right when. One moment of insight as to what is needed in the context of a particular dilemma that arises in the art making process might be the most important part of that studio time. Though it may be small in quantitative measurable Chronos oriented time, that moment is large in its Kairos oriented qualitative value.

In the cyclical education of the open studio there is a right time for total immersion, experimentation and creative intuitive problem solving and a right time to move out of this and to consciously reflect on lessons learned. The studio phase invites a Kairos oriented total immersion in experience. In order to learn from this qualitative experience, this is then followed by a phase of a Chronos oriented structured sequence of questions and discussion.

Four stages of teaching the open studio

A combination of our understanding of experiential teaching and of time have led us to our teaching structure which consists of four stages:

1. Participation in the open studio.

Art is made for extended periods of time. As previously described, choice of subject, technique and sharing are left up to each person.

2. Directed reconstruction of aspects of the open studio in response to set questions.

In response to specific questions about processes that happened intuitively in the studio, each participant consciously reconstructs these experiences in writing.

3. Extrapolation of learning from the responses.

Through group discussion led by the teacher these reconstructions are used to help participants to understand what has been learned about the open studio.

4. Integrative stage.

This final stage of internalization and integration of the intuitive practice and the theoretical understanding is ongoing and continues after the completion of formal studies. Over time the concepts learned form an internalized theoretical base which underlies the therapeutic responses of the students when they become professional art therapists.

The questions and their aims

The questions compiled for the students aim to facilitate the understanding of personal processes and of course the healing capacity of the open art therapy studio. The learning includes concepts specific to the open studio such as building the setting, the primary place of the art, imagination and the creative process, participant's relationship to art (often a sense of inadequacy in artmaking), the roles of the witness, the role of the facilitator and the group in the open studio context. Fundamental psychodynamic concepts, for example transference/countertransference and resistance (to name two), are studied in the context of the open studio model and their application to art therapy in general.

The questions direct the students to conscious recalling, recollecting and reconstructing of their unconscious, intuitive processes in order to reach understanding, insight and sometimes conclusions about the studio approach. While we tend to give between 1-15 questions to students, we include examples of 8 here. These 8 provide a backbone for the enquiry.

1. What did you feel when you first entered the studio?

This question is aimed at raising awareness of sensations, thoughts and feelings and leads to teaching different aspects of the open studio, depending on what the students answer. If the student was, for example, overwhelmed by the free choice and multiple possibilities, we may examine this. If the student was excited by the multitude of materials, we may teach about the role of the materials in stimulating creativity.

2. How did you choose your subject? Your materials? Where to work? How did having free choice impact on you?

Becoming aware of their process and what it was that stimulated their ideas and imagination is the motivation behind this question. We examine how students find out what they want to work on. Students learn ways of enabling participants (patients or clients) to find what they want to express, what subject is calling them or how to engage their imagination. They may come with a thought that has been occupying them or an idea in their pocket or with no idea at all. Sometimes it is the material that catches their curiosity or the work of someone else. This question invites the student to notice different ways of self – activating creative and imaginative work.

3. What do you most remember about the studio space? What elements of the studio facilitated your visual communication and creative process, and which inhibited it?

The formulation of this question suggests the importance of paying attention to the effect of the studio space itself, the arrangement and the nature of the furniture, the tools and materials and other concrete contents. This gives an additional opportunity to become conscious of the role of the space in self - activation.

4. What verbal/non-verbal interactions did you have with the facilitator, if any? How did these interactions affect you?

This question relates to the role of the facilitator – learning from the facilitator as a role model. It may address ways of being present including enabling the student to be alone in her presence, support, active and passive witnessing, responses, transference and counter transference.

5. What do you remember about what other participants were doing? How did this impact on your own process?

Becoming aware of the effect of the group even when there are no direct interactions is the focus of this question. It allows a conscious reflection on the role and influence of others working in the same space, whether the presence of the group supports or inspires or distracts or inhibits the participant. It also relates to awareness and understanding of the term *witness* in this context.

6. What verbal/non-verbal interactions did you have with other participants?

This question relates to the interactions that occurred, body language and facial expressions as communication, questions asked, spoken and unspoken responses, who initiated them and what role they played in helping or hindering the studio experience

7. What disturbed you or where did you notice resistance? How did you manage with the difficulty?

The first part of this question allows the student to consciously recall the moments of difficulty, challenge and resistance to the art making process, to the studio, to the facilitator or to peers. The second part asks that the students become aware of their responses to the resistance, if and how they managed to overcome this, ignore or work through it.

Resistance is used here in the traditional psychodynamic sense. It occurs when unconscious defenses try to block repressed uncomfortable contents from emerging into consciousness. In the studio, one manifestation of this sense of threat may be seen in difficulty in engaging in the art making process.

8. When did you notice you were most engaged and when least?

This question is about engagement in the creative process. Students explore what motivates them to feel alive, engaged and inspired. Was it the stimulus of materials, personal concerns, imagination, the art process? They are asked to remember if, and when, they became disengaged from the process and reconstruct what brought this about.

Additional questions asked may include for example: How did your choice of materials facilitate expression? What changes in your emotions did you experience during your time in the studio? How did what you chose to do impact on your sense of efficacy or insight?

Following are four examples of questions and responses. Through these questions, we illustrate how teaching occurs following the students' sharing of their reconstructions with the group.

Question 1: How did you choose your subject? Your materials? Where to work? How did having free choice impact on you?

Tali's Reconstruction:

I came into the studio and wandered around the room having no idea what I would do. I was standing wondering what was in the chest of drawers, noticing that the drawers were partially open but not sure if this was by accident or design. You said: "it's fine to look inside". This invitation to open the drawers opened something in me that had been hesitant, holding back. I began rummaging and underneath a heap of broken toys I found a small girl doll with a dirty dress and missing one arm. I knew immediately that she had been waiting for me. She became the center of my artwork which expressed a traumatic event in my early childhood that had come up yet again.

What was learnt?

Tali's process was encouraged when the therapist responded to her unspoken question while hesitating in front of the drawers. The students learned many lessons from this small, interaction: First, the importance of paying attention to body language and other non - verbal communications. When she opened the drawer and plunged her hands into the piles of muddled up toys, Tali's excitement was marked and the therapist's invitation to "look inside" was crucial. Second, the empowering aspects of discovery and choice are enhanced by *not* setting out all the materials in plain view. Discovering the broken doll made Tali realize that an old hurt was calling for attention. Third, that readymade objects may evoke associations leading to a choice of subject matter. The presence of damaged and abandoned toys, dolls and other objects is a non - verbal and non-intrusive invitation to project onto them hurt or neglected parts of self in need of healing.

Question 2: What do you most remember about the studio space? Which elements of the studio facilitated your creative process, and which inhibited it?

Yoni's reconstruction:

When I came into the studio, I found the beauty of the space breathtaking, the materials, tools and objects all attractively displayed. Working places with clean sheets of brown wrapping paper taped to the tables. The sink was clean, the rubbish bin empty. Obviously, you had invested a lot of energy in making the room look as it did. But I felt I couldn't make art in such a perfect environment. As if I would have to create something marvelous, as if whatever I did would spoil the aesthetics of the space, contaminate it. I felt paralyzed.

When other students started choosing materials and putting them on tables it helped. The fact that things were being touched, picked up, moved around made me feel less stuck. I collected various tools and materials and put them on the table too even though I wasn't sure that I would use them. Just to have stuff there made me feel less uptight.

What was learnt?

As the therapists and keeper of the studio space the therapist was taken aback by Yoni's description. In point of fact her studio had recently reached its lowest point of chaos, gradually over the past months. Knowing that a new group would be coming soon she had fired herself up with motivation and energy to tidy up. And as often happens with extremes she had taken to it with a vengeance and overdid it. When the art therapist shared this turnabout in her group discussion it led to learning about the need for finding a balance between an ordered studio that shows respect for the space and a certain amount of disorder that is liberating. The space should certainly not look neglected. However, it needs to be cared for without being so ordered as to deter using it freely.

Question 3: What do you remember about what other participants were doing? How did that impact on your own process?

Rina's reconstruction:

When I tried to do my own artwork alone at home, I would feel overwhelmed by emotion and after a short time would distract myself and busy myself with something else. In the open studio I felt I needed privacy and silence to discover what I wanted to do with my time there. I found a table separate from the others and began painting a disturbing recurring dream. I had tried painting it several times at home but hadn't ever managed to carry out my intention.

This time was different. Somehow the fact that I wasn't alone in the studio made me feel safe. Although I had created a bubble around myself, I was aware of other people in the studio. It didn't matter to me what exactly they were doing but it did matter to me that they were there and making art. I felt a sense of belonging to this group of individual working bubbles sharing a common space. Most surprising to me was that being in the group enabled me to immerse myself in extremely personal artwork.

What was learnt?

The main thing the students learnt from Rina's experience was that the presence of others working on their own art in the studio may make in depth personal creative work possible and that this may come about even when there is no direct interaction with them. This is an extension of Winnicott's concept of "the capacity to be alone in the presence of someone" as essential to authentic creativity. Here the presence is not only that of someone but of some others, not only the presence of the therapist but also of the other participants and their art.

In addition to the feeling of safety that enabled Rina to allow herself to be absorbed in what she was doing, she felt a sense of belonging. From this it was learnt that without any interpersonal communication a participant can experience herself as being a member of the studio community.

Question 4: What disturbed you or where did you notice resistance? How did you manage with the difficulty?

Lara's reconstruction:

When I came into the open studio, I felt anxious about making art, concerned it would not be good enough and worried about what others would think. I felt blocked and very anxious and I had a hard time getting into the creative mode. My unsure relationship with the creative world had begun in childhood and carried on into adulthood. It had led to my limiting myself to using only pencils and to copying photos as well as never allowing anyone to see my drawings.

Sitting in the studio overcome with self- loathing my old thoughts came up; that copying didn't count as I wasn't creating something original. I sensed a presence and looked up. You had sat down near me. I met your eyes and felt encouraged, as if you were telling me that you were aware of my vulnerability and wordlessly giving me support. Suddenly it felt ok to copy and use only pencil. I took out a photograph of my dad and began to draw, becoming absorbed. After a while I felt unsure and found myself seeking and finding eye contact with you. Again, I saw in your eyes empathy, support and curiosity. I sensed no judgement or expectation. At that point, I gave myself over to the process.

What was learnt?

The students learned the importance of accepting what emerges, without preconceptions, as to what is creative and healing and what is not. The non - verbal interaction between Lara and the art therapist was crucial as part of witnessing not only the emerging artwork but the process of struggling with her sense of self and her relationship with making art. Kairos was evident here - intuiting when a near presence and an empathic gaze was needed to help an unsure student get into creative work and sustain her engagement despite her misgivings.

Discussion

Preserving the art in academic art therapy trainings

We have described our understanding of the healing qualities of the open studio and how it can serve as a core for teaching both the open studio itself and psychological processes that also take place in other approaches to art therapy. The method we have developed is made up of active immersion in the studio experience followed by directed questions aimed at bringing the intuitive unconscious process into consciousness, allowing learning to be extracted. It is not by chance that there are multiple potential ways of understanding the set questions and responding to them. Often students ask for further clarification as to what is meant by a question. We reply that whatever they understood is what was meant. We don't intend a particular answer. The way each student understands the question is indicative of the aspects of the studio that occupies her thoughts. The different understandings offer different learnings.

While we list questions, this itself is not a linear process, but one which draws learning out of studying the *here and now* experience. For Tali the question "How did you choose your subject" brought up multiple lessons: the importance and nature of the attention of the therapist in facilitating expression, even with no verbal articulation; the effect of the studio and the way in which the room is arranged; as well as an understanding of how outer stimuli activate inner emotional content.

In the example of Yoni, the students began to understand the strong influence that the studio space itself can have, apart from the people in it. They learned how the studio may evoke transference to the space which may be perceived as an extension of the therapist facilitator or as a symbolic space representing the whole realm of art on a transpersonal level.

In Rina's example the students learned about the role of the group in the open studio in enabling a sense of belonging. The way in which individual work within a group makes it possible to be a member of a community even without direct interpersonal communication. This has valuable implications for those who suffer from loneliness and find the interactive social aspect of any group inhibiting or threatening.

Lastly the example of Lara allowed us to address a subject which is not uncommon amongst trainee art therapists, art therapists and participants alike. Lara felt resistance to creating due to strong feelings of inadequacy.

She found that external acceptance and a non-judgmental witness helped her feel that she was valid as was her choice of subject matter and style of art making. This allowed her to connect to herself on a deep level, accept what she was doing, and to change her relationship with her art and herself.

Allen (2013) identifies what she describes as the *clinification syndrome*, a process where art therapists gradually cease making art as clinical skills become the primary focus. This same tendency extends to art therapy training programs, where the field is developed more through scholarship and less through lived experience. Writing about making art is worlds apart from actively making art. In order to understand the process, it is essential that we do it. Through our physical sensations and interactions with the materials in the art making process we become aware of the nuances of the interaction. The attempt to academize art therapy by learning primarily through reading theory, fixed sets of rule and reduction to concepts not indigenous to the arts themselves is problematic. It means that we cannot guide people through their own process.

Academization can potentially bring about a new configuration within academia leading to a less marginalized status for art therapy. While this is an advance in the status of the profession we need to make sure that this progress is not at the cost of the deep connection to the heart and soul of our work – the art itself.

Including the open studio in the art therapy trainings not only ensures that art remains its center, but also that art therapists are deeply familiar with the arts and the creative process as well as learning its theory in a way that is indigenous through experience. This does not imply a compromise on rigor, understanding, theory or critical thinking. Indeed, in our experience, the opposite is the case. When understanding is embodied and internalized the art therapy can be engaged, documented and further researched in greater depth. The rigorous study of the processes in the open studio has a place in academia as does the study of visual language and arts-based research. The essence of the message, as seen from the examples above, is that teaching the open studio is a way of maintaining a balanced and fertile relationship between academization and the art experience.

Conclusion

This chapter describes an approach to teaching the open art therapy studio as fundamental to an art therapy education. It emphasizes the value of engaging in a deep creative hands-on experience followed by the exacting study of that intuitive process. The words of Kolb (2019) resonate with this approach. We recall that he wrote that dogmatic beliefs have the potential to close us off to new experiences, while "total immersion can cloud clear thought." (p57) We propose that timing is all, that there is a time for total immersion and a time for removing ourselves from the depths so as to retroactively observe, reflect and consciously learn. The structured approach we propose helps students understand the open studio as well as art therapy processes from personal, theoretical and academic perspectives.

References

Allen, P. (2005) *Art Is a Spiritual Path*. Boulder: Shambala.

Dewey, J. (1934) *Art as experience*. New York: Capricorn Books.

—. (1938) *Education and experience*. New York: Simon and Schuster.

—. (1986) "Experience and Education" *The Educational Forum*, 50(3), 241-252.

Finkel, D., Bat Or (2020) "The Open Studio Approach to Art Therapy: A Systematic Scoping Review" *Frontiers in Psychology,* October, 11, 1-16.

Friere, P. (2017) *The Pedagogy of the Oppressed*. London: Penguin Classics.

Jung, C. G. (1961) *Collected Works* volume 4. Freud and Psychoanalysis. Princeton: Bollingen.

Kalmanowitz, D. and Lloyd, B. (ed.) (2005) *Art Therapy and Political Violence: With Art, without Illusion*. London and New York: Routledge. (Chapter 6 Inside the Portable Studio: Art Therapy in the former, Yugoslavia 1994-2002).

Kalmanowitz, D. (2013) "Art, Imagination, Chronos and Crisis" *Journal of Applied Arts & Health*, 4(1), 313-324.

Kalmanowitz, D. (2016) "Inhabited Studio: Art Therapy and Mindfulness, Resilience, Adversity and Refugees" *International Journal of Art Therapy*, 21(2), 75-84.

Kolb, D., Joy, S (2009) Are there cultural differences in learning style? *International Journal of Intercultural Relations*. 33, 69-85.

Kolb, A., Kolb, D. (2005) "Learning Styles and Learning Spaces: Enhancing Experiential Learning in Higher Education" *Academy of Management Learning & Education,* 4, 193-212.

Kolb, A. (2019) "8 Things to Know About the Experiential Learning Cycle" Experience Based Learning Systems video, 8:07. August 3, 2019. 4:57 https://learningfromexperience.com/themes/experiential-learning-theory-videos/

McNiff, S. (1998) A*rt-Based Research*. London and Philadephia: Jessica Kingsley Publishers.

McNiff, S. (2015) *Imagination in Action: Secrets for Unleashing Creative Expression*. London and Boston: Shambhala.

Miettinen, R. (2000) "The Concept of Experiential Learning and John Dewey's Theory of Reflective Thought and Action" *International Journal of Lifelong Education*, 19(1), 54-72.

Moon, C. (2002) *Studio Art Therapy. Cultivating the Artist Identity in the Art Therapist*. London and Philadelphia: Jessica Kingsley Publishers.

Prior, R. (2018) *Using Art as Research in learning and teaching. Multidisciplinary Approaches Across the Arts*. Bristol and Chicago: Intellect.

Roberts, T.G. (2003) *An Interpretation of Dewey's Experiential Learning Theory.* ERIC. Retrieved November 20, 2020. https://files.eric.ed.gov/fulltext/ED481922.pdf.

Rubin J. (1999) *Art Therapy: An Introduction*. Philidelphia, Brunner/Mazel.

Scheverien, J (1992). *The Revealing Image. Analytic Art Psychotherapy in Theory and Practice*. London and New York: Tavistock/Routledge.

The Free university (2019) Retrieved Nov., 22, 2020. https://www.open.edu/openlearn/education/12-famous-confucius-quotes-on-education-and-learning

Waller, D. (1992) "Different Things to Different People: Art therapy in Britain. A Brief Survey of its History and Current Development" *Arts in Psychotherapy*, 19(2), 87-92.

Winnicott, D. W. (2003) *The Maturational Processes and the Facilitating Environment.* London: Karnac.

YouTube: *Experience Based Learning Systems LLC* (2020). https://learningfromexperience.com/themes/experiential-learning-theory-videos/

CHAPTER 9

MUTUAL VISUAL TRANSFERENCE: A GROUP SUPERVISION MODEL

YONATHAN SCHUR AND LIOR SCHUR

To approach a painting before
a title is given to notions
To depart from it prior to everything
that follows
Israel Eliraz (trans. Edna Shemesh)

Introduction

This chapter began with ideas introduced at a lecture which was given by the first author at the Ecarte conference in Italy in 1994, published as a paper 4 years later (Schur, 1998). We find that the materials presented there are even more relevant in light of the professional and personal development that we experience, as well as that of the profession as a whole. Thus, we wish to discuss these issues from an up-to-date perspective, stemming from the experience that we have accrued over the years in teaching and supervision.

The profession of art therapy, which was originally based on the language of art as a leading language (Kramer, 1971), has become over the years a profession in which art functions as an accompaniment to the dominant language of psychology. Various manifestations can be found for this, such as establishing a therapeutic framework of 50 minutes, as is customary in verbal psychotherapy and in treatment rooms that are not studio spaces. In addition to these, the demand placed on students who are in the process of supervision to become familiar with the language of art is diminishing.[1]

[1] In Israel, for example, 1,000 hours of practical art studies were basic prerequisite for starting the study program, whereas today only half of this number is required – and not all of it must be practical.

Many therapists find it difficult to offer suggestions from the language of art that will allow the patient to expand his or her range of expression and help him or her feel a sense of belonging to a broader cultural context (Schur, 2013). We share this feeling with Shapira (2014) who wrote, in the introduction to her paper, on the academicization that art therapy undergoes in general, and in Israel in particular, and mentioned Adamson and Allen. Adamson (1984) harshly criticized the trend of psychology becoming dominant over art in supervision programs, while Allen (1992) stressed the danger of making art therapy too clinical. The model presented here will describe the use of art as a leading, autonomous language in supervision[2].

The way art is brought into the treatment room – and, as a result, also for supervision – plays a crucial role during treatment. Dubowski (1985) argues that art should have its own advantages, and no attempt should be made to make it illustrative. He argues that art therapists, who also used to be (or still are) creators, are vividly and clearly aware of the unique relationship that exists between the creator and the art materials, forms, and images they create. Dubowski, like Allen, warns against the strengthening of the identity of the "therapist" at the expense of that of the "artist". Adamson, in a statement that seems extreme today, argues that only artists should be art therapists (Shapira, 2014). Dubowski (1985) argues that the artist-therapist can advance therapy where it gets stuck by intuitively changing work materials, out of an understanding of the artistic process and a deep familiarity with the qualities inherent in materials and techniques. Judd (1986) writes about the unique relationship that exists between artists and the images, symbols and forms they create and thus reinforces the claim that art itself should receive proper recognition as having an advantage in therapy.

In our work with mutual transference we rely on approaches that have been expanded by therapists from the British independent group, such as Winnicott, Little, Bollas, Coltart, Symington, Casement and Balint (for detailed information on countertransference see: Heimann, 1950; Laplanche & Ponalis, 1974). This approach considers countertransference as a tool for the therapist to understand his or her patients, and as an expression of communication between them. In art therapy, an investigation of visual

---

[2] Every therapist, especially at the beginning of their journey, is obliged to receive professional guidance – supervision. The purpose of the supervision for the therapists is to continue learning and training, to receive assistance in processing the treatment processes, to separate the contents of transference and countertransference, and to process the interpersonal processes that the therapist goes through within the relationships they form with their patients.

mutual transference creates an additional dimension of understanding the therapist's counter-transferential responses. In 1950, Paula Heimann introduced her revolutionary ideas. She argued that in countertransference, the patient "injects" into the therapist contents that the former is unable to recognize or verbalize. He "borrows" the therapist's unconscious, so that the latter may feel this content for him. Heimann defined the therapeutic encounter as one between two "unconsciouses", an encounter in which the therapist's unconscious perceives the patient's unconscious on a deep level. Kernberg spoke about the change in the concept of countertransference. For him, countertransference is accepted by most therapists as a total response to the patient's reality as well as the patient's own transference: "… these emotional reactions of the analyst are intimately fused, and that although countertransference should certainly be resolved, it is useful in gaining more understanding of the patient" (1975, p. 49).

Background to the development of the model

The model begins with work done with a group of therapists who sought to deepen their personal knowledge and experience of making art. The group met once a week, at the first author`s studio, and every third week one of the participants brought therapeutic materials to the supervision, while in the other two sessions the group members worked on their artistic process (Schur, 1998). At some point along the process, after the meeting ended, the supervisor watched the works of the supervisees in the studio. He had a feeling, not yet articulated, that he discern elements from the therapies to which he was introduced during the supervision, and that they resonate therapeutic content through visual cues and codes. It occurred him that the fact that the studio space serves both the supervision of the therapists on therapy and their work on their personal art processes, encourages inter-permeation of the two worlds. The works of art seemed to give visual expression to the mutual processes of transference and countertransference, which at that stage were not yet visible.

Curious to explore this nascent feeling with the group, the supevisor asked a supervisee in the next supervision to hang, alongside the works of the patient she presented, paintings she had recently made in the studio. During the group observation, similar colors and a similar laying of paint, common composition and content worlds that influenced the therapist's works were clearly perceived. The group repeated this work process in the following weeks, with the other supervisees and their patients. When it became clear that this phenomenon recurs with the supervisees, during the supervisions, the group began to refer to the art materials of both the patient and the therapist, and to examine the relationship between them and what happens in the therapeutic relationship. The supervisor and the supervisees sought to identify what is implied in the therapist's works and to understand through them the content that occupies the patient and that characterizes the therapeutic relationship.[3] The supevisor then conceived of the process as "visual countertransference" because the group referred to the very identification of the processes of transference through the visual materials. Today, in the spirit of the relational approach we feel we share, we conceive of the process as "mutual visual transference". Aron claims that,

> The term *countertransference*, though, obscures the recognition that the analyst is often the initiator of the interactional sequences, and therefore the term minimizes the impact of the analyst's behavior on the transference. The relational approach… views the patient-analyst relationship as continually established and reestablished through ongoing mutual influence… A communication process is established between patient and analyst in which influence flows in both directions" (1991, p. 33).

With the understanding that mutual transference is clearly and visibly present in the therapists' works having been established, the first author examined the possibility of introducing another change to the model: the therapist who brought the patient into the supervision presented the patient's works without the therapist's own works (although the group kept making art in a parallel process), and to present the patient without background explanations. The supervisor was curious to see if the impact they were witnessing occurs not only in the direct therapist, but also among the other group members – therapists who are exposed to the patient and his or her works in the supervision session. He invited the group members to respond to the artworks of the patient who was brought to the supervision, and not to his or her "life story" or "therapeutic narrative". This is how the model developed as it is taught today.

In working with the **mutual visual transference** model, a question sometimes arises regarding the introduction of the respondents' personal and seemingly irrelevant content. Ogden (1994) believes that in many cases, associations that seem "unrelated" arise with certain patients and at a specific time. He suggests thinking of these cases as a product of the "analytical third" and considering them as having potential value and meaning. Ogden suggests addressing all the associations, physical-emotional experiences, and sensations that the therapist experiences as

---

[3] We wish to thank Avi Berman for clarifying this significant point.

responses to the encounter with the patient's subjectivity. Ferro (1999) argues that the therapist should function as a receptor and interpreter for the patient's projective identifications. He believes that the experiences and impressions perceived by the therapist may be formed from the total personal experiences taken from the patient's life. Racker reminds us that the therapist's basic role is to create a substrate that will allow the patient to bring together his or her conscious and unconscious parts. He argues that the therapist can perceive the unconscious of his patients only from the components the therapist identifies in himself. This conception features a paradox to which he points: "… at times one perceives in the other exactly that which is very much rejected within oneself" (2018, pp. 16-17).

Today we can say with certainty that not only are substantial and enlightening connections between the supervisees' works done in reaction to the therapist's works, but the employment of verbalizations before using the art language impairs the group supervisory process and may cause a "blind spot" in relation to the patient. We can think of two examples of patients in psychiatric settings who were brought to the supervision. In both cases, the diagnosis and treatment were changed following what came up in the supervision session conducted according to the model presented here. In one case, a patient was brought in who had been diagnosed and has been treated as a schizophrenic for many years. By means of the reaction artworks, although schizophrenia could be accepted as a diagnosis, we hypothesized that the emergence of the illness was due to an undiagnosed combat injury (PTSD). In this case, despite the fact that indeed, his works could be seen as typical of schizophrenia patients, the supervisee accepted the additional hypothesis as optional. Considering what came up in the supervision group and the subsequent re-evaluation that was done at the hospital, the patient's treatment changed and later, he was moved to a rehabilitative treatment in the community. The second case occurred with a supervisee who worked in a psychiatric clinic with a patient who was diagnosed with a "personality disorder with psychotic episodes". During the supervision session, many reaction artworks related to sexual assault, a diagnostic direction that had not come up before. The supervisee took the insights that came up in the session, and when she raised the question directly in therapy, a new life story unfolded that had not been told before. As a result, the treatment focused on sexual assault and a door was opened to treating the patient as a broader human complex, outside the definitions of "personality disorder" and "psychosis".

Mutual visual transference in art

The tremendous importance we attach to the personal experience of the supervisees in the supervision process leads to an emphasis on continuous expressivity. During the supervision sessions in the supervisor`s studio, the therapists work in the same setting in which the patients work – in a room designated solely for making art. The room is large, spacious and full of various art materials, all within easy reach. This is a room where it is allowed to get dirty and make a mess. The floor is filled with deposits of previously made works, the smell of art materials is in the air and the whole arrangement is geared to creating a platform for a creative-artistic life.

The unique situation of art therapy allows for a therapeutic conversation that is different than usual. The therapist is required to overcome the initial urge to "understand" and express his or her insights. The therapist should maintain curiosity and alertness in himself while encouraging the preservation of ambiguity situations that lead the patient to develop their own language and be familiar with the ongoing dialogue that arises among the works in his or her creative process.

In the *mutual visual transference* model, emphasis is placed on phenomenological-structural observation, with the leading question being "what do we see?" (Betensky, 1995): We try to establish the artistic, formal and material elements used by the patient in his or her works; are they two-dimensional or three-dimensional? What is the format chosen for the work? Does it have figurative or abstract elements? Can patterns and templates be identified in it? What color characterizes it and is it possible, out of all these, to identify a "story" in the artworks? We pay close attention to the way the patient uses the materials. Milner (1987) refers to this by saying: "whatever its [work of art] content, or subject, whether a recognizable scene or object or abstract pattern, must be an externalization, through its shapes and lines and colours, of the unique psycho-physical rhythm of the person making it. Otherwise it will have no life in it whatsoever, for there is no other source for its life" (p. 191). In the supervisory sessions we experience a variety of artistic expressions in order to respond to the work we are observing. This ensues from the perception that familiarity with the language of art promotes the ability to connect to patients' works of art as aesthetic objects, thus strengthening the connection with the patients themselves.

The next question we ask in the supervision process, "*How do we feel?*", touches upon the observing therapist. Emphasis is placed on the therapist's experience in the presence of the patient's works: What somatic feelings arose in the therapist while observing the works that were brought in and with what feelings he or she worked during their artistic reaction? Next, we move on to the last question, "*What do we think?*", which seeks to create integration of the various stages of observation and discussion. We try to build the patient's image for ourselves and hypothesize the therapeutic themes in the room. We believe that the acquisition of the ability to analyze the works makes the discussion of artistic and therapeutic issues richer and more layered. The discussion makes it possible to discover the main difficulties that the creator faces. These are complexities that are often unconscious, and that are recognized only as vague areas of discomfort. Over time, discussions of a psychological nature about the works diminish significantly and the conversation focuses on art and its therapeutic "speech".

The *mutual visual transference* model calls for remaining in a vague domain, through which one can gain a more authentic experience of both the patient and the therapist. It relies entirely on the suspension of interpretation and thought. In the words of Ogden: "Rather, the patient who is presented in the supervisory session is a fiction created in the medium of words, voice, physical movements… unconscious communication such as projective identifications, and so on" (2005, p. 1267). Often, in the transition to the organizing and ordering mechanisms, there is a kind of defensive element in the face of a sense of general and threatening flooding that resonates the patient's experience with the therapist. The model relies on the deliberate suspension of these mechanisms and the real containment of the formation of feelings and emotions.[4]

It is important to clarify that this is not about free drifting in chaos. The art materials themselves as well as the artworks on display (both by the therapists and by the patients) form an infrastructure. During the work, the supervisees learn to regard their own art as a significant anchor that can be relied on in the therapeutic work. Ogden writes about it that,

[4] When art is not the principal language of therapy, a tendency may form to use structured exercises that make it hard to create a sense of continuity between sessions, since every session is experienced as a new beginning. The exercises prevent the patient from establishing an inner rhythm, and he or she may feel that there is a "goal" to achieve, a "lesson" with a certain purpose. Moreover, the tendency to swap different techniques and media within the language of visual art, or between the different arts, without the grounding of a therapeutic rationale, is a common response to the therapist's and/or patient's sense of anxiety that arises through the work.

> All the ways that the analyst consciously and unconsciously brings to the supervision his experience with the analysand do not add up to actual presence of the patient – rather, they issue in the creation of a fiction… creating the patient as a fiction – "dreaming up the patient" – in the supervisory setting represent the combined effort of the analyst and the supervisor to bring to life in the supervision what is true to the analyst's experience… (2005, pp. 1267-1268).

Delving into the non-verbal content gives the supervisees confidence in the potential communication inherent in the language of the materials. The therapist must allow himself to develop in unconscious ways. Thus, he will later be able to maintain a process parallel to the art therapy processes of his patients. This is a necessary development, which enables the growth of a deep and multi-layered understanding of the patient's artworks and psyche.

Mutual visual transference in a supervision group

The material accumulated during group supervision is much more than the sum of the participants' statements. The reaction artworks converse and resonate between them, exposing hidden elements in the works of both the patients and the therapists. The facets that are revealed to us during supervision constitute the basis for further work, first in the supervision group, and subsequently in the treatment rooms.

Group supervision creates a domain limited in time and space, where intuitive creation is possible, out of focused and unfocused attention concurrently. What comes to life in the room is as symbolic as it is concrete. Milner notes the need for a framework, "… a blank space, framed gap" (1987, p. 60). For her, this framed space makes it possible to perceive and interpret what is inside differently from what is outside it. We suggest thinking of Milner's words as an invitation to look at what is going on within the therapeutic space (or in the supervision space, for our purposes) as real and as symbolic at the same time. The feelings and thoughts of the supervisee responders are completely real, take place within the framed space and respond to what is created outside it. The artworks of the supervisees can be seen as metaphors and symbols for the therapeutic process and for the mental and emotional state of the therapist and the patient.

We are going back now, flipping through the first author`s notes on supervision, and things are getting clearer for us. We will give an example that illustrates the manner of supervision:

A supervisee brings some works of her patient to the supervision. She lays out a very large number of works in which lumps of paint, layers, stripes and vertical streaks of paint are seen on landscape-oriented sheets. Most of the works look muddy, and almost all are abstract. In each painting you can see the many layers inside it. Although the paintings contain a great deal of color, looking at the entirety of the works reveals monotony and repetitiveness.

From the picture unfolding before us, the supervisees approach their work areas and react through creation. At this point the supervisor feels the frenzy and restlessness that is strongly buzzing through the room. He notices a lot of covering and revealing that are intensely repeated in the various works.

In the following group talk, the participants recount that they responded to feelings of concealment, overload, flooding, pain, confusion, boundless mixing, "fog" and discomfort facing the patient's work. The supervisor finds himself pondering, "What's going on here? What are we dealing with? Where is all this going?" He feels confused, unable to gather the many pieces of information that overwhelm him. Any meaning that seems to begin to emerge immediately falls apart.[5] One of the participants also shares her feeling that "there is a membrane" that prevents her from feeling what is happening to the patient. To delve deeper into this feeling, she describes creating more and more covers and trying to observe what is going on beneath them. Each time she added another layer and another ready-made element. She wrapped it all in plaster bandages and later also in masking tape. During her work, she assembled and disassembled, in order to try and hold on to the experience of difficult ambiguity she had at the beginning of the work.

Another participant feels that the patient's works expose her to very uncomfortable situations related to sexuality. While working with the materials, she gets very dirty from plaster and red paint. She tries to clean herself up and fails, and the paint stays on her hands. She gets very wet while working and finishes her work with a hard feeling, "as if I'm dirty on the inside." The participant is very connected to the experience of harm that

---

[5] Goren (2015) relates to Bion's perspective and argues the even the supervisor should relinquish the knowledge he has in favor of a new understanding that grows from the greatest emotional intimacy possible to the group's experience of here-and-now. Inspired by Bion, she notes that the supervisor brings to the group all his life's knowledge, but that he must forget it all at the same time, in order to start afresh as if for the first time; only thus will he attain new experience without linking it to past experience: Without memory, without desire and without understanding.

the works convey, and her speaking about the mud and dirt expresses something of what the patient expresses in her work – a desire to tell and conceal at the same time.

The works of the entire group express conflict: they are clearly divided between clean, dry and well-kept works and dirty, saturated and muddy works. One describes an experience of panic during work, feelings of suffocation that afflicted her and a need to go outside and breath some fresh air. Otherwise she felt the need to build something. She began building a tower, but felt it was “too strong, masculine and aggressive”. She says she wanted to make it wet, but recoiled and made it very dry, like a “wound that can’t be covered”. The way the participants work corresponds to what is later found out about the patient who was brought in for the supervision, who comes from a violent home where there are many secrets with which she is entrusted.

Towards the end of the session, when the participants are supposed to organize the space and place their work on the drying racks, they leave the room with everything lying in the work areas and seems to have been hastily abandoned due to a dramatic event. It is important to note that this behavior is not at all typical of the group, which usually concludes the session with cleaning and tidying the room. I stay with the supervisee and she notes in amazement that what has just happened in the room accurately recreates her sessions with the patient, after which she is left surrounded by dirt and toils alone to clean and tidy up the room.

It can be seen that the work processes and the products all touch, directly or indirectly, the feeling of the heavy burden, secrecy and injury that the patient brings to the room through her works of art. The participants experience these feelings; however, each responds to the secret in a different, raw and intuitive way.

In the supervision model discussed here, the works of art create a kind of catalog of unconscious contents that are presented visually. In this context it is worth mentioning the writing of Foulkes, one of the developers of group analysis, who described the group process as one in which the participant encounters parts of him- or herself in the other participants. Foulkes (1964) referred to the group as a “hall of mirrors” and wrote about the group mirror as enabling the processing of conflicts reflected in the other, even though they are sometimes excluded from our own self.[6]

We need to examine when and where this content appears, and how it resonates in the participants' works. Together, we discover "families" of contents in those works to which everyone responds in their own way. When we aggregate the reactions, we obtain a stratified reference that expands the initial "catalog" that activated us without being deciphered or overt. The group encourages inquiry: the participants all deal with the same therapeutic issues, without their being formulated prior to the meeting. Each of them is required to meet with him- or herself and hence, with the therapeutic materials. As the group continues to evolve and become more sophisticated, participants deepen their familiarity with themselves and learn to distinguish between automated mechanisms they tend to activate and meaningful content for the specific patient brought in.

In therapy, there is always double attention – the therapist is in the experience, in the "here and now", but also observes it from the outside. In the proposed model, attention is simultaneously directed to the therapist's self-inquiry and to what the patient "says"; on the one hand, what interests me? How do I feel? What attracts or rejects me in the creative process? On the other hand, what is the patient interested in? What is she afraid of? What secret wishes does she express in her work?

The artwork made by the group participants may appear coincidental or unimportant to the supervision process. An example of the great significance of every nuance and the type of subtle attention that arises in group supervision can be found in a case study, as told in the words of a supervisee:

> One of the participants insisted on banging nails for a long time. The nailing provoked harsh reactions in the room due to the loud noise, but these did not prevent her from continuing. From her work process and the reactions of the group, I could mostly discern my patient's need to be seen and heard, to keep his presence from disappearing. He 'makes noise' through his anger and aggression. Only in this way does he manage to get his mother's attention.

---

[6] The hall or mirrors adds the idea of multiple viewpoints that today are considered as better deciphering the patient's concealed or outward-split worlds. Foulkes' "mirror response" does indeed yield the concealed in the following sense: the participant has reservations regarding another patient, and this very reservation indicates the domain with which he or she does not want to be acquainted.

During the supervision sessions, verbal and non-verbal dialogues occur frequently. These include technical consultations on matters related to art creation, or clarification of the artistic rationale behind a particular choice. Moreover, they deal with the formalization of issues and ways of dealing with difficulties. One of the most important aspects of the group's work is the discussion that takes place between the participants at the end of the work. These three aspects reinforce the participants' ability to assist one another in dealing with difficulties. An additional positive aspect is the inspiration and license to have new experiences, under the influence of others working in different styles or work materials.

One of the supervisees described the process in a way that sheds light on the amorphous and powerful feelings that characterize group supervision in its various stages:

> In the case studies I experienced both mental and physical reaction during the art creation and following the case study. Over time I realized that I am exposed to the patient's entire works and transference reactions as well as to the countertransference of each student therapist. My transferences were added to that complexity. The collective experience was most intense for me. Each case study means going out on a new adventure and into unique world; art leads to worlds that are fascinating, dark, magical, depressing, frightening and primary in direct manner; it is present and exciting each time anew (Turiski, 2008, p. 7).

Schaverien (1997) also refers to the transference and countertransference relationship. She argues that the work of art offers an alternative of external presence, because it is an object that exists outside the creator, while being part of him. Schaverien describes the creative process as one in which there is a split between "I-creator" and "I-observer". These two parts of the self may act simultaneously, but they have different priorities. Each of them performs its role and they alternate within the creative process itself. We can understand the process that Schaverien describes as a process of countertransference. The "I" of the artist creates a transference to the work while the "I" of the observer, like the therapist, responds more externally. It considers the meanings and implications and creates contexts shared between them. *Mutual visual transference* uses Schaverien's dual model "observer-creator/creator-observer" and expands the transferences to the respondents: the observers create from observing the patient's works, letting these suffuse them and thus trigger their personal creation.

In the creative process in supervision, exactly what Schaverien describes (Schaverien, 1997) takes place, to which the group dimension is added. In other words, dialogue no longer takes place only between the creative patient and himself as an observing creator, nor in the patient-therapist dyad, but is extended to the supervision group, which functions entirely as both creator and observer. At the end of the supervision in the *mutual visual transference* model, the respondents return to the position of "I-observer": in relation to both their individual works, the group and the patient. The "group self" collects, together with the supervisor, these understandings.

Foulkes (1964) emphasized the group's unique advantage as a hall of mirrors. Pines (1984), too, emphasized the importance of the multiplicity of reflections and the deconstruction of the experience of objectivity. In contrast to the experience in individual therapy according to the classical approach of psychoanalysis, where the therapist functions as a mirror perceived as the "truth", the group produces a multitude of mirrors. In so doing, Pines argues, it demonstrates the subjectivity and relativity of the mirror. Foulkes referred to the fabric of communication between the individuals in the group as the "Matrix", and treated it as having a triple meaning: a network of interpersonal communication messages, a common platform, and a uterine environment for nurturing new meanings (Avrahami and Berman, 2017).

In the model proposed in this chapter, personal reactions can be regarded as shards of a broken mirror that re-merge in the concluding assemblage. The group work is, in this sense, a restorative work, which reflects the patient's different self-states – "multiple self".[7] The group can bring a hidden trauma to the surface by presenting it in parts of pictures that appear scattered among the various participants. When the fragments are gathered, a painful picture emerges. The creators are not necessarily aware of the intensity of the harm they express in their works without the group context. In the very same way, even the supervisee who brought the case to the supervision is often unaware of the intensity of the trauma his patient is facing.

In the group supervision process, the participants echo the different parts of the patient's self. They respond to the meeting from a subjective position. The dynamics in which everyone responds allows for movement that shakes them out of fixation. This is a position that evokes a layered perception

[7] According to Bromberg (1999), the analytical encounter strives to attain a more flexible movement between the fragmented self-aspects. He sees the psyche as a latitudinal structure that consists of many self-states, which create an illusion of unity. The capacity to experience the self fully is conditional upon a validating encounter between the patient's consciousness and that of the therapist, in which they react to one another in a vivid and sometimes painful way.

composed of different points of view, which does not characterize ordinary observation, which tends to adhere to one prism. Rational use of the awareness of movement between different self-states expands the therapist's capacity to hear, in an interpersonal context, the echoes of the sounds of his patient's different self-states. A patient who is brought in to the supervision in the proposed model is accompanied and observed by a whole group of therapists, who look at his or her works with sensitivity and reflect hidden layers back to the therapist who accompanies him or her, so that the therapist can expand his perception and understanding in relation to the patient. In the model, the total number of experiences is also extended to those of the responding participants, who connect through their reaction works to the patient, the therapist and the experiences they have accumulated themselves, as therapists and as subjects in the world. Thus, even if the material that arises through the work sometimes seems irrelevant to the case, it is often found that what was seemingly planted in the respondent's inner world is closely related to the patient's experience that pervaded him.

Mutual visual transference: from therapy to supervision and back

In the process of supervision in *mutual visual transference*, a multilayered encounter takes place with the "enlightened" works and with the "shadows" hidden within them. As Bromberg (1999) writes, the purpose of this session is to recognize and expand the range of possibilities, rather than to amend or shatter the illusory space of therapy. The group allows the supervisee to touch the hidden layers that he or she will bring, in thought or action, to the renewed encounter with the patient. Regarding the role of the supervisor in the group supervision, we will quote Ogden: "The supervisor is responsible for creating a frame that ensures the supervisee's freedom to think and dream and be alive to what is occurring both in the analytic process and in the supervisory process... The supervisory frame is a felt presence that affords the supervisee a sense of security..." (2005, p. 1269).

Ferro describes therapy as "... a common emotional field, the vectors of which are made up of cross-cutting projective identifications" (1999, p. 181). Borrowing from this, it can be said that the group respondents' creations are in response to the relationship within the therapeutic dyad, to the intersection of vectors to which they are exposed in the works of the therapist and the patient. The reaction works prompt the supervisee to a re-envision familiar content, and to discover different ways in which the same tools and work materials chosen by the patient can be used. Many times, the supervisor can hear from supervisees that in the post-supervision meeting, the patients talked and created in reference to content and materials with which they had never worked before. Thus, for example, one of the supervisees put it in her post-supervision meeting: "I had a strange feeling that my patient was with us in the room when we talked about her. She created a work very similar to what one of the participants in the supervision has created."

The willingness of the supervisee to get to know her (or his) patient through contact with the materials that have been processed and "digested" among her group members also encourages contact with parts of her own psyche. It can be said that sharing opens up, for all concerned, an opportunity to observe, recognize and create unexpected reactions. The supervision evokes the unconscious dialogue that takes place between the inner worlds of the therapist and the patient. It is a "contact" between one unconscious and another unconscious, which Aron describes as "...ongoing mutual influence in which both patient and analyst systematically affect, and are affected by, each other" (1991, p. 33).

The question "what do you feel" about the works of art calls for direct, exposed and physical responses. The therapist may feel nausea, headache, weakness in the legs, hunger, thirst and so on, without being able to explain at that moment why he experiences these bodily reactions intensely. Rieck writes: "The patient produces in us the bodily sensation he requires so that we can process it toward represented feeling and then thought" (2014, p. 141). Physical responses may be perceived as a "disturbance," something that should be eliminated to stop it from interfering with the therapeutic understanding. We found that holding to and welcoming these feelings effectuate for the therapist a deep and meaningful encounter with the hidden information that the patient has transmitted to the therapist through a bodily message. The mental content assumes physical form and thus seeks to rise to the surface of both the therapist's and patient's consciousness. This is the reason for the great emphasis we place on the supervisee's physical reactions during the supervision session.

Concluding the group supervision session and returning to the patient

During the group session the therapist relinquishes control, "hands over" his patient to the group by means of the works of art he or she has created. The therapist must accept the fact that the other participants in the room now see a face that he himself does not necessarily notice. The artworks brought by the therapist constitute a close and personal "analytical third",[8] now expropriated from the therapist-patient dyad. These are moments when the supervisee should trust the group members to support him, without judging his weaknesses or failures as a therapist, yet without ignoring them.

The supervisee is in an exposed and vulnerable position that can provoke anxiety and evoke other contents typical of group dynamics: competition, envy, anger and so on. The therapist, who usually sits in his room with the patient only, is now exposed to the gaze of the rest of the group and the supervisor. They can see the therapeutic processes, sometimes with a critical eye. What did he see? What did he not notice? What therapeutic interventions did he choose? What difficulties did he encounter and how did he deal with them?

Apart from relinquishing control, it is important to remember that the therapist in supervision also has an important role as part of the group process, and that he possesses first-hand knowledge that no one in the group but himself holds. Aron (1991) reminds us that just as it is important to consider the huge role of the group in supervision, it is also important that the individual is not swallowed by it. This is also the key in returning the "ball" to the hands of the therapist-supervisee in the supervision process.

While creating the reaction in art, one of the students is busy trying to burn pieces of cardboard in order to create a pile of ashes, as a reaction to the patient who was brought in. It costs her a lot of effort. At the end of the first part, when the group bring the works to the center of the room for collective observation, she decides to place a glass of water next to the pile that she has created, and smells of burning. As she places the glass on the floor, the water

[8] Ogden (1994) stresses the possibility to use the analytical third experience in order to gain deeper acquaintance with the patient's emotional experience. He notes that the patient should be attentive to his reverie processes, and to acknowledge them as part of the analytical third. He explains that often, "unrelated" associations that come up for the therapist are assigned to distraction and lead to an effort to focus on the patient. Ogden suggests regarding all the associations, bodily-emotional experiences and feelings experienced by the therapist as a reaction to the encounter with the patient's subjectivity. Nevertheless, it is important to note that using the products of the analytical third requires the therapist to distinguish, sensitively, between instances where his reactions are indeed related with the formation of the analytical third, and those where his reactions stem from his excessive preoccupation with himself.

is spilled on her work. She brings in paper towels and tries, to no avail, to soak up the little puddle as the whole group, to her embarrassment, looks on.

The student who brought the patient to the supervision observes, captivated, all that is happening. When it's his turn to share, he tells the group that what happened now accurately recreates what happened at the school where he treats that child. The week before our supervision session, the patient arrived late at the treatment room and in a cold and distant tone shared with him what had happened: that day he "peed in his pants" and tried to soak up the wetness to no avail, by shoving more and more toilet paper into his pants, in a failed attempt to hide his shame. The therapist shared that in those moments he himself was filled with sadness and pain over what had happened to the child.

When the student was about to throw the paper towels into the bin, he asked her to leave the wet paper as part of her reaction work. He was not sure he was interested in sharing the fresh situation with the class. However, when he witnessed the student's failed attempt to absorb in the very same way the water she spilled, he felt he had to share what he intended to keep inside the treatment room.

What occurred in the supervision was a kind of reconstruction of the missing therapeutic incident. The therapist shared the patient's affectless recounting what had happened before. What took place in the supervision can be seen as "enactment" (Perelberg & Levinson, 2003) – an embodiment in action that was a new path into the unconscious and a means of entering the symbolic processes. The student's unconscious response and her feverish attempt to find a "solution" to the sense of failure that gripped her allowed the therapist to vividly witness what was missing in the patient's description. He could feel with her and through her the shame that the patient could not express in those moments.[9]

For the therapist, what he experienced through the supervision allowed him to organize the feelings of confusion and frustration he faced when he was unable to help his patient at the right time. The "enactment" of the trauma in the supervision created another opportunity for verbalization for both the patient and the therapist.

---

[9] For further details, see the review of the discussion following Ellman and Goodman's lecture (Ellman & Goodman, 2017), which dealt with trauma representation, and the possibility of the act of exchanging words with states in which the ego remains stunned in the face of trauma.

By connecting to the events that occurred, the therapist could help gather the materials that had accumulated during the supervision and give them meaning.

At the end of the supervision, the supervisee can decide which of the materials presented will be used by him later on, and he can also give up suggestions that he deems unsuitable. And in the words of Aron: "it is only by thinking in terms of both autonomy and mutuality, both the individual and the social, both independence and dependence on others that we can best understand creativity" (1996, p. 158). Sometimes, the insights revealed during the supervision can be used by the therapist immediately. At other times, the therapeutic occurrence needs to mature in order to allow for effective intervention in accordance with the suggestions made.

Conclusion

This chapter presents a model for group supervision in art therapy, based on the language of art as a leading language. The model seeks to reinforce trust in the ability of art to expose unconscious content. Mutual transference contents are always present in therapy, however instead of forcing them "through the back door," in the supervision we seek to invite them as our guests, out of respect and attention to what they have to offer us. The use of the language of art is expressed both in the phenomenological examination of the works that are brought to the supervision and in the creation of personal artistic reactions, which are created without prior acquaintance with the patient. It is important to encourage art therapists to believe in their ability to "listen" to the works of art, by connecting with themselves and by identifying and discovering deep emotional processes that guide the creative trajectories of their patients. In Ogden's wonderful words: "it is important that at least occasionally the supervisor and supervisee feel that they have 'time to waste'. Such a state of mind allows for a less structured, more freely associative type of thinking that is akin to the analytic state of reverie. Thinking of this sort often generates fresh perspectives on what the supervisor and analyst felt they 'already knew'" (2005, p. 1278). Symington (1996) believes that curiosity and imagination are essential qualities for psychotherapists in their work, and even mentions in this regard Bion, who wondered in the seminar he gave why we write the main points of our session with the patient after the session, instead of trying to draw a picture of the next session.[10]

Supervisees are exposed to raw content, leading to confusion and uncertainty. In this chapter, we wanted to show that paradoxically, it is precisely these feelings that allow the mutual transference relationship to powerfully surge in a way that can be used in the supervision process. Ogden (1994) suggests taking into account all the associations, physical-emotional experiences and feelings that the therapist experiences in response to an encounter with the patient's subjectivity. In this spirit, the feelings that arise during the supervision are understood as products of the analytical third and therefore – as meaningful for the patient.

The stages in the model are:

1. The group of supervisees meet the patient only through his or her works, while allowing the visual and emotional materials to be absorbed in them by viewing.
2. Participants choose the art materials through which they will "converse" with the works they have seen, without speaking. The reaction works are made as the personal studio work of each respondent, in the company of peers.
3. Phenomenological examination of the reaction works in order to delve deeper into the patient's and respondents' artwork from the artistic and psychic aspect.
4. Striving to refine common elements in the reaction works, before the individual deep examination.
5. Focused observation of selected reaction works.
6. Integration of the artistic expression and the patient's understanding and, hence, thinking about the further development of the treatment.

The various steps in the model are designed to help create order, from the position of staying in the necessary chaos. Following Corry (1997), it can be said that from observation of the various philosophical approaches that developed in ancient Greece, one can discern a recurring assumption in them: behind the chaotic world of phenomena hides order that can be

[10] We wish to thank Dr. Amit Fachler for bringing this source to our attention, part of a seminar that Bion gave in 1978 to the Kleinian group in the British Psychoanalytical Society, and which was never published. Symington (1996) attended the seminar and includes a citation thereof in his book, at the end of the chapter titled "Imagination and Curiosity of Mind".

attained through inquiry. Similarly, the more the discussion of the supervision develops, and the observation deepens, the clearer the picture becomes out of the chaos and a certain hierarchy of the content is created. The work in the room, as part of a large group of respondents, also encourages effects of transference between the participants, in a way that layers the work even more. All the supervisees, and in particular the therapist who brought the patient to the supervision, respond to the same set of works. At the same time, their emotional and physical presence has an effect on others: breaths, creaks, movements and noises of work tools and also "being infected" with mental and physical sensations. This subject is not discussed at length in this chapter, and we believe there is room to continue studying it in the future.

It is important to pay attention to the complex and difficult action required of the respondents: on the one hand, to dedicate to and immerse themselves in the contents that flood them, and on the other hand, to separate the patient's content from their personal content so that they can serve as a sensitive filter of feelings that arise in them vis-à-vis the patient's artworks.

In the chapter we wrote that we believe that observation by a creative therapist sharpens the attentiveness and the sensitivity to nuances. Therapists who continue to create art independently are, in our view, more sensitive to the artworks of their patients, not only from the content aspect, but from the aspect of identifying the way the work was created. It is important that art therapists develop a personal artistic language that will ultimately project to their patients the belief in their ability to create and evolve without words.

References

Aron, L. (1991) "The Patient's Experience of the Analyst's Subjectivity" *Psychoanalytic dialogues*, 1(1), 29-51

Adamson, E. (1984) *Art as Healing*. London: Coventure.

Allen, P. (1992) "Artist-in-Residence: an Alterntive to 'Clinification' for Art Therapists in Art Therapy" *Journal of the American Art Therapy Association,* 9(1).

Aron, L. (1996) *A Meeting of Minds: Mutuality in Psychoanalysis*. Hillsdale, NJ: Analytic Press.

Avrahami, L., Berman, A. (2017) "Tree and Rhizome in Group Therapy Space" *Psychology*. Retrieved Nov., 12 (Hebrew). https://www.hebpsy.net/articles.asp?id=3609

Betensky, M. G. (1995) *What Do You See? Phenomenology of Therapeutic Art Expression*. London: Jessica Kingsley.

Bromberg, P. M. (1999) "Shadow and Substance: a Relational Perspective on Clinical Process (pp. 379-406) in S. A. Mitchell, L. Aron (eds.). *Relational Psychoanalysis: the Emergence of a Tradition*. Hillsdale, NJ: Analytic Press.

Corry, L. (1997) *The Literary World of Jorge Luis Borges*. Tel Aviv: Ministry of Defense Publication.

Dubowski, J. (1985) *Who Took the Art out of Art Therapy?* [Unpublished paper], presented at the international review of the arts in therapy, Goldsmith' College, London.

Eliraz, I, (2012) *Poetry Looking at Painting: Following J. Borkovsky's Paintings*. Tel Aviv: Keshev Leshira (Hebrew).

Ellman, P. L., Goodman, N. R. (2017) "Finding Unconscious Fantasy" (pp. 1-21) in P. L. Ellman, N. R. Goodman (eds.) *Finding Unconscious Fantasy in Narrative, Trauma and Body Pain: A Clinical Guide*. London: Routledge.

Ferro, A. (1999) *The Bi-personal Field: Experiences in Child Analysis*. London: Routledge.

Foulkes, S. H. (1964) *Therapeutic Group Analysis*. New York: International Universities Press.

Goren, N. (August 2015), "Between Bion and Foulkes" (supervision lecture in Lev Hasharon Hospital, Pardessiya) *Israeli Institute of Group Analysis*, http://iiga.org.il/?page_id=1708 (Hebrew).

Heimann, P. (1950) "On Counter-Transference" *International Journal of Psycho-Analysis*, 31, 81-84.

Judd, C. (1986) "Book Reviews" *British Journal of Psychotherapy*, 2(4), 145-151.

Kernberg, O. F. (1975) *Borderline Conditions and Pathological Narcissism*. New York: Aronson.

Kramer, E. (1971). *Art as Therapy with Children*. New York: schocken Books.

Laplanche, J., Pontalis, J.-B. (1974) *The Language of Psycho-Analysis*. New York: Norton.

Milner, M. (1987) *The Suppressed Madness of the Sane Men: Forty-Four Years of Exploring Psychoanalysis*. London: Routledge.

Ogden, T. H. (1994) "The Analytic Third: Working with Intersubjective Clinical Facts" *International Journal of Psycho-Analysis*, 75, 3-19.

Ogden, T. H. (2005) "On Psychoanalytic Supervision" *The International Journal of Psychoanalysis*, 86(5), 1265-1280.

Perelberg, R. J., Levinson, N. A. (2003) "Panel on 'Acting out and/or enactment'" *The International Journal of Psychoanalysis*, 84(1), 151-155.

Pines, M. (1984) "Reflections on Mirroring" *International Review of Psycho-Analysis*, 11, 27-42.

Racker, H. ([1968] 2018) *Transference and Countertransference*. London: Routledge.

Rieck, M. (2014) "The Therapist's Corporeality as a Matrix for Deep Analytic Work" *Sihot – Dialogue: Israel Journal of Psychotherapy, 28*(2), 137-145.

Schaverien, J. (1997) Transference and Transactional Objects in the Treatment of Psychosis (pp. 13-37) in K. Killick, J. Schaverien (eds.). *Art, Psychotherapy and Psychosis*. London: Routledge.

Schur, L. (2013) *The Cultural Context of Art as a Significant Tool in Therapy* [unpublished thesis]. Lesley University.

Schur, Y. (1998) "The Personal Artistic Process of the Art Therapist as a Basis for Supervision" *International Journal of Art Therapy*, 4, 32-36.

Shapira, G. (2014) "Open Studio: A Model of Visual Art Therapy Based on Spontaneous Creation and Acting from an Open and Unguided Therapeutic Position" (pp. 135-158) in R. Berger (ed.). *Creation – the Heart of Therapy: New Theories and Models in Art-Based Therapy, Developed by Israeli Therapists.* Kiryat Bialik: Ach (Hebrew).

Symington, N. (1996) *The Making of a Therapist*. London: Karnac Books.

Turiski, R. (2008) *Studying the Patient: Art Therapy Supervision Model as Basis for the Dialogue woven between the Patient's Artwork and the Art Works of Students Responding to him* [unpublished thesis]. Lesley University.

CHAPTER 10

CO ∞ FIGURATION FIELD IN ART THERAPY SUPERVISION AND TEACHING

REUMA WEINBERG AND RONIT AMIR

In this chapter we examine the different meanings that coexist within the learning and training space of art therapy, a discipline based upon the creation of art. We focus on a state that endorses 'not knowing,' which serves as a catalyser for the experience of seeking acquaintance with the self through artistic practice in therapy, in supervision, and in the training of therapists.

Uncertainty and lack of knowledge are co-present in every creation-engendering process, as well as in each therapeutic encounter. Art therapy patients often find themselves, in a concrete and literal way, vis-à-vis the 'white page' situation; facing a blank page.

At the onset of the creative process, patients sometimes do not know how and, at times are unclear about, where their work will originate and develop from. Neither do they possess the foreknowledge of where they will be led by the dialogue between emotions, thoughts, ideas, mode of expression, materials, colours, composition, and their interrelationship.

Therapists are also subject to the mysteries of not knowing. They have no idea either of what will emerge during work with the patient and the art that will be created. Which issues will arise, be revealed, and gestate, and what they are likely to encounter within the patient and within themselves during the therapeutic process.

During art therapy sessions and while studying this method, similar processes take place, that affect the development and deepening of treatment. They can be the patient-therapist relationship, the connection between guiding supervision and guided tutorial group, in the attention paid to relationships of transference, development and growth, bound up with processes triggered by uncertainty and awareness respectively. All these constantly evolve, not only in the course of studies but also throughout the years of practicing art therapy.

We seek to ask how, during treatment and art therapy studies, one can provide students who are new in the field and veteran therapists with opportunities to seek something unknown, and how to grapple with feelings of anxiety-related ambiguity associated with a shapeless unknown.

In the concept we have coined, co ∞ figuration field, we aimed to illustrate how the intimidating place of not knowing can become a creative and inviting experience. The co ∞ figuration field acts as a processing ground for germinating and growing a raw layer of meaning. It entails the use of concrete and diverse art materials, possessing both unique and real qualities, and during treatment structures a platform on which the soul seeks, experiences, practices, discovers, and embodies the self.

The various forms of expression, as well as the primary and secondary processes of the individual human experience, are manifested and cooperate in creating meaning. In tandem, they enable the weaving of a lasting, vibrant therapeutic fabric, nourished by the bilateral movement of conscious and unconscious psychic matter. In that way, a prolific field is created, which invites both therapist and patient to partake in a process oriented toward the patient's growth and search to figure out himself or herself.

An essential tool for art therapists is the ability to enter a creative space and create with art materials, to observe and experience their patients through the eyes of an artist who bonds with an intuitive experience through their chosen medium; in the course of the therapeutic encounter, they also observe the art work and its creative process. As individuals who have experimented with the materials of art and their relation to the mental content, therapists must be in touch with the feelings and emotions generated and apply them in order to enhance the treatment process. They create with what arises from the encounter and in its wake, and experience a 'talking with one's self'; firstly through art, and only then via observation.

When an art work comes into being as part of a training/supervision group in which all the participants respond to the encounter with the work, the experience of the encounter is powerful in terms of the contact that therapists achieve with the patient and with themselves. It develops the therapist's ability for reverie, and sheds light on countertransference mechanisms, thus enabling a closer knowledge of the patient.

Not knowing, art, and self-acquaintance

The process in which patients and therapist acquire self-awareness amounts to a never-ending journey. The oscillation between knowing and not knowing is ever-present, as well as a wide range of discoveries, embodiment of creation, and self-fashioning which are made possible under the right conditions.

Questions pertaining to what we know, the possibility of being aware, the ways to explore and make acquaintance with the self, form the essence of emotional therapy. In the Socratic dialogue *Meno* (Plato, 1997), Plato unfolds the paradox that Meno sets out before Socrates - the possibility of learning something which was hitherto unknown to us. If we do not know what we are seeking, how can we look for it, and how can we tell when we have found it? Knowledge depends upon the existence of the unknown, but in what way can we seek something we have no clue about?

The question of humanity's self-knowledge, as it emerges from art, culture, philosophy and psychoanalysis (there are countless examples: the story of the Garden of Eden, Oedipus, Plato's *Politeia,* Aristotle's *Ethics* and epistemology at large, as well as Hamlet and Macbeth, and T.S. Eliot's *Four Quartets*), conjures up a complex picture. It presents the contradictory forces operating within the human psyche, and the striving for knowledge that will reveal to individuals their self, and the nature of their existence, knowledge that satisfies the longing to decipher one's own, and others' existential code, as well as other forces intent on maintaining the status quo. The great difficulty in the face of uncertainty co-exists with the fear of learning the truth, and concerns about what could arise out of that knowledge.

As we sought to identify the various meanings that coexist in a therapeutic space that allows one to seek out the acquaintance of the self through artistic creation, we underwent an experience resembling a process in which blurred objects are transformed, and begin to take shape (Ogden, 1989) and to receive a name (Bion, 1962). We wanted to find a concept that could give names to experiences and forms which are partly nonverbal in essence. We became aware both of the challenge posed by this enterprise, as well as our concern that the definitions might actually distance us from the essence of the experience that takes place in the creative act.

Creation in a therapeutic setting, as we aim to present here, includes work conducted throughout the therapy session, and discussing it later during individual or group training and supervision. Creativity's essence is manifested through the language of personal and subjective experience, which is difficult, and sometimes impossible, to translate faithfully into a communicative verbal language. This language is primarily based upon the experience of sensory absorption, the foundation with which we perceive the world. Stemming from that experience is pre-verbal emotional communication that develops through touch, texture, form, voice, vision, and movement.

This type of communication accompanies us throughout our life as a significant sensory experience, comprising a very significant layer of our existential experience. In verbal communication we employ a pool of arbitrary, dictated signs, each of which seeks to be generalized (Noy, 1999: 42) and which might, therefore, distance us from experience. Ultimately, we found an answer to that query in the compound we coined, co ∞ figuration field, which combines a linguistic term with a graphic sign.

Let's take a closer look at the choice of the elements that make up this concept, and the connection and meaning interwoven between them.

We chose the prefix co, whose primary meaning is 'common' or 'mutual.' This choice reflects our belief that individuals need the presence of others who know them and may help them in the process of achieving self-awareness.

Bion ([1962] 1967) emphasizes the experience of knowing entailed in mental pain. He refers to the need of the soul for the nourishment deriving from the support of another soul (mother or therapist) who can help tolerate and organize that experience. It may lead to a transformation in knowledge – K - a link between ourselves and what we know.

The transformation in K occurs during a shared process: the patient projects onto the therapist raw, 'undigested' sensations and nameless, unrepresentable sensory impressions that he cannot fathom, and which he tries not to know or come into contact with due to the pain involved ('beta-elements'). The therapist absorbs the raw sensations of the patient, thinks them through, and returns them, once processed (alpha-function): this is made possible by the emotional knowledge combined with experience and previous knowledge.

Art is inextricably intertwined with the experience of sharing and reciprocity, in that it brings about an encounter between artist, artwork, and viewer: what happens in that encounter is the outcome of the union between them. The same is true for the art therapy process. In the triangle formed between the work, the therapist, and the patient (Schaverien, 2000), a mutual dialogue emerges, nourished by each participant's contribution to forging an experiential and conceptual togetherness on the road to mental growth.

An artwork constitutes an unconscious touch that gives shape to any sensory data involved in it, and infuses meaning through its bond with the creator's self-experience. Observing the artwork, understanding it and discussing it, as well as the process in which it is construed together with the therapist, grants these experiences a meaning that may also be subject to the reality testing of the external world.

These two often coalesce as separate circles of meaning. Accordingly, their interactions, which we represent through the prefix co, enables the launching a dialogue in which each side of the triangle contributes to creating the patient's self-identity from the encounter with his or her different facets. The mirroring that art helps bring into the world is geared here toward a meeting-point of parallel processes between therapist and patient. It exposes them to a broader emotional and cognitive 'colour palette' of self, patient, and what transpires along the therapeutic encounter, and thus affects the therapeutic process.

In the same way that the work of art affects the therapist consciously and subconsciously, the therapist's artwork similarly impacts on the patient's experience and on the contents, which are fashioned through the therapeutic process. The sharing of artmaking is also a means of support and awareness for the therapist in the therapeutic process and enhances the therapist's facet in the therapeutic triangle.

The sign ∞ represents, for us, the power inherent in the relationships between the various components of the concept in order for change to take place in the wake of treatment. The sign 'confiscates' the term from the purely verbal sphere, thus implying the movement which transpires between the pre-verbal loci which emerge as the work of art is created during treatment, and the verbal loci which are phrased out of its contemplation. It indicates the space where the meaning of the inner emotional world is experienced before it is defined.

Out of this potential infinitude, the patient's perceived emotional experience emerges and crystallizes. Bion (1967b) links infinity to the unknowable. The therapy session opens with 'the abyss of the infinite unknown'; the therapist must begin it unhindered by any previous memories, desire, and understanding, and must openly listen to the unknown, absorbing it before it becomes known. It was not coincidental that Bion borrowed from the poet John Keats (Keats, [1817] 1958) the phrase ‘negative capability,’ to reflect the therapist’s capacity to bear the pain, confusion and opacity entailed in not knowing.

Lack of knowledge is inherent to the province of art, as attested by Keats and other artists from various disciplines. When one dares to remain in a state of not knowing, the therapist has a chance to open up and encounter the ultimate reality of the patient (o). The o is not to be found within the precincts of knowledge or learning; it is a state and process of becoming, of genesis (Bion, 1970).

The concept of figuration comprises various dimensions of grammatical and linguistic ‘states of matter’ that are co-present in the creative work. In various dictionaries it features both as a verb or action and as a noun derived from the verb. As a verb, to figure or to figure out, means to solve a problem, to understand or reach an understanding, make sense, to be a part of, but also to give representation through shape or figure and to give an image or metaphor of something (Cambridge Dictionary; Merriam-Webster Dictionary).

Through the art-making activity itself, new and unknown contents are revealed through forms of expression. Lefort (2004) maintains that an artwork is an ongoing, infinite exploration that generates the ability to understand through the act of painting, which summons the visible. On the one hand, the encounter with the artwork enables the exposure of patient and therapist alike to the experience of close and intimate contact with it. Concomitantly, it creates a safe distance through the awareness of art as an ‘external’ object, which enables meaningful observation and the discovery of personal aspects.

By its very nature, an artwork serves as a tool to express that which usually precedes conscious knowledge and, therefore, permits the ‘unthought known’ (Bollas, 1987) to emerge through the actions embodied in the work. It makes possible a process of discovery and shape-giving, which leads in turn to developing self-knowledge grounded on experiencing the here-and-now of therapy. During the creation and crystallization of the artwork, the sheer raw art materials are transformed into psychic raw materials. The embodiment of the psychic materials in a work of art that is tangibly present outside the patient’s inner world, renders it both container and reprojecting object. Both the work of art and the therapist echo the patient’s search for meaning.

The learning which emerges from the creative process, as well as reflections on the work, foster the patient's and the therapist's ability to build a bridge between the experiencing and the observing self. Patients not only express the self through art and thus become acquainted with themselves, through observation they also express discover, organize and decipher their inner code.

It is the broadening, deepening, and internalization of the experience and its conceptualization which allow the patient to bring together and embrace the two types of knowledge: self-knowledge, and knowledge about oneself. Through the shared process of creating and reflecting with the therapist, patients create themselves by discovering new inner experiential dimensions. The same goes for the therapist, in the mental working-through of the continued reverberation of the contents which have germinated in the field extending between her and the patient.

The artwork expresses a dialogue between the two worlds; inner and outer, giving leeway to the different tasks to be performed through that dialogue.

Outwardly, the task requires developing the ability to absorb stimuli from the environment and organize them into an inner picture that faithfully represents reality. Inwardly, the mission entails developing the capacity to organize and embed new experiences into a cohesive sense of self (Noy, 1999). This combination of inner and outer worlds affords an opportunity not only for encounters with unconscious experiences, including their visual and real manifestation. It also enables searching, discovering, and creating meanings throughout the creative and the reflective retrospective process.

The dictionary definitions of field are 'plot of land,' 'yard', and 'area or discipline.' The first meaning refers to an open area where natural vegetation grows. When the land is cultivated, the earth provides the nutrients for growing crops to nourish people. Since we believe that the goal of therapy is to bring about the patient's mental growth, our initial association of the term comes from the field of agriculture. A further overtone comes from the disciplines of mathematics and physics, in which 'field' indicates the forces acting on entities located in the same arena, and the interaction between these forces.

In psychoanalysis, the notion of field refers to the interpersonal analytical space in which a bond is forged between the therapist's subconscious and that of the patient. The imagery and emotions which awaken and the events that occur during treatment stem from that inner field. The actual existence of the artwork as part of art therapy sessions led us also to conceive of field as the 'visual field' to which Merleau-Ponty (2004) refers. He argues that in such a field the ability to see is the ability to exist and be involved in the world. The basic power of vision amounts to its ability to express more than itself. The seer is the visible, and visibility, just as much as physicality is an integral part of its essence.

Merleau-Ponty quotes Cézanne as saying that a life spirit is infused in the painter when he 'thinks in painting' not when he expresses his views, but as soon as his vision becomes gesture. In the visual field, an encounter with the world takes place through sensory perceptions and the meaning people give them. Merleau-Ponty reveals an ancient and primeval intermediate space, 'a concrete, invisible, mysterious field' (Kenaan, 2004, pp. 12-13)

When art is employed in a supervision group, whatever transpires in the field expands the conscious and unconscious connections that are fashioned in the therapeutic triangle. Foulkes (1964) refers to the space formed in the group which allows mental movement between the group's participants. He defines it as a matrix, a network of communication created between group members at the conscious and unconscious level.

The resulting field gives meaning to verbal and nonverbal connections, enabling experiences to be extracted and processed not only through the eyes of the therapist but also from other angles and forms. Phenomena such as resonance and reflection take place in a hall of mirrors.

These phenomena describe the conscious and unconscious influence which the individual exercises on the group and vice versa. The shared examination of the patient's artwork, the artistic feedback of each group member, and the reflection on it, enlarge the inner sense of being from the therapy session which is presented to the group.

This sense of being is simultaneously projected and mirrored, moving back and forth between patient and therapist. A similar movement coexists on a different level, as the contents of the therapeutic field are projected onto the field of the supervising group and mirrored back. The matrix is like an imaginary uterus, nourished by the body of the group and can constitute a holding 'envelope' for the therapist, preparing the conditions to approach the patient's o, and thereby enabling an insight that can contribute to the treatment.

Let us turn now to experiencing the co ∞ figuration field through the attempt to paint which transpired during one therapy session of Reuma with Ronnie (a pseudonym), as well as the therapist's evolving reverie following the encounter with the art therapy supervision group. We will see how glue and pasting – art materials provided in a therapeutic context – metamorphose into psychic materials that reflect the patient's experience of connection and bonding. Then we will show how, in the supervision group, Reuma and the group's members placed particular emphasis on how the choice of cardboard, canvas, and silk paper constitute a different platform for working than Ronnie's flimsy paper base. The choice of these materials raised thoughts concerning the containment necessary for the patient and the ways that mental contents are held and worked through during treatment. Their work process, the artwork itself, and the ensuing feedback, affected the way Reuma considered the meeting with Ronnie and her understanding of patient and therapist's needs, as well as their mode of being present throughout treatment.

A therapy session: seashells, sharks, and glue

Ronnie arrives after his holiday in Australia, at Shell Beach in the Shark Bay area. He shows me pictures and a video filmed at the beach which is composed entirely of shells, and describes it with excitement. His enthusiasm, however, is tinged by a note of sadness, a sense of distress, as he unfolds the relationship with his partner. Again, as in other meetings, he describes the uncertainty that he senses about their relationship. He craves to feel loved; she is distant and unable to show love. He feels that "it's impossible to form a partnership with her; she is simply egocentric," he declares. Right away, as he utters these words, he starts to create an artwork.

Asked which materials he needs in order to execute the artwork; he pauses for a moment: "I have no idea; I don't know. Show me." "I don't know either yet; what if we wander through the room together and look at the art materials?" I suggest. He nods affirmatively, and roams around, inspecting, and then splits away for a moment. He allows himself to linger and observe, then chooses materials from one area of the room, while I bring miscellaneous materials from the warehouse. The seashells I found there had caught my attention, recalling the beaches he had just returned from. I place them among the other collected items.

As I look at the objects on the table, I'm surprised to find out that among the materials he chose for work were the 'worry dolls' which I had brought back from Guatemala. They are not used in clinics as creative materials, but as a means of projective working-through. I feel uneasy about the way he might use them. Think to myself that maybe I should give them up for his sake, let him create with them and feel guilty for not having guided him properly, and made clearer which materials are available. I feel it's hard for me to simply say: 'They are not meant for artmaking.' Almost in the same breath, I am overcome by a sense of ownership and a desire to keep them solely for myself. I am angry at him for having put me in such situation. I wonder which actual reaction of mine might be appropriate for him right now. Just intensely feel this gap wedged between us. Feel that its origin lies elsewhere, beyond the immediate concrete situation.

I tell him: "These aren't creative materials; they are worry dolls." "Oh, sorry, I didn't know," he replies. I feel that a cloud of embarrassment shadows his face, and that the space in the room has become less safe. The border has been pushed out, the territory has been marked as mine, and I become the landlady who has the power to grant or withdraw, while he is totally subject to my will. I feel that protecting my space has rendered me distant, cold and arbitrary. A sense of insecurity suffuses the room.

His face softens as he sees the shells I brought him. He asks for hot glue and at once selects two shells and fixes them, squeezing a generous amount of glue onto the middle of the paper he has chosen as the base. Only after completing that action, he touches the rest of the shells, sensing their texture and character, chooses some more, and scatters them on the base. For a moment, he scatters them randomly, and then meticulously shifts their location in relation to the two first shells he glued. He moves, fits, examines and then, in a gesture of consent, sprinkles a tiny drop of hot adhesive on them and glues them in place.

Observing the delicacy with which he glues them, my feeling changes. The distance I sensed before begins to fade. I feel with him more and more, watching, fascinated by his creative process, wide-awake and slightly disturbed by the feeling of something permanent, very powerful that suddenly shifts into a transient state. I'm beginning to sense that there's a connection to what transpired between us about the worry dolls, but still cannot quite put it together and phrase it in words. The way he's attaching these shells is very different from his tight cementing of the first two. I'm not sure which of the shells he placed on the base were glued and which ones were merely scattered there. As he continues to affix them, my tension increases as he looks for the shells that are not yet attached to the paper base. The hot glue leaves burns on his fingers, but he ignores them and keeps working.

I am amazed that he remembers precisely which of the shells placed on the base are affixed and which ones are not yet glued. I feel as if we were playing a memory game. As he tries to locate shells, he finds suitable for attaching to the paper base, I sense that even though he is working and I'm observing, I am completely with him in my mind, comprehending the memory of the gluing experience; wondering where the connections to the surface are located, and where the shells are unattached. I am immersed in a sort of suspense story: on the one hand, the shape is developing, but, on the other, it's not entirely clear how it will continue growing, what's really going to happen beyond the first two shells that were laid in place and glued so quickly and meticulously.

In tandem, I keep wondering about the connection between us and what is happening now, at the session, in light of his work. I think about the sense of insecurity which permeated the room previously, and the closeness that prevails right now. My thoughts returned associatively to a memory-game I recalled, a game in which one must find a partner, the other. I feel that the initial action of affixing the shells vis-à-vis the detection, pasting, and searching operation contains a wealth of memories, emotional attachments and imprinting, as well as a novel exploration of what is suitable to be attached to what, and when to do so.

The experience of bonding and the relationship taking form on the paper becomes so real that, for an instant, the sound of the waves and shells on that Australian beach seems perceptible in the room. At that moment, a question arises about the relationship with sharks. I wonder whether there is a significance to Ronnie's choice of that particular beach. Is there a sense of unconscious danger lurking beneath the magnificent seashore?

Ronnie decides to stop. Leans towards the work, feeling it all at close quarters, then moving away from it a little as he declares "Not f i n i s h e d yet." Rising from his chair, he lifts up the work and leans it against the wall. I stand next to him. From that angle, the work looks different; it stands there like another entity. With an astonished expression, he exclaims: "Wow, there are seashell couples here! I didn't even notice I was gluing them like that."

A tense silence fills the room. Then Ronnie starts describing his surprise upon discovering the clustering of the shells, and that, unwittingly, the artwork seems to refer to his relationship. I bring to his attention the choice of hot glue and the way he used it. His work now breathes life into his description of the connection and bonding with his partner, that he brought up at the start of our session. How he immediately felt committed to the relationship, despite sensing her unequal commitment to him. His realization that she was unwilling to devote herself to him, accompanied by a sense that she is not generous towards him.

I check if he expected something similar from me as well when he brought the worry dolls. He nods, confessing that he assumed that what was in the room was being offered to him, and then found out that it wasn't quite so. "Maybe it would be better if I checked," he muses aloud.

He shares the insight that reflecting on the work process has led him to reassess his relationship with his mother. He perceived her great devotion to him as warm, that it "had done him a world of good." The artwork made it clear that he nurses expectations from the 'other' which do not withstand the test of reality. That realization is permeated by feelings of frustration, disappointment, grief, and the fear of pain associated with severance.

Ronnie discovers that the longing to cement the relationship was too impulsive, too quick, too 'glued' and automatic. It left him no freedom to create a gradual process of becoming acquainted, testing and adapting to his needs. The two of us return to his choice of hot glue, and in the process, we attain a further insight into the significance of selecting this material, beyond its potential for rapid adhesion. We realize that his choice of fast and scalding glue is bound up with the scorching cost of burns and pain and yet he keeps using it, without flinching or stopping to explore other options.

At this point, both Ronnie and I feel that an opportunity had opened up to explore and understand further the relationship between an immediate solution and pain. He seems to have grasped something new about himself.

Supervision group meeting: cardboard, canvas, silk paper, glue, watercolour and acrylic paint

We set up an art supervision group that gathered to try and unravel the enigmatic encounter between Ronnie and myself, to generate resonance for the story of the therapy session and the artwork created there. Everyone in the group responded through her artwork and reflections on the encounter.

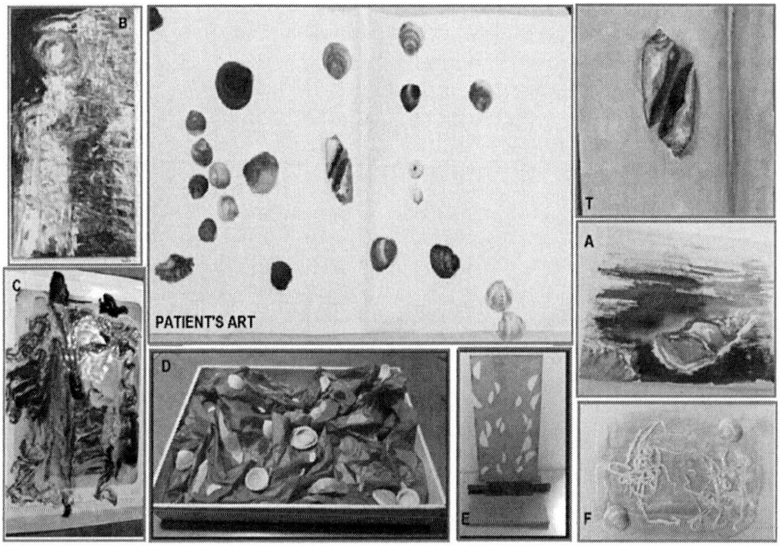

The artworks that the group members created were composed of different art materials:

Reuma (T): used different types of paints: acrylic markers, pencils and pastels on cardboard (20/21cm).

Ne'ama (A): watercolour on paper (12/10 cm).

Einav (F): hot glue drawing on water, sand and sea shells on cardboard (25/35 cm).

Nili (E): three-dimensional illustration of a small pinball machine, a painting of flying heads of garlic on a base of Bristol paper sheet, with watercolours, clothespins, a base of coloured paper and cardboard (30/21/16 cm).

Sara (D): cardboard box, burgundy-coloured tissue paper laid out in such a way as to create dents, wrinkles and protrusions, pieces of torn paper and sea shells laid out in various shapes (27/19 cm).

Hadar (C): coloured Panda pencils, glue, and nail polish on aluminium foil (40/60 cm).

Shani (B): acrylic paint and pencils on canvas (40/25 cm).

I felt as though I were part of a field that continued to exist even after the supervision session ended. I was within it, and felt how myself and the others continued to be attracted by it. How the meanings deepen, grow and emerge through the art encounter. Following the session, for example, Einav sent me a poem by T. Carmi titled Attention

> It's hard for two seashells to have a real conversation.
> Each listens to its own sea.
> Only the pearl diver or antiquities dealer
> Can determine without fear: 'It's the same sea.'

I was excited to realize the extent to which the poem echoed my response through art to the session with Ronnie. I focused on the two main shells that he glued immediately. I chose them because of the tensile shape created between them, they looked like two mouths facing each other. During the work, I felt a strong need to plunge deeply into each shell, to try and unravel the secret of its being.

The attention I gave each one of them made me sense the dissonance wedged between the desire to talk, and the longing to listen to that inner sea. I identified with the pearl diver and the antiquities dealer, but unlike those professional figures of knowledge in the poem, mine was accompanied by a fear of not knowing. That concern always arises from understanding the mental complexity manifested in therapy in general, and in Ronnie's difficulties experienced at that particular time, which surfaced during his therapeutic process.

The poem also echoes the sense of loneliness that arose in the encounter with Ronnie. Shani confessed that in her renewed observation of the work she executed in response to Ronnie's, she realized that she had avoided relating to the emptiness, scarcity, helplessness, and loneliness she'd felt as she gazed at Ronnie's work. Her words and those of Carmi's poem led me to think that his loneliness had indeed not won the place it deserved, that I did not accompany him in this predicament.

My sense of emptiness was exacerbated by the fact that everyone in the supervision group addressed the question of the basis that Ronnie chose for his artwork, which we all thought too flimsy, lacking strength and stability. It was interesting to realize that everyone in the group chose for their response work a more stable and containing base, like cardboard, canvas, or a tray.

Concomitantly, the sense of constriction significantly increased. Both Nili and Shani said they could not take time to linger over their artistic response, because of the feeling of constriction and lack of space that emerged from their work. Hadar told us that she had breathing difficulties as she finished the work, because the air in the room was impregnated with the adhesives she had chosen for her work, which gave off a quite unbearable odour.

Sara shared the insight that the concave inner surface of the seashell always remained untouched, thus creating a gap, a blank space. She compared the shell to the human body, to a soft stomach that remained neglected vis-à-vis an empty space. Her analogy helped me connect with the emptiness that Ronnie must have sensed.

The dissonance that arose between the emptiness and the density made me realize that the construction is an attempt to automatically fill the emptiness that ultimately left Ronnie with a sense of emptiness and loneliness. It created a sense of stickiness, which does not allow the breathing space indispensable for a reciprocal relationship. This feeling was also transmitted to me through the way we behaved during the therapy session itself, and it became more acute in the supervision group.

Einav established a dialogue with the glue in Ronnie's work: "I wanted lots of that glue, but I wanted it to be in motion, sometimes connecting, sometimes gently moving away." In her artwork, glue became a means of adhesion to design a space where there is movement between two shells.

In my encounter with the work of the group members, I began to discover another layer of relationship between the nature of Ronnie's attachment to his loneliness and aggressiveness, and the connection between the two. In art, this is reflected in the work of Ne'ama, Shani, and mine. None of us used glue at all; we formed an organic connection between the base and the painting, selecting colours that could be absorbed into the base and which, in turn, it could contain. Encouragingly, we realized that a connection can be formed other than by using rapid and scorching glue.

During the therapy session with Ronnie, the issue of his relationship with his mother came up, as well as its effect on his expectations from his partner. Throughout the meeting, I thought that their relationship had not altered over time, and that Ronnie's arrival at manhood had not affected the nature of his relationship with his mother. Her endless devotion to him was attuned to the early stages of his development: he remained her little boy.

I thought that perhaps the weight of the shells represented his growth. At the end of the session, I picked up the paper. I saw that it was too weak and could not hold the shells without support and I felt that he himself needed holding. There was no match between the base and what he had placed on it. When the work was transferred, a fold was created on the sheet; it engaged my thoughts, and I expressed that in my art response, but was unable to fathom its significance.

In her work, Sara created a platform on which the shells were placed in many different shapes; some slightly hidden, some revealing the concave part, and some liable to slip off. They are located in the folds of soft and flexible burgundy silk paper that leans on a sturdy cardboard bed. The silk paper made dents and protrusions in a way that invited different modes of meeting between the shells and the base. Sara's work let me regard the folds in another way, not only in the mode that I had experienced the base as both tight and foldable, but as a possibility for a multidimensional base, consisting of both soft and hard, container and holder.

As long as the paper was placed on the table, it was impossible to tell how relatively thin it was as a container for the shells. When I picked it up, Ronnie had already left the room. This raised more thoughts about his entrusting me with the responsibility for keeping his work safe, for his seashell work to remain whole.

Afterwards I wondered about the matrix that Ronnie needed from me in therapy at that moment, and the materials which would help him to create, express, and hold the sense of loneliness and aggression that came up in the encounter which could provide him with a more organic connection between background and figure, between container and contained (Ogden, 2004).

Training/Supervision model

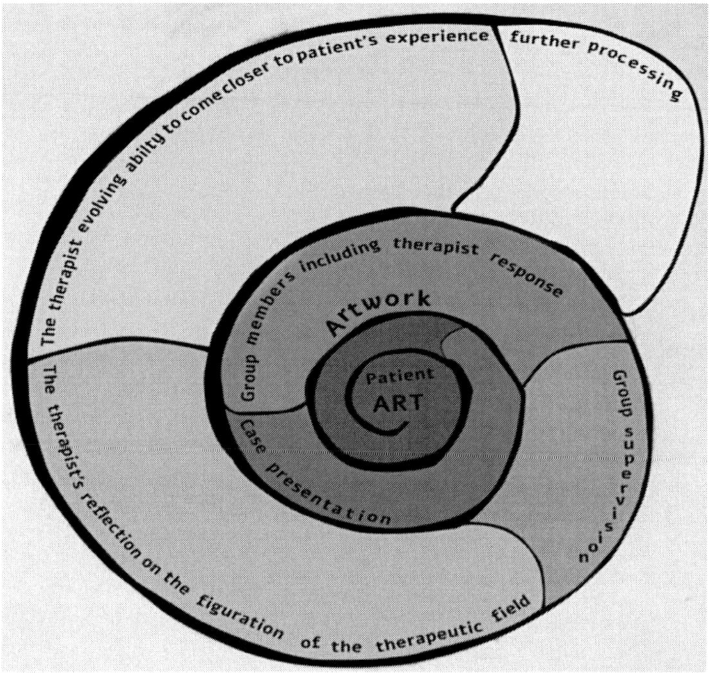

Fig. 2

The model employed is based on art created within the framework of a supervision and training group itself, as a tool permitting a multidimensional space for learning, reflection, and processing of the contents that came up, in tandem with the artwork created during the therapeutic process, which was presented in the supervision. It is a kind of spiral that originated in the co-figuration field between therapist and patient, and continued in the co ∞ figuration of the training field.

In the first stage, the therapist presents the group with the patient's case description and artwork (patient art and case presentation). In the next stage, each member of the group including the therapist, responds by making art related to the case study and the artwork presented (artwork response).

Upon completion of the artwork, a group discussion is held (group supervision), in which each member of the group presents his or her artwork and the meanings emerging from it while making the work, in a way likely to bring the therapist closer to the patient's experience.

In the following stages, the therapist shares his/her thoughts on the therapeutic field, drawing on the contents raised in the supervision group, and the implicit connection to the patient presented at the training session. Room for expression is allotted to this stage through further processing in the next session of the supervision group; this enables the therapist to bring additional thoughts, dreams, the patient's holding of his or her soul, and how the guidance has impacted on the therapy.

From not knowing to co ∞ figuration field

Through the description of the therapy session with Ronnie and the ensuing supervision, we aimed to convey the different dimensions of the co∞ figuration field, which originates from an intuitive art work. In the creative process that Ronnie already underwent in his choice of art materials, psychic contents emerged from his inner world. Via the artwork, its fashioning, the experiences that accompanied the various modes of adhesion of the seashells and the ways of using hot glue, he gave expression and form to his world.

Once he had finished the work, and contemplated it together with Reuma, he noticed the pairs of shells scattered on the page. The work of art which had previously been part of him, became an external independent object – an object which has a say, an object that allows self-mirroring communication and enables new insight.

His shared reflection with the therapist on the newly created artwork and on the fresh symbols that arose from it (through the tangible working process) allowing a view of the self as part of something else. It opened up a space for both a novel awareness, and the sense that there is something inside which knows the patient better than he himself does (Marion Milner, 1987).

In view of the tangible manifestation of shape signification and primary relationship patterns, Reuma also sensed his difficulties in establishing close contact and a relationship that would develop naturally. She witnessed the scorching burns from the hot glue and also the way he ignored them. As she looked at the artworks created by the group members in the supervision session, and responded to the session with Ronnie and his artwork, she discovered her own difficulty in encountering his loneliness.

The return to the artwork after the meeting with Ronnie and the sense of emptiness that emerged from the work hit her close to home. She felt that he was lonely even during the meeting. Suddenly, she realized that perhaps the same speed with which the first shells were glued was mirrored in the hastiness of their insights. Perhaps it might have been better to linger with his loneliness, making room for it.

It was a moment when the therapist experienced the difficulty of meeting the emotion concealed beneath the surface. It was a moment of surprise, fraught with sadness and pain, but also with the joyous realization that the encounter with such feelings created something new, an insight shared by Ronnie and herself.

Landau (2009) refers to Bion and Meltzer's remarks when he mentions that mental development is a never-ending process of discovery. Suddenness and surprise accompany the revelations. The realization process creates something novel, and is accompanied by an experience of inner expansion.

Supervision through artmaking affords a promising space for growth and for enhancing professional abilities, skills, and conceptualizations essential for developing clinical abilities both for professional art therapists, as well as for art therapy students. Such a training and learning process lets the therapist access additional meanings and perspectives on the therapy session which they present to the supervision or training group. The group's members enjoy the benefits of learning processes through the use of art as a meaningful supporting tool for live treatment, the very same tool offered to the patients, alongside its rewards and disadvantages.

The model we suggest lets the supervision group grapple with the dynamics of transference, counter-transference, and aesthetic counter-transference in a supportive environment that affords the time and space indispensable for a dialogue between primary and secondary languages, for an encounter with the outer world as also for tunnelling into the self, the patient's sensations, and emotional experiences.

Ongoing group instruction according to this model allows trainees or students to develop an awareness of their response patterns and the meanings they attach to different therapeutic situations. The feedback that group members give each participant in the training session, in which they present a case study for supervision, is likely not only to shed light on the case-study they present, but also to introduce them to the multiplicity of response modes, and the different interpretations which other therapists suggest.

This training/supervision method fosters the possibility of achieving a more conscious and broader personal awareness of the therapist's self-state as a professional, as well as a realization of his or her unconscious self-activated states. That awareness may thus broaden the therapist's world in highly significant ways.

References

Bion, W. (1962) *Learning from Experience*. London: William Heinemann.

—. (1967) "Notes on Memory and Desire" *Psycho-analytic Forum*, II(3), 271-280.

—. (1967) *Second Thoughts*. London: William Heinemann.

—. (1970) *Attention and Interpretation*. New York: Basic Books.

Bollas, C. (1987) *The Shadow of the Object: Psychoanalysis of The Unthought Known*. London: Free Association Books.

—. (2011) *The Christopher Bollas Reader*. London: Routledge.

Ferro, A. (1999) *The Bi-Personal Field: Experiences in Child Analysis*. London: The New Library of Psychoanalysis.

Foulkes, S. (1964) *Therapeutic Group Analysis*. London: Karnac.

Keats, J. (1958) *The Letters of John Keats*. H. E. Rollins. Cambridge, MA: Harvard University Press.

Kenaan, H. (2004) "What Lies between Eye and Mind?" in Merleau-Ponty M. *Eye and Mind*. E. Dorfman (trans.) Tel Aviv: Resling (Hebrew).

Landau, M. (2009) "Thoughts, Meaning and Anti Meaning" Retrieved October 10, 2019 (Hebrew). https://www.hebpsy.net/articles.asp?id=2358

Lefort, C. (2004) "Introduction" in Merleau-Ponty M. *Eye and Mind*. E. Dorfman (trans.). Tel Aviv: Resling (Hebrew).

Merleau-Ponty, M. (2004) *Eye and the Mind*. E. Dorfman (trans.). Tel Aviv: Resling (Hebrew).

Levy, I. (2006) "A Voice of her Own: Marion Milner and the Independent School" in *The Suppressed Madness of Sane Men: Forty-Four Years of Exploring Psychoanalysis*. D. Ruppin (trans.). Tel Aviv: Tola'at Sfarim (Hebrew).

Noy, P. (1997) "The Normal Processes for Maintenance of a Sense of Self: Art" Extended version of the Professor Ruth Yaffe Memorial Lecture. *The Psychoanalyses of Art*. Shalvata Hospital (Hebrew).

—. (1999) *The Psychoanalysis of Art and Creativity*. Tel Aviv: Modan (Hebrew).

Ogden, T. (1989) *The Primitive Edge of Experience*. New Jersey: Jason Aronson.

—. (2004) "On Holding and Containing, Being and Dreaming" *The International Journal of Psychoanalysis*, 85(6), 1349-64.

Plato, (1977) "Menon" in *Plato, from the Collected Works Vol. 1*. J. Liebes (trans.). Tel Aviv: Schocken.

Schaverien, J. (2000) "The Triangular Relationship and The Aesthetic Countertransference in Analytical Art Psychotherapy" (pp. 55-83), *The Changing Shape of Art Therapy: New Developments in Theory and Practice*. Gilroy, A., McNeilly G. (eds.). London: Jessica Kingsley.

—. (1992) *The Revealing Image Analytical Art Psychotherapy in Theory and Practice*. London: Tavistock/Routledge.

CHAPTER 11

EXPERIENTIAL TEACHING OF AN ART-BASED PARENTAL TRAINING COURSE: PRINCIPLES AND OUTCOMES

LIAT SHAMRI-ZEEVI AND ANAT GILAD

Introduction

Recently, there has been increasing acknowledgment of the need to develop art-based parental training courses (ABPT; Shamri-Zeevi, Regev & Guttmann, 2018), in response to issues in the clinical settings and challenges students face in their interactions with their clients' parents.

For many years, parental training was perceived as an "extension" of emotional therapy for children, and received scant attention in the clinical field or in training programs. Entry-level therapist-students often state that they lack the first-hand experience and the skills to conduct parental training although it constitutes an integral part of therapy for children. Students often feel scrutinized when they are required to discuss a child's progress in therapy with the child's parents. In addition, in cases where students identify with the child-client in parental training, they struggle to form a therapeutic alliance with the parents and understand their difficulties from a containing and empathetic stance.

To respond to these needs, this chapter describes an innovative ABPT course that was developed at The Academic College of Society and the Arts. The course is designed to integrate a theoretical-psychotherapeutic body of knowledge that students can use and build upon, which also provides hands-on experience in art-based interventions that can be applied in parental training. Our experience shows that the combination of the theoretical and the practical helps expand students' therapeutic repertoire and allows them to make use of the techniques they learn in the course when working with parents in the clinic, thus leading to a better, deeper relationship with parents, and therefore with the child.

Art-based parental training

Parental training is a broad field which is now considered to include many different components of the therapeutic intervention. It focuses on difficulties in the parent-child relationship, and aims to associate the parents' inner world, their parenting experiences and goals with their behavior in the encounter with their child's inner world and behavior.

Art-based parental training (ABPT) is a form of training that uses creative processes and the observation of artwork as part of the parental training process (Deaver & Shiflett, 2011). Art therapy refers to the creative processes and the artistic product as a text that contains in itself the story that the client tells, as well as the transference relationship between therapist and client (Schaverien, 1999; Steinhardt, 2017). The prime theoretical notion underpinning art therapy is that the creative process inherently has a therapeutic effect on the creator (Pratt, 2006). In the last twenty years, a broad theoretical and research foundation has been established based on the therapeutic potential of art therapy (e.g. Cohen-Yatziv & Regev, 2019; Maujean, Pepping & Kendall, 2014) which rests on the idea that artistic expression does not only concern the end product, but that the process of creation and the end product together can promote significant mental processes.

There are several advantages to including artistic interventions in clinical interventions in parental training. The first is that art, as a projective tool, allows the art maker to reveal suppressed feelings and other unconscious content in a less controlled manner (Schaverien, 2008; Snir & Hazut, 2012). This may foster the emergence and exposure of emotional content the parent may struggle to articulate. Art can bypass verbal narratives and allow for internal observation and the emergence of different experiences, thus connecting the parents to their past experiences and their children through the play-experiential dimension of the creative process (Shamri-Zeevi, Regev & Snir, 2019). The artistic activity can hence lead to a better understanding of the therapeutic process their child is undergoing.

Learning modes – experiential learning

Art Therapy training programs aim to develop and implement experiential learning. Studies in recent years (e.g., Brownell & Swaner, 2010; Heinrich

& Green, 2020; Kuh, 2008) have shown that different formats of Experiential Learning (EL) in higher education programs provide good quality, meaningful learning outcomes. Rainey and Kolb (1995) developed a model of experiential learning consisting of several components that can be implemented in varying order depending on the context and setting in which learning takes place. In this model, the learning cycle includes *active experience*, which then moves to *abstract conceptualizations* and to *the generalization of the principles* beyond the specific context in which the encounter was experienced. Progress in learning and in conceptualization generate *reflective observation* or critical observation of this knowledge and the process by which the changes in understanding occurred. This culminates in the learner's ability to *apply* this knowledge while experiencing and processing the content in new situations. The assumption is that meaningful learning is primarily directed by the students' tangible experiences in the program. Learning grounded in experience is thought to be more fully embodied by the learner in this process, creating the possibility for cognitive, but also emotional and affective gains (Rivera & Heinrich, 2016).

Rainey and Kolb's (1995) notions of experiential learning are consistent with Winnicott's (1971) ideas on the critical role of creativity in the human psyche and its developmental processes. Winnicott emphasized the importance of the ways in which individuals glean insights from the internal processes that take place in the therapy room, rather than from their responses to the therapist's interpretations (regardless of the therapist's insights). In this way, understanding is accompanied by a creative exploratory experience and joy. Similarly, in experiential learning in the ABPT course, students "create" their insights from their experiential encounters in class and as a result acquire theoretical knowhow. The theoretical material studied in class in an experiential-creative manner becomes associated with the students' prior knowledge and consolidated into a deep and meaningful knowledge base. This forms an integrative learning experience in which the students are active participants in the "creation" of the new material that they have assimilated in a creative way.

The learning process in the course (as depicted in the flowchart) progresses in parallel axes and includes experiential and theoretical learning. The theoretical learning axis reflects *theoretical conceptualizations* of emotional content that focus on the parent-child relationship and the art therapist-child-parent relationship. This type of learning is consistent with the components of the *active experience of experiential artwork* on the *experiential learning* axis.

Table 1: Flowchart of the learning process in the art-based parental training course

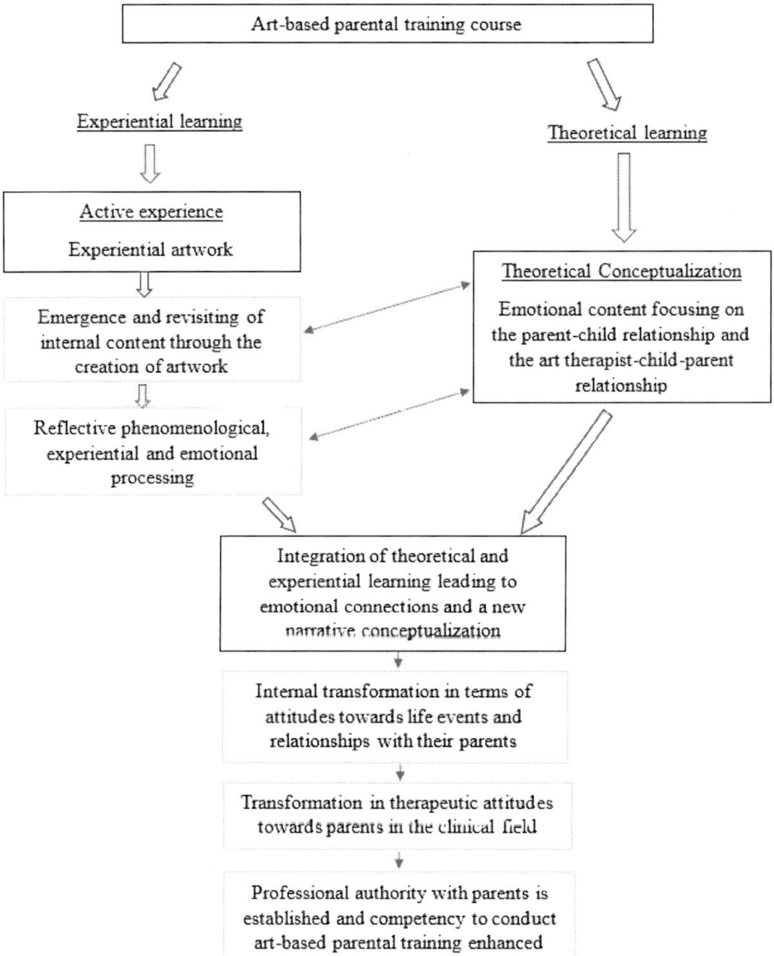

This leads to the emergence and revisiting of internal content through the creation of artwork and reflective processing at different phenomenological, experiential and emotional levels. The combination of the two axes leads to the *integration* of theoretical and experiential learning, which produces *experiential* and *personal-emotional processing*, which in turn leads to *emotional connections* and a *new narrative conceptualization*. Students undergo an *internal transformation* in terms of their attitudes towards life events and relationships with their parents. There is a *transformation in the students' therapeutic attitudes* towards parents in clinical practice, where the student-therapists' *professional authority with parents is more firmly established* and their competency to conduct ABPT is thus enhanced.

Main content of the ABPT course

The course is divided into six main sections:

The personal component: This section deals with the students' own childhoods in terms of their internalized and real parents, the children they were, their imaginary children, and their actual children (if any).

The transition to parenthood: The developmental stages in adult life where individuals become a parent, the projections, fantasies and the meaning of this transition in their lives.

Being a parent: The parental experience at the beginning of the development of the parent-infant relationship.

Ghosts from the past: The many ways that life, with its low points (deprivation, loss, divorce, war, transitions and immigration, economic crises, etc.) and high points permeate parents' mental states and constitute a critical component of their lives that influences their parenthood and their expectations and needs that are directed towards their child. These psychological factors are often projected onto children and are embedded in their psyche and self.

Breaking the cycles: The ways in which an opportunity is created to break vicious pathological cycles and transform the parenting experience into an opportunity for rectification and modification for both the parent and child.

Therapeutic perspectives: The different methods of training and dealing with parents and parenthood from a variety of theoretical-clinical perspectives.

The course is made up of 14 four-hour sessions. Each section is taught on the theoretical and experiential levels. The theoretical part involves presentations, academic material and the analysis of clinical cases. The experiential part involves art making (typically using structured interventions that students can implement during ABPT in the clinical field) and viewing films, as well as processing individual and group reflective artworks.

Examples of the interventions and their purposes as a function of the course topics are presented in the table below.

Table 2: Brief outline of art-based sessions and interventions in the course

No.	Main topic of the session	Art-based intervention	Art materials	Purpose
1	My parents and myself during my childhood	Make a drawing of the child you were (at a significant age when you can remember yourself). Make a drawing of your parents in the same situation.	Open buffet of art materials	Developing the students' ability to reflect and observe themselves as children in order to spark an emotional connection to the course topic.
2	Parent-child relationship (mother-child, father-child)	Make two sculptures representing your early relationship with your parents (choose ages 0-5), the first mother-child; the second father-child.	Cardboard, Clay	An observation and separation of the different relationships that can exist in the child-mother/ child-father relationships.
3	Becoming familiar with the students' nuclear families	Make a family drawing that includes figures, animals, plants or other objects.	Oil pastels	An observation of preliminary information in terms of how students perceive the family unit.
4	Ghosts in the nursery – An exploration of the students' own families	Make a chart of your own family by drawing circles, where each circle represents a family member (by color and size). Students are asked to	Cardboard circles of different sizes and colors, markers, oil pastels	Identifying and observing behavioral patterns, thoughts, beliefs and values from the students' own families.

No.	Main topic of the session	Art-based intervention	Art materials	Purpose
		place the circles on the page according to their different relationships and write down a prominent feature related to each family member.		
5	Breaking the cycle - describing, expanding and understanding the difficulties and patterns in the relationships which parents need to cope with in their daily interactions with their children.	Our home – each student creates his/her home and invites us in. What will we see and whom will we meet?	Open buffet of art materials	An expansion and understanding of different patterns, thoughts and ways of coping (both successful and unsuccessful) in the students' relationships with their parents.
6	Summary and integration session - the child I once was and what I can give that child today.	In relation to the first intervention, students are asked to make their inner parent (existing within them) who, after undergoing a process in the course, is able to give the internalized child the same deep needs which served as the basis for the artwork in the first session.	Open buffet of art materials	Observing the changes and progress that took place during the course.

An example of the first intervention in the course and the emotional process that followed can be seen in Michal's reflection. In the first lesson, Michal (pseudonym), a 35-year-old mother of three children and a third-year Art Therapy student, was asked to draw the image of the girl she once was, and then an image of the mother of that girl. Michal described her experience as follows:

I created an image of myself at the age of three standing in the sandbox in nursery school, looking up at my mother who was on the third floor. My hands were outstretched towards her and expressed a longing for her to come and take me away. My mother, who suffered from postpartum depression as of my birth, stands with her face behind the half-closed window with the shutter down, and does not acknowledge my pleas. As a result of the work in the course and the perspective of observing the two artworks from above (I placed my image on the floor and hung my mother's image on a chair. For the first time in my life, I was able to look at my mother with compassion and acceptance, and notice *her* helplessness. As I recalled this incident from the past, it stirred up a great deal of anger inside of me, since I continued to view it through the eyes of that little girl, whose desire for her mother's maternal gaze and responsiveness remained unrequited. The course was the first time in my life that I was able *to be* and view the scene from an external point of view, to observe the image of the girl I was and the image of my mother who had been depressed since my birth, and *hold the two perspectives and conflicting emotions that they aroused in me.* This also had implications for my parental training in the clinic, where my therapeutic capacity underwent a transformation and I was able to feel compassion for parents who struggle to have feelings of love for their children, and work with them with empathic acceptance of their difficulties. The ability to work with art materials refined my childhood experience for me and allowed me to understand its bias, which at times had remained a stumbling block in my life until adulthood (Image 1).

Michal's description emphasizes the strong transference that took place during the course, and the mental fusion that occurred later between her memory of the event and her experience of it, which changed her perspective on this traumatic childhood event. After this experience, the nature of her work with parents changed, as well as her relationship with her own parents.

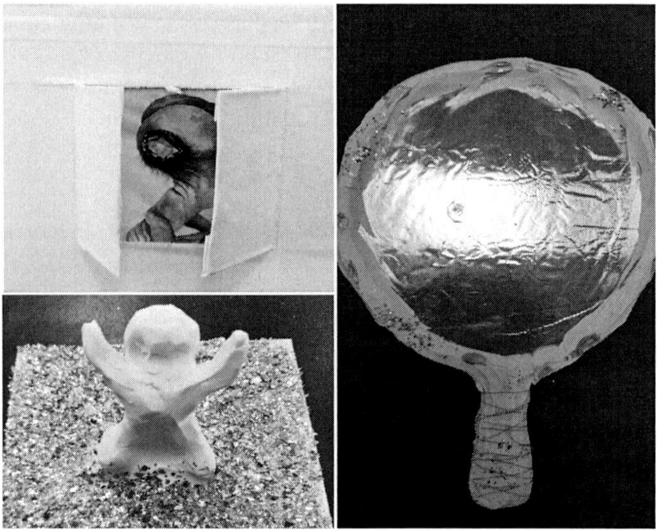

Image 1 – Michal and Mother - In the first session of the course mother behind the half-closed window (Watercolor paints on cardboard), Michal calls for her mother (plasticine).

In the last session Michal's mirror (plasticine on cardboard).

Parents' experiences occasionally require adjustments and adaptations from both the parents and the therapist (Shamri-Zeevi, Regev & Snir, 2015; Shamri-Zeevi & Regev, 2020). Understanding the parents' experiences in therapy is crucial to making these adjustments in the best possible way. The same principles can be applied to art-based parental training teaching. Our clinical program incorporates creativity into the learning process in an effort to train therapists who will make the therapeutic engagement into a creative encounter on the part of both therapist and client. The use of art and reflection helps students see the situation from multiple perspectives, some of which cannot be perceived without the use of art. This form of learning allows for the expression of the students' unconscious content that comes to the surface through creation in art and its processing, and in dialogue with their colleagues and the lecturer. For example, Noa (pseudonym), aged 28 and married without children, is in her third year of the program and shared her story:

At the beginning of my internship, I felt very judgmental of the clients' parents, particularly regarding their blind spots in terms of their relationships with their children. For example, a client who suffered from emotional dysregulation whose father was also not regulated only saw the problem in his child without being aware of his own issues and the effects of his emotional state and behavior on his son. I became angry and critical of the father who could not see or engage with his son, and I could not feel any empathy for him. During the course and through the artwork, I understood that my major childhood wish was for my parents to see me and relate to me as an equal (Image 2). I realized that there is a whole spectrum between full recovery and full adoption of new patterns and I learned to appreciate the efforts parents make to improve their parenting, rather than repeating patterns from their past. I have developed the ability to identify and empathize with the parent and the child at the same time and as such contain complex and conflicting emotions.

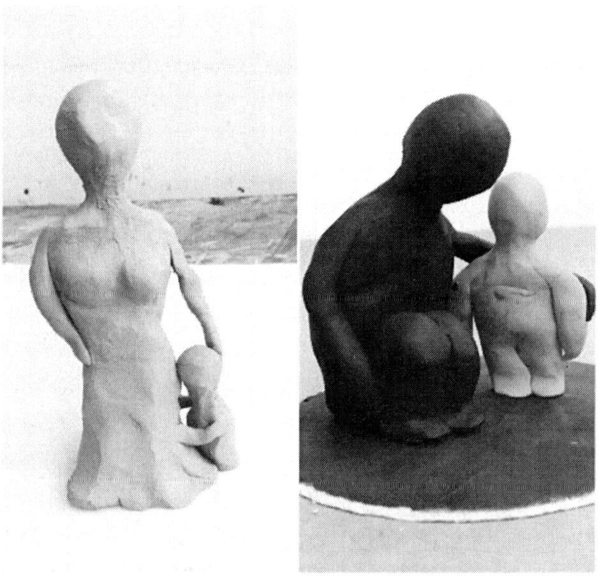

Image 2 – Noa and Mother – in the first session of the course Noa hiding behind her big mother (clay). In the last session as equals (plasticine).

Two substantial sections in the course cover the subject of intergenerational transmission and the breaking of cycles. These sections evoke memories and personal-emotional and familial content at high intensity and encourage a renewed observation and re-examination of past events, which are identified, acknowledged, and "reset" from childhood (Fraiberg, Adelson, & Shapiro, 2003; Ogden, 2017). The process is supplemented by important insights that establish ways of thinking and working with parents in the clinical setting.

Some of the students are parents and occasionally feel that the course affects their parenting behavior with their own children, particularly in terms of the development of their awareness of intergenerational transmission and the breaking of cycles. Tali (pseudonym), 32, a third-year student and mother of one daughter, expressed her feelings on the subject:

The concept of breaking the cycle acquired a new meaning when I first became pregnant and I found myself troubled by the possibility that I would repeat patterns from my nuclear family that had harmed me in the past, and pass them on to my own children. The difficulties I experienced during the course surprised me and made me view my role as a mother as a way to break the cycle. In the first artwork at the beginning of the course, I made a picture of a mandala with a healthy and peaceful self-core, into which my parents' suffocating hand (experienced as threatening and invasive) was penetrating.

At the end of the course, when I looked at the collection of my artworks, I noticed that in the lesson when we discussed the mother-child relationship, I made a sculpture placed on an open hand that allows the baby girl to rest on it, but also allows her to leave when she wants, unlike the deceptive symbiosis I experienced with my parents. This artwork symbolizes the potential for breaking the cycle for me, so that I can form a pattern for my children through which they can establish their unique imprint.

One of the focal areas for parental training in the curriculum is the development of the reflective function of the parent and the child. Fonagy & Target (1998) described a process of mentalization or the reflective function that develops during therapy as a result of the therapist's readiness to contain and give a name to emotional processes occurring during the therapeutic process. A person's reflective ability is the product of this mentalization process and constitutes the organizing element in the individual's experience, by structuring the behaviors of the self and others in terms of mental states. The development of a reflective ability appears to give students and parents feelings of control, emotional regulation, an understanding the self and others, and a sense of responsibility for their actions (Becker-Weidman & Hughes, 2008; Bleiberg, 2002). In a study by Regev & Snir (2014) on parent-child art psychotherapy, the therapists reported that they believed that the use of art in parental training helped parents become engaged in a process of mentalization and develop mental processes that enabled them to observe themselves and the relationships with their children, similar to the process that students go through in the course.

Experiential teaching triangle: Art-student-lecturer

During experiential learning, transference and counter-transference processes take place throughout the course between the lecturer and the students, in the dynamic classroom space. *Transference* refers to the patient's/student's inner emotional experience, which originates in the past and is thrown in the 'here and now' into the therapist/lecturer interaction (Freud, 1912), and includes anxieties, defenses, and internalized object relations (Klein, 1952). *Countertransference* occurs when the therapist/lecturer transfers emotions to the patient/student, often as a reaction to transference. The relationship that develops between the student and the lecturer in relation to the contents that arise in the course (usually those that deal with early relationships within the family), may cause transference and the transfer of self-images, which is known as projective identification (Klein, 1946).

When applying these terms to ABPT course, the concept of transference takes on a different quality, since art emerges as the third factor that enters into the delicate dynamics forged between the student and the lecturer. Art is present as an "analytical third" (Ogden, 1994), and as an object containing deep mental content, which is revealed during the course. The artwork is an intermediary and a means of communication between the two, and constitutes a significant component in terms of the nature of the transference relationship as well.

ABPT courses may evoke deep emotional content and dynamic processes, some of which are released and processed in the classroom setting (as shown in the examples above). The transferential relationship between student and lecturer can be elicited by student self-roles, and by the position of the lecturer as witness/observer. Transference and projective identification are contained and deciphered by the lecturer, and are then returned to the student as part of the learning process by providing modeling techniques for containment as well as intervention methods.

Thus overall, this transference is manifested in the students' artworks, where the art contains the content that emerged as a result of the topics learned in the course both theoretically and experientially, as well as the transference relationship with the lecturers. This boosts their ability to understand and use this approach as therapists. Honig (2014) coined the term 'pentagonal potential space', which refers to five components: the lecturer, individual students, the core group, the art materials/artworks and the learning space created by the lecturer. All these interact uniquely within a dynamic relationship in response to the course topics. The experiential learning allows students to assimilate and internalize the nature of the lecturer-art therapist relationship and use it to enhance their own strengths, which may reinforce their professional authority and their sense of competence in parental training sessions in the clinical setting. For example, Michal described her experience:

In the last lesson when we were asked to review our first artworks from the course from our current perspectives at the conclusion of the course, I used white plasticine to create a hand mirror that was facing me. I asked the lecturer to bring me a new package of white plasticine. The pure white color of the new plasticine package was significant; it needed to be fresh and untouched. The lecturer's response and availability were important to me. Much like the mirror in which I was reflected, I also felt seen and visible to the lecturer (Image 1). This experience during the course accompanied me through all the parental training sessions, particularly with parents who were *unable to truly see* their children and believe they were valuable. *They needed me to modify and adjust the mirror so that they could see* the value of their children, and their value as parents.

This student's commentary suggests that a combination of art-based experiential learning and theoretical learning allows for the processing of personal issues and emotional content. These experiences generate a transformation in the way the student-therapists relate to parents, who become aware of the countertransference process that was generated in their relationship with these parents. In this way, they are able to understand the projected emotional content in the transference relationship and contain and respond to it. This further allows for flexible thinking and a sense of freedom in terms of offering more knowledgeable and therapeutically processed responses.

Resistance among students

Sometimes, experiential-emotional learning may evoke resistance among students. This is often directed towards the artworks or towards the lecturers, who contain and work with this content in the classroom space by creating connections that allow students to be present with their own emotional intricacies. Bion (1962) referred to the "container" as a central function of the mother for her infant and of the therapist for their client. The mother's containment for her infant plays a central role in the infant's normal development. Similarly, the lecturer plays the same critical role for the student. The contained material is the content, such as the feelings, thoughts and behaviors of the infant (or student), which become tolerable through the mother's/lecturer's facilitation. The nature of this facilitation is to give meaning to the student's particular situation by offering containment and the lecturer's ability to bear this load.

The containment of the resistant reaction and the processing of this issue in class is internalized by the students and allows them to apply this experience and knowledge in the clinic when parents object to training or to the integration of art in parental training.

Room setup and materials

Space. The spaces need to be designed for learning. This can include opportunities to learn from and through previous esthetic, spiritual, cultural, and kinesthetic experiences while mediating a current learning moment (Seaman, 2007). The classroom in which the course takes place should be spacious and equipped with a sink, storage cabinets for the art materials, shelves for storing the artworks and a table which contains the "open buffet of art materials".

Art materials. The organization of space and the way the art materials are arranged in the classroom, as well as in the therapy studio, should make them accessible and welcoming, even for individuals who do not experience the language of art naturally. The layout of the work environment and art materials in the "buffet" should convey a visual message and encourage the creation of images using materials that are offered in a preliminary and indirect way (Steinhardt, 2000). This variety of creative materials allows students (as well as clients) a wide range of creative tools to express their inner worlds based on the assumption that art as a language consists of colors, shapes, lines and images that serve as tools for expression where words fall short (Malchoidi, 2007). In some classes, the lecturers choose to use specific art materials; for example, when discussing the mother-child relationship they use clay, whereas in other classes, the "buffet of art materials" is offered in a more open manner. The choice of art materials in the course is based on the variety of materials found in the art therapy room and includes painting materials ranging from more easily controlled materials (such as different pencils, pens, markers, oil pastels, chalk, etc.) to less easily controlled materials (such as finger paints, gouache paints, watercolor paints, beach sand, glitter, etc.). There is a selection of paintbrushes, papers, glues, collage cutouts from magazines, materials for three-dimensional work, sculpture and assemblage (such as clay, plaster, wooden cubes, wool), natural materials and various junk/found/recycled materials. This assortment of materials allows each student to select what best suits his/her emotional state in the classroom, and learn about his/her ability to become attentive to and “flow” with the work, as well as the need to be in control (Steinhardt, 2000).

Sink. In each classroom, there is a sink and an area that allows students to work freely with water and different liquids and smearing materials. The presence of a sink in the classroom encourages students to work with water, and with “dirty” liquid and regressive materials without fear. This allows for the containment of primary processes in the mutual group space, without having to leave the room to rinse their hands or the utensils they worked with. The course may evoke repressed memories and emotions that are difficult to process, and often students are inclined to leave the room “for a breather” to disconnect from the emotional load they experienced in the classroom. At a concrete and visual level, the way in which the classroom is laid out conveys to the students that any content that materializes and emerges in the room can be contained both emotionally and creatively.

Conclusion

Overall, this teaching approach assumes that the encounter between the world of art and the world of therapy fosters a rich triangular relationship between the lecturer, the student, and the artwork. The presence of art materials in the classroom provides students with the opportunity to take part in a visual creative experience that utilizes their imagination and enables the symbolic and non-verbal expression of unconscious content (Case & Dalley, 2006; Schaverien, 2000).

This art-based parental training course uses artistic techniques as an integral part of the learning process. As presented in this chapter, the various facets of experiential learning allow for a broad assimilation of the content taught in the course. Art-making in clinical training appears to encourage conceptualization, integration, and self-awareness in the students.

Academic programs may benefit from using ABPT throughout the whole curriculum, since a transformation takes place in the personal and professional realms which merge and allow students to hone their professional identity as art therapists. The personal relationship to creative work enables the students to become involved in learning on a deeper level, and their autonomy and sense of achievement enhance the development of confidence and self-esteem important to the novice therapist.

References

Becker-Weidman, A., Hughes, D. (2008) "Dyadic Developmental Psychotherapy: an Evidence-based Treatment for Children with Complex Trauma and Disorders of Attachment" *Child and Family Social Work*, 13(3), 329-337.

Bion, W. R. (1962) *Learning from Experience*. Karnac.

Bleiberg, E. (2002) *Treating Personality Disorder in Children and Adolescent: A Relational Approach*. Guilford press.

Brownell, J., Swaner, L. (2010) *Five High-impact Practices: Research on Learning Outcomes, Completion, and Quality*. Association of American Colleges and Universities.

Case, C., Dalley, T. (2006) *The Handbook of Art Therapy: second edition*. Routledge.

Cohen-Yatziv, L., Regev, D. (2019) "The Effectiveness and Contribution of Art Therapy Work with Children in 2018 – What Progress has been Made so far? A Systematic Review" *International Journal of Art Therapy*, 24(3), 100-112.

Deaver, S., Shiflett, C. (2011) "Art-Based Supervision Techniques" *Clinical Supervisor*, 30(2), 257-276.

Fonagy, P., Target, M. (1998) "Mentalization and the Changing Aims of Child Psychoanalysis" *Psychoanalytic Dialogues*, 8(1), 87-114.

Freud, S. (1912) Recommendations to Physicians Practicing Psycho-analysis. *The Standard Edition of the Complete Psychological Works of Sigmund Freud*,12, 109-120.

Fraiberg, S., Adelson, E., Shapiro, V. (1975) "Ghosts in the Nursery: A Psychoanalytic Approach to the Problem of Impaired Infant-Mother Relationships" *Journal of the American Academy of Child Psychiatry*, 14, 387-422

Heinrich, W. F., Green, P. M. (2020) "Remixing Approaches to Experiential Learning, Design, and Assessment" *Journal of Experiential Education*, 43(2), 205-223.

Honig, O. (2014) *Post-graduate Art Therapy Training in Israel: Personal and Professional Transformation through Dynamic Artwork-based Experiential Transformative Courses* [Doctoral dissertation] University of Sussex.

Klein, M. (1946) *Notes on some schizoid mechanisms In Envy and Gratitude and Other Works 1946-1963*. Delacorte Press/Seymour Laurence

Kuh, G. D. (2008) *High-impact educational practices: What they are, who has access to them, and why they matter*. Association of American Colleges and Universities.

Rainey, M. A., Kolb, D. A. (1995) "Using experiential learning theory and learning styles in diversity education" (pp.129-146) in R. Sims., S. Sims (eds.). *The Importance of Learning Styles: Understanding the Implications for Learning, Course Design, and Education*. Greenwood Press.

Malchiodi, C. (2007) *Art therapy sourcebook*. McGraw Hill Professional.

Maujean, A., Pepping, C.A., Kendall, E. (2014) "A Systematic Review of Randomized Controlled Studies of Art Therapy" *Journal of the American Art Therapy Association*, 31(1), 37-44.

Ogden, T.H., (2017) "Dreaming the Analytic Session: A Clinical Essay" *The Psychoanalytic Quarterly,* 86(1),1-20.

—. (1994) "The Analytic Third: Working with Intersubjective Clinical Facts" *International Journal of Psycho-Analysis*, 75, 3-19.

Pratt, R. R. (2006) "Art, Dance, and Music Therapy" *Physical Medicine Rehabilitation Clinic in Northern America*, 15, 827-841.

Regev, D., Snir, S. (2014) "Working with Parents in Parent-Child Art Psychotherapy" *The Arts in psychotherapy*, 41(5), 511-18.

Rivera, J. E., Heinrich, W. F. (2016) "Assessing Multiple Dimensions of Significant Learning" (pp. 418-448) in L. Wankel, C. Wankel (eds.). *Integrating Curricular and Co-curricular Endeavors to Enhance Student Success*. Emerald Publishing Group.

Schaverien, J. (2008) *The Mirror of Art: Reflections on Transference and the Gaze of the Picture.* https://aras. org/sites/default/files/docs/00037Schaverien. pdf.

—. (2000) "The Triangular Relationship and the Aesthetic Countertransference in Analytical Art Psychotherapy" (pp. 55-83) in A. Gilroy, G. McNeilly (eds.). *The Changing Shape of Art Therapy: New Developments in Theory and Practice*. Jessica Kingsley Publishers.

—. (1999) *The Revealing Image: Analytical Art Psychotherapy in Theory and Practice.* Jessica Kingsley Publishers.

Seaman, J. (2007) "Taking Things into Account: Learning as Kinesthetically-mediated Collaboration" *Journal of Adventure Education & Outdoor Learning*, 7(1), 3–20.

Shamri-zeevi, L., Regev, D., Guttmann, J. (2018) "The Efficiency of Art-Based Interventions in Parental Training" *Frontiers in Psychology*, 9, 1495.

Shamri-Zeevi, L., Regev, D., Snir, S. (2015) "The Usage of Art Materials in the Framework of Parent Training" *The Arts in Psychotherapy,* 45, 56-63.

Shamri-zeevi, L., Regev, D., Snir, S. (2019) "Art Based Parental Training (ABPT) – Parents' Experiences" *International Journal of Art Therapy.*

Shamri-Zeevi, L. Regev, D. (2020) "Parental Responses to Artistic Processes in Art-Based Parental Training" *Art Therapy.*

Snir, S., Hazut, T. (2012) "Observing the Relationship: Couple Patterns Reflected in Joint Paintings" *The Arts in Psychotherapy*, 39, 11-18.

Steinhardt, L. (2000) *Foundation and Form in Jungian Sandplay: An Art Therapy Approach*. Jessica Kinglsey Publishers.

—. (2017) "From Dot to Line to Plane: Constellating Unconscious Imagery in Art Therapy" *Art Therapy*, 34(4), 159-166.

Winnicott, D. W. (1971) *Playing and Reality*. Basic books.

PART III:

RESEARCH

CHAPTER 12

CREATIVITY: THEORETICAL ASPECTS AND THEIR IMPLICATIONS FOR THE TEACHING OF ART THERAPY

DALIA MERARI

... Few realize that any human being can be creative and that life circumstances may stimulate creativity.
(Erika Landau, 1973)

Introduction

This chapter was written at the times of the Coronavirus pandemic. The whole world is still under quarantine. Students, lecturers, patients and therapists – the entire population was demanded to undergo change.

Two principles of creativity became manifest in the aftermath of the swift change: *brainstorming* and *divergent thinking* (Yu and Subramanian, 2017). These principles will be addressed in the theoretical review further in the chapter. The crisis of the Covid-19 period demonstrates the importance of creativity in teaching under situations whereby change is compelled by external conditions; but even in the ordinary course of events, creativity plays a significant role in teaching.

The concepts of "creation" and "creativity" have been adopted in many areas. In this chapter, which will focus on creative teaching, I shall first aim to examine the concept in its theoretical aspect, which highlights the creative processes. Theories on the subject constitute a basis of knowledge which opens up a window to understanding the central theme of the chapter.

Theories on creativity stem from the realm of psychology, which constitutes a theoretical basis for the art therapy profession: the existing theoretical corpus of art therapy was crystallized mainly on the basis of psychological theories. However, it should be emphasized that extensive research is being conducted in the field of art therapy, which has evolved, over the years, into a professional identity which focuses on the language of art. Concomitantly, when examining the central theme of this chapter – creative teaching – one may receive the impression that most of the literature on this discipline is based upon sources from the domain of education. Most researchers in this realm are themselves educators.

Literature on the subject is rich with manifold works on the role of creativity in the teaching of different fields of study (for instance, Mullen, 2019; Fayer & Collins, 1991; Gardner, 1982; Jeffrey & Craft, 2004; Gustina & Sweet, 2014; Cremin, 2009a, 2009b; Chan, 2007; Yu & Subramanian, 2017). However, it seems that in the pedagogical field of art therapy, creativity assumes special importance. This stems from the fact that the artistic medium is intrinsically creative.

The concept of creativity is often mentioned among art therapists, who focus on art as a therapeutic language. However, the meaning of creativity in teaching art therapy must be understood and interpreted in a far broader context. The very act of artmaking is a creative process which is manifested in the representation of the synthesis between the patient's inner subjective world and outer reality. This creative process has therapeutic value (Jung, 1964; Winnicott, 1971).

Creative teaching and education for creativity

A distinction must be made between creative teaching and education towards creativity, that is, whether the focus is on the creative lecturer, or on the lecturer's abilities to teach the student creativity (Yu & Subramanian, 2017; Chan, 2007; Brinkman, 2010; Cremin, 2009a; 2009b; Jeffrey & Craft, 2004; National Advisory Committee on Creative and Cultural Education, 1999).

The distinction between creative teaching and creativity-promoting education has concerned educators over the past few decades. This division related to creative teachers versus teachers who teach creativity – abilities which may coexist in the same individual – making it difficult to distinguish between these two concepts (Jeffrey & Craft, 2004). Teaching creativity entails encouraging students to develop self-thinking on the subject-matter under discussion, discovering new ideas and novel perspectives that the student develops beyond the material delivered by the lecturer. The connection between teaching creatively and teaching for creativity lies in the fact that creative teaching serves the student as a model for developing his or her own creative approach (Cremin, 2009a).

The importance of creative teaching in any field is self-evident, as far as the effective method of delivering content to students is concerned. Nevertheless, in the case of teaching art therapy, creative teaching assumes particular importance as a way of developing the creative approach of the future therapist. The aspiration to cultivate the student's (and would-be therapist's) creativity stems from the awareness that the patient population presents a wide clinical diversity, which calls for the implementation of the widest possible range of means. The term "creativity," in its therapeutic context, refers mainly to the promotion of mental flexibility, whose purpose is an analysis of the array of factors and a synthesis of the set of approaches that would lead to an optimal solution-focused therapy.

As previously stated, this chapter will focus on the teaching-instructional aspect. In the first part of the chapter, I will engage with definitions of creativity, as well as with some theories relevant to the subject. It should be emphasized that there are numerous theories of creativity, which stem from the relevant topics they deal with. In this chapter, I have chosen to present theories that relate mainly to the applied psychological aspects. I shall subsequently refer to these theories in the section on creativity in teaching art therapy. Finally, I will furnish examples from a survey I conducted among art-therapy lecturers at the Academic College of Society and the Arts, which addresses creativity at large, and creative teaching in particular. I wish to emphasize that the chapter will not delve into the motivations for creativity that many theories have engaged with, including those of Freud, Jung, Kris, Bellak, Rogers, Rollo May and others. The choice of creative teaching as the subject of the chapter stemmed from a deep appreciation for the creative developments of the lecturers and their contribution to the special curriculum of the college.

Definitions of creativity

The definitions of creativity are context-dependent, in the sense that they reflect the starting point and area of expertise of the definer (Amabile, 1996). I will address three accepted definitions of creativity:

Landau (1973), an educational and clinical psychologist, defines creativity as a trait inherent – to some degree – in every person. This feature enables to forge associative connections between information, materials and experiences that are independent from one another. Landau's approach is relevant to the training of art-therapy students, as it underscores the development of new approaches to familiar situations. The student's ability to go through a process of reframing situations, that is, to shift to a new perception of a familiar situation, is an essential development required for the training of an art therapist.

Arieti (1976), a psychiatrist, argues that Creativity must be such that – sooner or later – may be understood and accepted through ordinary thinking and be evaluated according to known tools, otherwise the result will be bizarre. As a psychiatrist, Arieti fears the bizarre. However, there is extensive literature which shows that many artists suffered from a wide spectrum of mental illnesses and were hospitalized in mental institutions at various times in their lives. The ability to express emotions in an original way through graphic, musical, literary images and the like has led to the realization that the image, like the dream, expresses an instinctual-mental-spiritual power, which, being different from the conventional, is creative in essence (Stack and Lester, 2009; Sass, 1992; Ludwig, 1995).

Amabile (1982), a social psychologist specializing in business administration, offers two definitions: a consensual and a conceptual one. According to the consensual definition, a product or response is creative, insofar as skilled observers independently concur that it is creative. Skilled observers are those who are familiar with the field in which the product or response was created. Creativity may, therefore, be regarded as the trait that characterizes a product or response that was valued as creative by "a reliable subjective assessment technique" (Amabile, 1982, p. 1001), or, alternatively, creativity is the process that led to that which was valued as creative. It should be noted that this definition refers primarily to the product rather than the process, as up to this day, there is no consensual description of the creative process.

According to the conceptual definition, a product or response will be assessed as creative if a) it is innovative, appropriate, useful, accurate or valuable in terms of its field of existence; b) it is formed in a *heuristic* rather than an *algorithmic* way. In this respect, the adjective "algorithmic" refers to a solution characterized by a predetermined trajectory (Hilgard and Bower, 1975; McGraw, 1978), whereas "heuristic" refers to the existence or development of trajectories which lead to solutions in accordance with external circumstances and inner (personal) ability.

Theories of creativity

Components of creativity, no matter how minimal, are probably accessible to everyone. Creativity develops from the person's experience, the information available to him or her and, especially out of the daring to abandon the familiar and the safe for the sake of the new and the unknown. When attaching the epithet "creative" to a person or work, we consider its characteristics as well as the totality of individual circumstances. For instance, the age of the creator, cognitive abilities, previous training in the field, the mental state at the time of creation, the ability to withstand failure, and so forth. We are, thus, grappling with a very complex concept which incorporates elements related to different aspects, including the creative product, the creative process, the creative personality and the role ascribed to the environment regarding the chances for creative development (Slabbert, 1994). In the late 1980s, the anthology *The Nature of Creativity: Contemporary Perspectives* (Sternberg, 1988) was published, which included chapters by the best psychologists researching the field of creativity, representing theories from different perspectives on the subject. From this collection one may realize how rich this field is. Among the researchers, particularly worth mentioning are Howard Gardner, Teresa M. Amabile, and Mihaly Csikszentmihalyi.

Another group that has worked in the field are psychoanalytically-oriented theorists, who have studied the motivation behind the development of creativity. They formulated various theories as well, each with his/her special outlook. These include Jung, Rollo May, Freud, Winnicott, Kris, and others. The specific research field of creative teaching, which is the focus of this chapter, draws mainly from the psychological theories and applies them to the learning environment.

Creative ability has been studied for over a century. However, the first general theory was proposed by psychologist Graham Wallas in 1926. It is based upon a four-stage sequence of processes common to all artworks and in all fields. These include *preparation*, *incubation*, *illumination* and *verification*.

—The *preparation* phase refers to the segment of time whereby the creator is engaged with the preparation elements; that is, meditating freely, collecting information or data, paying heed to others and allowing himself to "wander" mentally.

—The *incubation* phase derives from the fact that a time span elapses between the preparation and the illumination phases. This period can be very short—even a few minutes—and also very long—it may last months or even years. In fact, it is a process whereby the material gathered during the preparation stage is processed in a way that may be active or passive. The passive form entails an unconscious elaboration process of the material and its organization.

—The *illumination* phase occurs when the creative person discovers the solution to a problem. This solution may spring out of a sudden and/or intuitive clear insight, although a sophisticated product may require the investment of further continuous endeavor.

—The *verification* phase is the fourth stage, whose role is to grant the stamp of approval, based upon a critical evaluation of the creator himself.

In later years, Rossman (1931), Osborn (1953) and Taylor (1964) proposed expansive models of the original theory. In 1956, Guilford proposed a different theory which analyzed the components of creativity and, in tandem, developed a creativity test (the Guilford Test of Creative Thinking). According to his approach, creativity, as a cognitive function, is based on a large number of factors and is not one and the same as intelligence. These factors are defined by him as "primary mental abilities." According to this theory, thinking is the most important component in creativity. Thinking may be focused (*convergent*) or ramified-heuristic (*divergent*); the latter amounts to creative thinking. It is a type of thinking that is not conformist or conventional, but which progresses in search of unconventional solutions. The components of divergent thinking are flexibility, originality and a fluency that describes the ability to create a stream of ideas that meet certain requirements.

Since the emergence of these theories, additional works have been published, including the model of Amabile (1996), which addresses the components of creativity and the creative process. According to this model, the three components of creativity are: Domain-relevant skills, creativity-relevant skills, and task motivation. These are described below.

Domain-related skills relate to the scope of knowledge in the area and to the technical qualifications and/or special "talents" required for its implementation (Schank & Abelson, 1980). These skills depend on cognitive abilities, perceptual and motor skills, and formal or informal training and factual knowledge of the field in question; that is, facts, principles and opinions concerning the area and the ability to grapple with relevant problems. Indeed, in regard to scientific creativity, Newell and Simon (1972) found a high correlation between the ability to be creative and the degree of professional training, at least as far as fairly routine tasks are concerned.

Creativity-related skills refer to what is known as appropriate cognitive style, overt or covert heuristic knowledge to create new ideas, and an appropriate work style. These depend upon training, experience in fashioning ideas and personality traits. The skills associated with creativity are sometimes difficult to define and are expressed in the fact that as a result of the creative process, a product or response will exceed in quality what was hitherto known in the same field. It is important to note that even if a particular individual is gifted with exceptional field skills, in the absence of creativity-related skills, the product of his action will not be considered creative by expert judges. What do these skills include? This is what is known as the "creative style," characterized by the ease in understanding the complexity of the situation or problem, alongside the ability to disengage from predetermined conceptions when solving the problem.

Creativity-related skills combine the following abilities:

1. Disengagement from a perceptual setup: Using a means for a different purpose than the designated one.
2. Disengagement from a cognitive setup: Employing a different cluster of possible solutions.
3. The ability to understand complexity.
4. Maintaining response options open for the longest time.
5. Suspending decisions.
6. Efficient memory.

Task motivation

Amabile (1996) emphasizes the importance of *intrinsic motivation.* Individuals will be more creative if their motivation stems from self-interest, satisfaction from the task and the challenge posed by the job itself, rather than if they are impelled by external pressures, such as managerial demands. Previous researchers have also emphasized the importance of intrinsic motivation. Koestler (1964) advanced a postulation according to which the highest creative ability is manifested under conditions of absolute freedom, since only under such conditions may the realms of intuition be reached. This return to an unconscious and playful mental level is essential for the creative process.

Rogers (1954), as well, attaches particular importance to independence from an external audit factor and emphasizes the need for an inner focus of evaluation. This type of focus places the individual as the primary evaluator of the creative action and ascribes but a secondary role to the environment. Crutchfield argued that "conformity pressures tend to elicit kinds of motivation in the individual that are incompatible with the creative process" (1962, p. 121).

Ostensibly, according to these three researchers, independence from external constraints encourages creativity. Nevertheless, Amabile 1996, adds to the expanded theory the dimension of the environment as a significant component in creativity. Erika Landau, who has been thoroughly involved in creativity-promoting education, also emphasizes the importance that she ascribes to the environment as an element which encourages creativity. However, the lessons drawn from the period whereby the whole world is fighting the coronavirus, which poses a physical and mental existential threat, demonstrate that the claims that the optimal conditions for creativity are stress-free and that creativity necessitates complete freedom do not stand the test of reality. Undoubtedly, inner freedom is required for creativity but, at the same time, the environment sets conditions that generate the need for change and, in many cases, this need becomes the source of the basic motivation for creativity. Manifestations of such creativity-promoting incentive may be discerned in various fields, including education. I will expand on the last aspect in the second part of the chapter, which focuses on the teaching of art therapy.

Robert J. Sternberg, a social psychologist, has developed a theory that expands the perception of creativity and underscores the ability of every person to be creative. This requires a number of conditions for the development of creativity, described in what follows:

> Creativity is a decision in the same way investing is. People are not born creative or uncreative. Rather, they develop a set of attitudes toward life that characterize those who are willing to go their own way. Examples of such attitudes toward life are willingness to (a) redefine problems in novel ways, (b) take sensible risks, (c) "sell" ideas that others might not initially accept, (d) persevere in the face of obstacles, and (e) examine whether their own preconceptions are interfering with their creative process. Such attitudes are teachable and can be ingrained in students through instruction that encourages students to think for themselves. (Sternberg, 2013, p. 1)

The central emphasis in this expansive theory lies on the human being's abilities and desires. Although Sternberg addresses some of the elements that feature in earlier theories, such as risk-taking and the like, he lays particular emphasis on education, especially in the context of the potential inherent in the creative lecturer. According to Sternberg, creativity comprises several aspects which need to be addressed: a) abilities, (b) knowledge, (c) styles of thinking, (d) personal attributes, (e) motivation, especially intrinsic motivation, and (f) environment.

It may be argued that a person endowed with creative capacity will not be able to realize the potential if he/she is unwilling to embrace some risk, or in a situation whereby the environment does not lend minimal support to creativity. According to Sternberg, this is especially valid in the case of teaching. The creative lecturer will set up learning conditions and a supportive environment not only in speech but in everyday deeds as well.

Creative teaching

We find in the literature a vast number of references to the subject of creative teaching in various fields, such as teaching languages in a creative way, teaching mathematics creatively and the like. Studies have been conducted as well, demonstrating the contribution of art to the creative dimension in the medical professions, such as among nursing students (Meggs & Greer 2011) and medical students (Edmonds and Hammond 2012). In the latter study, medical students were exposed to artworks at a gallery and were asked to relate to them in focus groups. According to Gustina and Sweet (2014, p. 50), as a result of experiences of this kind, "students appear to have gained or enhanced observational, analytic and interpersonal skills, and to have applied these skills to their clinical practice." This study, like the abovementioned others, advances the realization that the creative aspect of teaching endows an additional dimension to the formal knowledge imparted in the studies. The assumption was that the development of an artistic channel would improve the students' creativity and their professional ability. The creative lecturer is the one who implements novel, compelling, original and intriguing teaching methods to convey the material in an effective and appealing manner, and finds ways to adapt the teaching methods to the characteristics of the students and to changing learning situations.

An extreme approach to the relationship between formal information and "creativeness" was adopted by Maslow (1967). In his article on the creative approach, he argued that there is no point in learning facts or techniques and that the purpose of teaching is to cultivate in the individual the ability to grapple with problematic situations without resorting to approaches or consensual predetermined rules and independently from the influence of others. In this way, the individual will be able to become a self-confident contestant who is not afraid or deterred. Regarding Maslow's approach, it may be argued that – although the importance of intellectual freedom in creative teaching is undisputable – no discipline can be taught without conveying a basis of prior knowledge. Over the years, Maslow expanded and altered his theories on creativity. His critics even noted that his theory of creativity somewhat contradicted his well-known theory of the hierarchic pyramid of needs.

Creative teaching in the psychotherapeutic professions

In teaching psychotherapy professions, the lecturer grapples with a built-in contrast between two conflicting demands: on the one hand – the need to teach the subject while abiding by and focusing on the essentially rigid theoretical bodies of knowledge; on the other – the need to afford the student with intra-psychic and inter-psychic observation abilities, which are not part and parcel of the formal learning curriculum, and are based upon the student's curiosity concerning an overall understanding of human situations in a flexible and variegated environment.

The ability to combine the fixed and the flexible elements is one of the defining characteristics of creative teaching in art therapy. This mode of teaching allots considerable weight to the experiential element. In order to be assimilated on both cognitive and emotional levels, the theoretical material should be presented in combination with experiential learning, which is mainly based upon the world of symbols and images of lecturer and student alike. This experiential basis provides a connection between the cognitive and the emotional planes.

That is, teaching art therapy requires a combination of theoretical and creative skills on the part of the lecturer. The creative skills are manifested in the lecturer's ability to transmit the two distinct areas which comprise the subject-matter of the profession – mental health and the arts. The ability of the lecturer to constitute a model for students in the field is an important component in cultivating creativity in therapy, as attested by the lecturers in the survey to be described later.

Like any other academic profession, teaching art therapy has undergone a process which does not necessarily promote creativity. The demands from the profession have led to the awareness that it is essential to base the academic curriculum upon a solid theoretical basis. The emphasis on academicization has posed a dilemma mainly with regard to the theoretical courses. To what extent may these courses incorporate creativity, that is, divergent, critical, and experiential thinking? To what degree is it possible to teach in a way that will not entail just memorizing material, but rather enable the learner to create value himself – stimulate thinking, cultivate criticism, and spur the student to generate insights of his/her own? How to motivate a student to imagine and think?

In her analysis of creativity, Amabile (1996) emphasizes, among other things, the importance of disengagement from existing perceptual and cognitive systems. According to this view, it is paramount to transfer existing knowledge in a way that allows for criticism and open-mindedness to other avenues of thinking, beyond the content conveyed in the lesson; that is, encouraging "divergent thinking" (Wang and Nickerson, 2017). It is our aim that throughout a structured academic lesson, students will be trained to apply skills, such as creative and critical thinking, that would pose a challenge for the lecturer. Moreover, we seek to encourage the students' ability to discern opportunities to activate these skills even beyond the framework of formal teaching; that is, at the clinic. A further element which has become particularly important in recent years is the need for creative teaching that would suit a world of changing environment, characterized by migration and a mixture of cultures and languages.

The level of ambiguity occasionally posed by complex problems in a therapeutic profession such as art therapy – even in areas that apparently seem comprehensible – is highly noticeable. Hence, traditional answers to such complex clinical situations, which rely only on the application of field-related skills, will narrow the range of therapeutic options, and may, therefore, obstruct its improvement. I shall mention in this context Brull's position (1973), who argues that success in therapy lies not only in scientific knowledge and experience, but also in the ability of the therapist to release mental powers and hope for the future. This is possible if the therapists allow themselves to look inwards. By doing so, they will overcome their anxiety by the willingness to constantly create new patterns to understand the patient, that is, by way of the creativity inherent in them.

Obviously, an exclusive resorting to creative thinking in teaching does not guarantee its quality. The essence of creativity is the ability to break free from familiar patterns and, by so doing, making it possible to cope with complex problems within an innovative framework that exceeds the lecturer's knowledge base. Success based upon a creative approach may encourage the development of the personal motivating factor within lecturer and student alike, which also holds true for the therapeutic process. In this respect, it is worth mentioning Landau's view (1973) that the creative approach to therapy amalgamates the fields of science and art. From the artist one may learn the naive gaze, a primary outlook on the patient's problems, which makes it possible to reach his/her uniqueness. From the artist one can also learn the handling of details without losing touch with the whole. From the scientist one can learn the way of setting up the deliberate and proactive question, the modesty required in order to cope with circumscribed problems and the tolerance in face of a sense of frustration. From both one can learn openness vis-à-vis the surroundings, the daring – despite the anxiety – to go out into the open, unfamiliar and unknown world, the inner freedom to choose from a wide world a certain alternative and the playfulness with elements and information items known to us, while setting them in new contexts.

The lecturers at the Academic College of Society and the Arts in Israel developed a creative system, according to which the teaching of the theoretical courses incorporates plastic imagery, which enriches and visually illustrates the theoretical materials. These images create a linkage between cognitive learning and sensory perception, adding an experiential dimension to concepts, which leads to an active and creative involvement on the part of the students. In addition, the theoretical lesson is accompanied by a practical session whereby the content learned in the theoretical framework is applied and conceptualized through diverse images and art materials. The practice takes place in creation workshops, which allow the student freedom in the selection of materials, as well as a choice between individual work and work with a group of colleagues.

The lecturer, in the practical session, allows each student a latitude that calls for creativity. Beyond consisting an emotional space of expression, the power of the artwork allows for a student who experiences difficulty in putting his/her feelings into words – or is unaware of the spontaneous content projected onto the work – a further channel of expression beyond the verbal one. The triangle created between the student, the artwork and the lecturer resembles, to some extent, the classical therapeutic model whereby transference and countertransference processes take place, but the lecturer's significant role in distinguishing between a therapeutic situation in a clinic and practice in an academic class should be emphasized. We do not seek to treat students, but rather to teach and train them toward a therapeutic profession.

Challenge and creativity under the Covid-19 pandemic

During the outbreak of the coronavirus, all lecturers were requested to switch to zoom instruction. The sharp transition generated stress and uncertainty. Experiential learning and the employment of art materials, tailored for teaching art therapy, became particularly jeopardized under zoom teaching, but this challenge brought with it a host of novel and wide-ranging ideas. The unfamiliar teaching technology was speedily acquired. The creative abilities of the lecturers, their mental-flexibility training and their rich teaching experience enabled the drastic change. The conceptual transformation of the teaching staff was catalyzed by brainstorming and mutual inspiration.

Even prior to the outbreak of the pandemic we had resorted to a type of "peer instruction" (Crouch & Mazur, 2001; Cortright, Collins & DiCarlo, 2005), but the employment of this method was increased during the epidemic, due to the urgent need to find solutions to an alien situation which affected staff members and students alike. According to the devised strategy, a supervising student was appointed for each exclusive student meeting. The supervisor presented a topic and conducted its discussion and, at the end of the meeting, summarized the insights raised in the discussion. The method helped to crystallize creative ways to solve the difficulties posed by the new situation, both in terms of the variety of ideas proposed and in terms of boosting the motivation of the entire learning community to deal with the crisis, by actively mobilizing them to chart the path.

The independence provided by this teaching method increases the students' involvement in the individual and group-learning process. The crisis triggered by the outbreak of the coronavirus pandemic is exceptional in terms of the changes it demanded in all areas of life, including teaching. However, even during routine periods, teaching poses an ongoing challenge, and it is necessary to renew, update and redesign the curriculum and adapt it to the environment.

Lecturers' survey

For the composition of this chapter, I deemed it pertinent to record the views of art therapy lecturers on creative teaching. The survey questions were answered by eighteen (female) lecturers at the Academic College of Society and the Arts in Israel, most of whom have seniority and extensive experience in this field. Beyond the importance of the insights themselves, which emerge out of their vast experience in the field, it was also interesting to realize the extent to which these insights are in line with the theories reviewed above.

The survey consisted of six open-ended questions which the lecturers were requested to answer. There was a degree of overlap in some of the answers. At the end of the survey, I summarized the answers to every one of the questions and underscored major themes. Below are the summaries of the lecturers' responses to each and every question.

What is creative teaching?

In the answers to this question, two main themes arose, one relating to the lecturer and his/her personal qualities, the other – to the recourse to means and technologies. The characteristics of the creative lecturer branched into four parameters: (1) emotional flexibility and tolerance for different opinions and approaches; (2) the lecturer's ability to improvise and adapt the content and the teaching method to the classroom situation, as well as to the students' level and cultural background; (3) the willingness of the lecturers to learn and reinvent themselves; and (4) challenging students to develop intellectual independence.

The second theme described creative teaching as that which invents novel venues, methods and means that will enable conveying the material in an experiential way.

Is creative teaching of special importance for the teaching of art therapy?

All the respondents believed that, indeed, in teaching art therapy, creativity assumes special importance. A main reason for this – mentioned by all the respondents – is that art therapy itself requires a creative approach on the part of the therapist due to the variety of patients, the range of problems and the multiplicity of possible forms of making contact with them. In his/her way of teaching, the lecturer instantiates a model for the creativity expected from the future therapist. A further rationale pointed out by the respondents is that since the field of art therapy is interdisciplinary, combining psychology with the language of art, its teaching requires even higher creativity. In fact, the nexus between the two areas, which the lecturer is required to establish in each lesson, is essentially creative. In the opinion of some of the respondents, not only is creativity of special importance in teaching art therapy, but the teacher must also be a creative artist him/herself.

How does creativity manifest itself in teaching art therapy?

In the first question, the teachers were asked to address the importance of creative teaching at large. The second question focused on the special importance of creativity in teaching art therapy, whereas in the present question the respondents were asked to specifically describe how creative teaching is conveyed in this field.

Beyond the characteristics relevant to creative teaching in any field, one respondent noted that creative teaching of art therapy should comprise three aspects: experiencing the sensory and symbolic aspects of art, reflecting on the experience, and connecting the experience to the theoretical material. The importance of learning the theoretical material by way of experience and artistic experimentation was noted by most respondents. Additional respondents emphasized the importance of engaging in sensory experience when working with materials and resorting to visual images in order to teach and internalize concepts.

Enabling versus interfering conditions for a creative teaching of art therapy

In their answers concerning the promoting versus the hampering conditions for a creative teaching of art therapy, the respondents addressed two types of factors: the atmosphere in the learning environment and the physical conditions. The mentioned atmosphere factors referred to the prevailing spirit in the institution, especially creative academic freedom, expressed in the approval, encouragement and appreciation of the management and staff with regard to a creative approach.

Although the question addressed the *conditions* that affect creative teaching, some of the respondents referred, once more, to the characteristics of the lecturer as an influencing factor, and some also noted the openness of the students as such a factor. The physical conditions noted as encouraging creative teaching were an ample workspace, the availability of diverse materials for creations of various kinds and learning in small groups (allowing for more intimacy between teacher and students and between the students themselves).

As might have been expected, the conditions enumerated as interfering with creative teaching were the opposite of those that encouraged it. However, some of the respondents also regarded restrictive conditions – referring to the coronavirus period as an example – as a factor that could promote creativity, as a way of dealing with the restrictive learning environment. Among the respondents were those who mentioned anxiety (of the teacher and/or of the students) as a factor that hampers creativity, as well as insufficient preparation, lack of motivation, judgmentalism, reductionism, concreteness, and burnout.

Can you provide, out of your personal experience, examples of creativity in teaching art therapy?

Most of the examples offered by the respondents based upon their personal experience in creative teaching related to their coping with crisis situations. One teacher described her dealing with a particularly antagonistic group through a creative approach that completely changed the patterns of communication with the group and turned resistance into a fertile ground for learning. The teacher adopted an approach that surprised the students, both in terms of the working materials and in her conduct throughout the lesson, and in this way rendered the aggressive elements of the group non-threatening and inclusive. A crisis situation described by another teacher related to a group which was in a state of stagnation and performance anxiety. In this case, the teacher's creative intervention entailed resorting to humor: she attached crayons to the broomsticks that were in place and asked the students to draw with them. This act led to a relaxation of tension, release and relief from stagnation.

Teaching during the Covid-19 pandemic constituted an unusual crisis and posed a massive challenge to teachers. It is not surprising, therefore, that most of the examples cited by the teachers referred to this period. It is worth noting here that adapting the teaching of art therapy to distance learning is far more challenging than adapting teaching methods in subjects based solely upon frontal lectures, since art therapy classes involve the use of different art materials and active interaction between students. Learning in front of the screen a profession whose essence consists in contact with materials, creation and understanding of therapeutic processes through empirical experience, posed a special difficulty. The creative solutions specified by the teachers were based upon unconventional uses of homes and their contents as a substitute for the physical conditions and art materials found in the college, as well as the use of remote communication – computer and mobile phone – as a substitute for the teacher's physical presence. Under these circumstances, joint work of teachers assisted in creative coping strategies in the preparation of the lessons.

Can you point out a further aspect of this issue?

Several lecturers' answers to this question expressed a concluding view on the importance of creative teaching. One of the lecturers wrote:

> The creativity of lecturers at large, and especially in the field of art therapy, is a most significant issue, in my view, that affects the quality of learning. The lecturer's sense of mission, high motivation and deep connection to the profession are indispensable for creative and interesting teaching. All these can be significantly enhanced by a meaningful teaching environment; namely, communication between staff members, institutional support, and constant enrichment.

Another lecturer pointed out:

> Creativity, in my eyes, is the heart of learning. Deprived of it, the individual will memorize learning material without fully understanding what is written in the books. A learning experience which includes all five senses is the ultimate learning experience in my view. We may remember some of what we read, but we will always remember that which we experienced.

One of the lecturers gave a concise expression to her feeling about creativity in teaching: "Creativity is what renders teaching art therapy a fun thing..."

Synopsis of the survey

The emphasis on the qualities of the teacher as a central component in creative teaching stands out in the lecturers' responses. Environmental factors – including the prevailing atmosphere in the institution, the freedom granted to lecturers and students – and the physical conditions, such as workspace and availability of material, are auxiliary elements that enable creative teaching. Content-wise, most respondents emphasized the importance of the experiential component in creative teaching, and the combination of the psychology field and the language of art, unique to art therapy. The survey highlighted the impact of the teaching experience during the coronavirus period, especially in examples on the implementation of creative teaching under stressful conditions and at times whereby a drastic change in teaching methods was essential. However, the prolongation of such periods may probably exert a negative impact on the capacity for creative teaching.

Summary and concluding remarks

The psychological theories mentioned in this chapter are cornerstones for understanding the essence of creative teaching. I have put forth theories that have discussed creativity from the outset of the academic engagement in the subject, out of a wish to trace the developmental process of fathoming the concept. The concept of creativity was initially referred to in the context of exceptional individuals, geniuses in their field, to include pioneers and the great innovators in the spheres of science and art. Only later did the notion develop that in every person there lies the ability to be creative in one way or another, granted the favorable conditions for expressing creativity.

By its very nature, teaching as a whole – and teaching art therapy in particular – is a creative process. The processes described in the theories on creativity are surprisingly similar to the lesson-developing phases. The stages of preparation, incubation, illumination and verification which characterize the creative process as described by Wallas (1926) and, more broadly, by Amabile (1996) and others, are also the processes that the lecturer goes through. In the preparation phase, the lecturer is actually "mentally wandering" through materials related to the field. A long or a short incubation period is required up to the illumination point. However, the verification phase is critical in this process, as it amounts to a transitional stage between the maturation of the idea and its implementation in the classroom. At this stage, the creative lecturer is required to reinvent himself anew each time in light of the changing and unpredictable classroom dynamics. These theories may elucidate the mental processes attributed by the responders in the survey to the qualities required from the creative lecturer. Hence, it may be deduced that the linchpins of the creative process are an integral part of the essence of teaching art therapy. The classical steps of the process – unfolded in the theoretical part – often take place without the lecturer's awareness. Nevertheless, they are of particular importance to the teaching of the profession, whereby these processes apply in the fashioning of theoretical lessons and in the creative expression in workshops.

Thinking about the quality of teaching throughout my years at the academy has led me, over time, to put in writing my thoughts on this challenging subject, which demands innovations and, at times, even actual revolutions (Merari, 1997). In recent years, in the wake of the technological developments that have transformed many areas, novel studies have been added to the literature on the necessity for creative teaching. Probably, this need stems from the experiential dearth created by the speedily evolving power of technology. Apparently, the computing environment and the internet, which open up many possibilities for communication, fail to create the intimacy forged through personal contact.

The question is whether teaching might be brought to a place whereby it would enjoy the technological benefits of the new age without sacrificing the important value of experiential learning; whether these two concepts – technology and experiential learning, which involves all the senses – are necessarily contradictory or, as we have realized in the recent period, may complement each other. Here, the creative aspect has a most significant contribution, in its capacity to integrate and create a new "product."

Acknowledgements

I wish to extend my gratitude to the entire teaching community of the Academic College of Society and the Arts, for maintaining an atmosphere which encourages creativity, involvement and collaboration. Special thanks are due to the teachers who participated in the survey: Anat Eindor, Anat Wolf, Daphna Finkelstein-Yaakobi, Dana Shaham, Dr. Elana Lakh, Gili Navoth, Janice Shapiro, Dr. Liat Shamri Ze'evi, Dr. Michal Lev, Michal Weller, Noa Danziger, Dr. Noga Ariel-Galor, Orly Balasha Ilan, Pazit Dushy, Reuma Weinberg, Roxana Sztyglic, Sharon Papay, Shevy Medzini. Their ideas and insights echoed the theoretical concepts presented in the chapter and added their rich personal experience in teaching art therapy. Working with them has been a great privilege. I also wish to thank my old friend Talia Graveh, for her long-lasting encouragement and my husband Ariel for his constant support, patience and help.

References

Amabile, T. (1982) "Social Psychology of Creativity: A Consensual Assessment Technique" *Journal of Personality and Social Psychology,* 43, 997-1013.

Amabile, T. (1996) *Creativity in Context.* Boulder, Co: Westview Press.

Arieti, S. (1976) *Creativity: The Magic Synthesis.* New York: Basic Books.

Brull, F. (1973) "Divrei Ptiha" [Opening Remarks] in *Yetsiratiut [Creativity]*, edited by Erika Landau. Tel Aviv: Gomeh (Hebrew).

Brinkman, D. (2010) "Teaching Creatively and Teaching for Creativity" *Arts Education Policy Review*, 111(2), 48-50.

Chan, D. (2007) "Creative Teaching in Hong Kong Schools: Constraints and Challenges" *Educational Research Journal*, 22(1), 1-12.

Cremin, T. (2009a) *Teaching English Creatively.* London: Routledge.

Cremin, T. (2009b) "Creative Teaching and Creative Teachers" in *Creativity in Primary Education*, A. Wilson (ed.). Exeter: Learning Matters.

Cortright, R., Collins H., Dicarlo S. (2005) "Peer Instruction Enhanced Meaningful Learning: Ability to Solve Novel Problems" *Advances in Physiology Education*, 29(2), 107-111.

Crouch, C., Mazur E. (2001) "Peer Instruction: Ten Years of Experience and Results" *American Journal of Physics*, 69, 970.

Crutchfied, R. (1962) "Conformity and Creative Thinking" in *Contemporary Approaches to Creative Thinking*, H. Gruber, M. Wertheimer (eds.). New York: Atherton.

Edmonds, K., Hammond M. (2012) "How Can Visual Arts Help Doctors Develop Medical Insight?" *The International Journal of Arts & Design Education*, 31(1), 78-89.

Fryer, M., Collings J. (1991) "British Teachers' Views of Creativity" *The Journal of Creative Behavior,* 25, 75-81.

Gardner, H. (1982) *Art, Mind, and Brain: A Cognitive Approach to Creativity*. New York: Basic Books.

Guilford, J. P. (1956) "The Structure of Intellect" *Psychological Bulletin,* 53, 267-293.

Gustina, C., Sweet R. (2014) "Creatives Teaching Creativity" *The International Journal of Art and Design Education*, 33(1), 46-54.

Hilgard, E., Bower G. (1975) *Theories of Learning* (Fourth ed.). Englewood Cliffs, NJ: Prentice-Hall.

Jeffrey, B., Craft A. (2004) "Teaching Creatively and Teaching for Creativity: Distinctions and Relationships" *Educational Studies*, 30(1), 77-97.

Jung, C. (1964) *Man and His Symbols*. New York: Anchor Books.

Koestler, A. (1964) *The Act* of *Creation.* New York: Dell.

Ludwig, A. (1995) *The Price of Greatness: Resolving the Creativity and Madness Controversy*. New York: Guilford Press.

Landau, E. (1973) *Yetsiratiut [Creativity]*. Tel Aviv: Gomeh. (Hebrew).

Maslow, A. (1967) "The Creative Attitude" in *Explorations in Creativity*, R. Mooney, T. Razik (eds.). New York: Harper & Row.

McGraw, K. (1978) "The Detrimental Effects of Reward on Performance: A Literature Review and a Prediction Model" in *The Hidden Costs of Reward*, M. Lepper, D. Greene (eds.). Hillsdale, NJ: Erlbaum.

Meggs, S., Greer A. (2011) "Perspectives on Interdisciplinary Pedagogy" *Design Principles & Practice: An International Journal*, 5(2), 205-218.

Merari, D. (1997) "Creativity: Theoretical Aspects and Their Implications in the Teaching of Occupational Therapy" *The Israeli Journal of Occupational Therapy*, 6(2), H51-H62 (Hebrew).

Mullen, C. (ed.) (2019). *Creativity Under Duress in Education?* New York: Springer.

National Advisory Committee on Creative and Cultural Education (NACCCE) (1999) *All Our Futures: The Report of the National Advisory Committee on Creative and Cultural Education*. London: DfEE/DCMS.

Newell, A., Simon H. (1972) *Human Problem Solving.* Englewood Cliffs, NJ: Prentice-Hall.

Osborn, A. (1953) *Applied Imagination: Principles and Procedures of Creative Thinking.* New York: Scribner's.

Rogers, C. (1954) "Towards a Theory of Creativity" *ETC Review of General Semantics,* 11, 249-260.

Rossman, J. (1931) *The Psychology of the Inventor.* Washington DC: Inventors Publishing.

Sass, L. (1992) *Madness and Modernism: Insanity in the Light of Modern Art, Literature and Thought*. New York: Basic Books.

Schank, R., Abelson R. (1980) *Scripts, Plans, Goals and Understanding.* Hillsdale, NJ: Erlbaum.

Slabbert, J. (1994) "Creativity in Education Revisited: Reflection in Aid of Progression" *The Journal of Creative Behavior,* 28, 60-69.

Stack, S., Lester D. (2009) *Suicide and the Creative Arts*. New York: Nova Science Publishers.

Sternberg, R. (ed.) (1988) *The Nature of Creativity*. Cambridge: Cambridge University Press.

Sternberg, R. (2013) *Investment Theory of Creativity*. Retrieved Aug. 31, 2020.
http://www.robertjsternberg.com/investment-theory-of-creativity.

Taylor, C. (1964) *Creativity: Progress and Potential*. New York: McGraw-Hill.

Wallas, G. (1926) *The Art of Thought*. New York: Harcourt Brace.

Wang, K., Nickerson J. (2017) "A Literature Review on Individual Creativity Support Systems" *Computers in Human Behavior*, 74(7-8), 139-151.

Winnicott, D. (1971) *Playing and Reality*. London: Tavistock.

Yu, C. X., Subramanian G. (2017) "A Mentoring Approach for Developing Creativity in Teaching" *Malaysian Journal of ELT Research*, 14(2), 1-19.

CHAPTER 13

PAINTING AN ART-BASED RESEARCH OF INTIMACY

MICHAL LEV

Introduction

Sit with me
on a garden-bench
the hours are ours to spend
Feel the grass,
tickling the toes
hear my silence interludes
Recall how close we used to be
how far we are,
my dear

I have written and painted for as long as I can remember. When I immerse in artmaking, some force of energy takes control over me, with the capacity to make me calmer, more serene and connected to myself. During my art therapy studies, I identified these experiences as intimate. Working with couples and families, through art psychotherapy, I have witnessed art's similar effects on my clients' connection to self and their relations to others. However, quite surprisingly, within the arts and therapy fields, in-depth attention has not been given to the linkage between artistic expression and the phenomenon of intimacy.

The positive relationship between intimacy and well-being was established over the years, suggesting that high levels of intimacy are linked to the quality of relationship and to one's sense of self (Kabat-Zinn & Salzberg, 2018). Several researchers highlighted the significance of increased intimacy in the success of therapy and claimed that the therapeutic space, and relationship between therapists to patients, facilitated, aspired for, and honored the creation of intimacy (Schaverien, 2020). I was surprised to find a connection between intimacy and sexuality, one that may explain its exclusion from proper therapeutic discourse, mainly rendering it taboo.

Despite the importance of intimacy to well-being and in relationships, I found multiple definitions for intimacy within the literature, among which were closeness, familiarity with, warmth and affection (Collins, 2012). However, rather than defining the concept of intimacy, these definitions explored the intimate experience and suggest that certain conditions, which include elements of trust, deep knowing, empathy, and consent, must be present for humans to achieve intimacy with each other (Blass, 2017; Wieden, 2018).

Perhaps the value of intimacy for well-being and relationships, together with its various definitions, lead to the multiple assessment models that strive to understand the phenomenon better. These models use quantifiable measures and rating scales, and approach intimacy as an inter-personal phenomenon, between close people and mainly couples (Leonard, 2014; Schaefer & Olson, 1981; Sinclair & Dowdy, 2005). I found these approaches and scales to be limiting in understanding intimacy's deeper sense.

This chapter presents my art-based research of intimacy as an intrapersonal phenomenon. My research inquired if and how the process of painting and drawing, together with witnessing and reflection on the process and imagery, further an understanding of intimacy. I also asked whether particular qualities and features of artistic media, processes, and reflection through video footage editing, could further intimate experience.

The research was built on findings from a pilot study (Lev, 2016) where I approached intimacy as a temporary experience of body and mind, in which we feel closeness and familiarity within certain conditions. It suggests four qualities of painting, video editing, witnessing and reflection on the creative process, and artworks as facilitators of intimate experiences: (1) persistence and continued immersion, (2) physical proximity and zooming in, (3) attention to detail, and (4) sensuousness.

Methodology

Choosing the paradigm for my inquiry of intimacy, I postulated what is research? To me, it means an ongoing search for meaning. Research should facilitate my understanding of a topic and bring about a renewed vision. It hypothesizes, or plants questions and then tills the ground to enable growth and development in unpredictable ways. It presents examinations and explorations thoroughly and with a constant congruence to context (McNiff, 2018). How knowledge is developed and formed and who it serves and for what purpose were questions I aimed to address through the method of my research study.

It has already been established, empirically and scientifically, that creativity and art can lead to other ways of knowing in research (Allen, 2016; Fried, 2019; Kalmanowitz, 2018). When it comes to exploring social and psychological phenomena, the arts have access to places where words do not and can act as a mediator for deep exploration of self (Lev, 2020b; Summer et al, 2017). The solid ground of quantitative research methods makes us step out of our comfort zone to make way for innovative inquiry (McNiff, 2019), as in Bachelard's (1964) method of taking knowledge apart, breaking up concepts, and then constructing and rebuilding them in a new way.

I used art-based research methods, involving me as the researcher and participant co-researchers (hereinafter: "co-researchers"), in the process of drawing and painting as a mode of inquiry. The study was assembled incrementally, with respect for the way in which new knowledge and discoveries emerge from the creative process.

Four adults, between the ages of thirty and eighty, who are familiar with the creation of visual art, participated in the study. They varied in their socio-cultural characteristics, such as age, gender, economic status, ethnic and religious roots, sexual orientation, and marital status. Among them were two males and two females. Before their participation in the study, I approached each of them by phone and presented the research topic, the research questions, and settings. Five individual sessions were held with each participant: three experimental sessions and two reflective sessions of approximately ninety minutes each. I informed the co-researchers that the first three sessions would take place in their private studio places, where I would witness them drawing and painting using their choice of media and materials. I would then conduct a verbal discussion about their reflections on the painting process and imagery, in order to explore their understanding of intimacy. The two reflective sessions with each participant (sessions four and five, in sequence) included the viewing of edited videos, followed by a verbal discussion about the research questions and findings.

I, the researcher, a secular Jewish woman in my mid-40s, live and practice art and psychotherapy with couples and families in central Israel. For practical reasons, the research was conducted mainly in my country of residence, which may have inherent sociocultural consequences and biases. Despite these conditions, I made every effort to recruit widely from all groups living in Israel and respect the co-researchers' rights and the integrity of their unique experience and backgrounds.

To further comfort, ease and support authentic expression, the setting of the study included multiple locations, which were the personal workspaces of each participant. Co-researchers were recruited through self-referrals and acquaintances, drawn from the general public, artists, and mental health professionals.

The Research process

The research was constructed of six modes of inquiry as interdependent elements:

1. ***Drawing and painting by the co-researchers in three experimental sessions lasting approximately 90 minutes***

This phase took place in the private studio space of each co-researcher while I was present as an active witness, similar to my presence during art-therapy sessions in which the client creates art while the therapist witnesses the process. The co-researchers wore a head-mount video camera while they drew and painted to enable direct focus on their hands and imagery during the process (image 1). They were free to choose their own media, art materials, and subjects of painting. Their relationship and gaze were centered on the painting. I sat on a chair a little behind them, trying as much as possible not to interfere or affect their process.

My position as an active witness made use of my emotional openness and a felt sense that provided information in answering the research questions. Without my being explicit about it, my "baseline" position signaled to the co-researchers that they were free to become intimate with their work. Most of the co-researchers' studio spaces included numerous artworks that had been painted by them in the past. The imagery of their artworks also functioned as silent witnesses to their painting process and reflections.

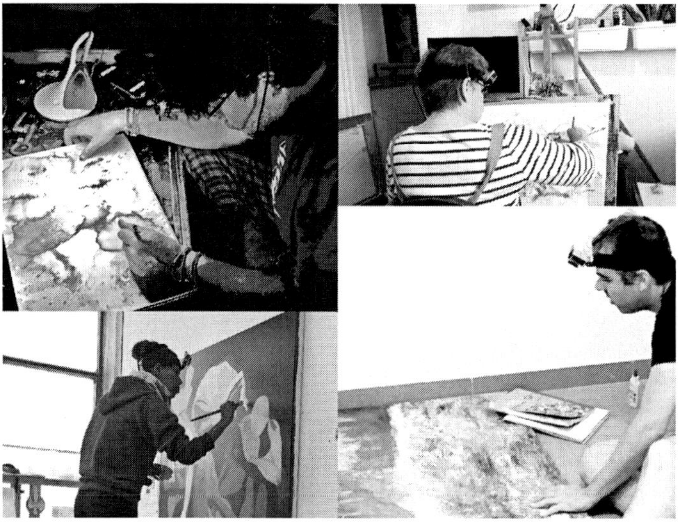

Image 1. The co-researchers wore a head-mount video camera while they drew and painted © Michal Lev.

2. *Reflective discussion with each co-researcher immediately after the experimental sessions*

The discussion that followed each painting session was conducted while the two of us were seated in the studio space, looking at the painted artwork of that session. I was interested in the co-researchers' experiences and reflection with the eventual goal of discussing their understanding of intimacy. I directed co-researchers' attention to physical, visceral information, inquired about their definition of intimacy and discussed if, and how it was affected by their painting session and reflections. The discussion also asked about specific qualities of their art materials and techniques, as furthering the intimate experience.

The experimental sessions were documented by audio and video recordings, which were then uploaded to my computer and saved on the cloud. Since all the co-researchers were Israelis, the discussions were held in Hebrew. After each session, I transferred the recorded files to my PC, played the files aloud, translated them from Hebrew to English, and transcribed them to Microsoft Word documents. I was careful to maintain the accuracy of the co-researchers' ideas, to keep information from getting lost in translation. The printed English transcriptions served as an additional mode of inquiry. Multiple readings of the documents allowed me to become intimate with the texts, while devoting time and attention to the words, in search of essential passages that addressed the research questions. During the systematic analysis of the transcriptions, recurring elements and motives stood out as identifying qualities.

3. ***My artistic responses to individual sessions and the process of inquiry as a whole***

I used painting as a mode of interpretation for my experience as a silent witness to the co-researchers' painting processes. I utilized the same painting media, materials, and techniques that the co-researchers used in each experimental session, as I painted alone in my own studio space. My attempts to trust the natural flow of conversation with each co-researcher led to the primacy of my artistic response, because the participants did not necessarily articulate qualities of intimacy and the discussions did not yield direct answers to the research questions. I looked for ways to help me get closer to the participants, to understand them and their painting processes. Therefore, I used art's manifold ways of knowing.

Process guides from my pilot research (Lev, 2016) were used to further my examination of the artistic experience and the co-researchers' understanding of intimacy. The following seven questions focused on the process of painting and the artworks that resulted: *What is the nature of intimacy? What do I see (i.e., what painting materials I used, their characteristics, the technique used)? How comfortable do I feel now? Were there moments of intimate experience during the painting process? What do I feel toward the artwork? Did I have any insights? If it could speak, what would it say to me?* It is important to note that not all the questions presented necessarily required a verbal or written response, but did offer an open platform for responsive expression.

In addition to responding to each session with the research questions in mind, I waited at least one week following the third experimental session with the co-researchers, and responded artistically to the whole body of work that each one generated. The rationale behind this stage was to explore the effect that many artworks-as-witnesses might have on intimate experience.

I also videotaped, journaled, and then systematically reviewed the sessions of Phase Three.

4. *A private exhibition*

The exhibition, which took place after the three experimental sessions with the co-researchers, and my own response-art sessions that followed, consisted of 28 artworks (the co-researchers' artworks and my own response art). I arranged the artworks in the studio space so as to dedicate a specific area per participant, hoping to assimilate a community created by families of artworks (image 2). Presented for myself alone, the exhibition continued for a couple of weeks, with the goal of reflecting upon the research questions, relationships between the artworks and their possible impact when they are viewed and experienced together. I photographed, videotaped, and examined this part of the process as well.

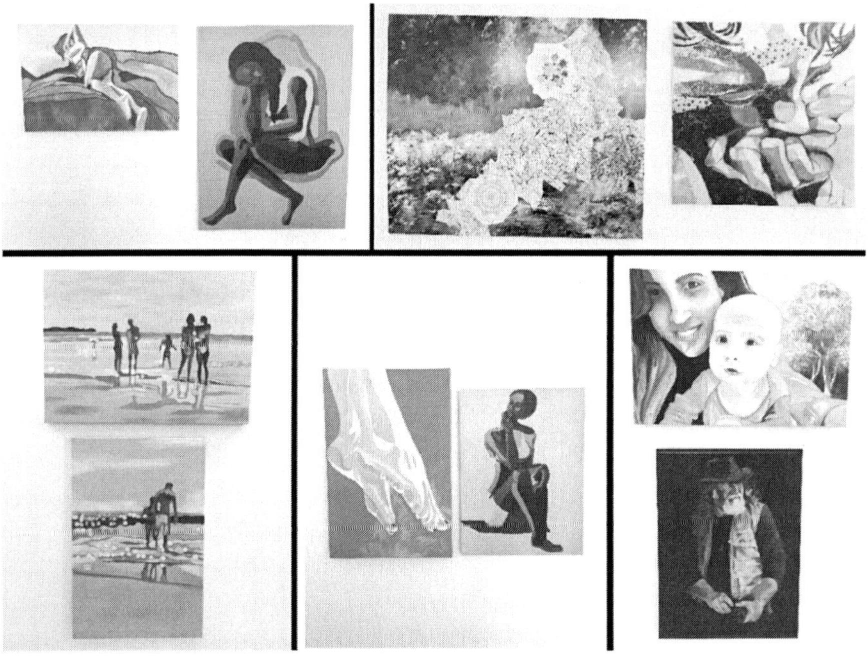

Image 2. The private exhibition © Michal Lev.

5. *The creation of edited videos*

For each participant in the study (the co-researchers and myself), I created five edited videos, approximately ten to fifteen minutes long. The process of editing the video footage included multiple viewings of the video files produced during the experimental painting sessions of the co-researchers. It also included my response-art to their sessions, photographs of the processes and artworks, the transcribed texts, and my journals. My careful examination of video footage included being intimate with the body of work, while cropping and organizing videotaped moments that seemed to echo ideas from the verbal discussions and response art sessions, informing the research questions.

I devoted attention to the participants' use of art materials and their hand and body movements, by noting the time and duration of significant repeated gestures. I noted what their painting routine included and how much time they spent on preparations and readying themselves for the painting process. I examined how long it took them to become encapsulated within the process, as well as what encouraged their persistent immersion in painting, and what interfered with it. I looked at how attentive they were to their environment, to my presence, how they used each material, how they held their painting tools, and so on.

Since I did not initiate or encourage any conversation during the painting sessions, it was easier to direct my attention to their hands and their head movements. I noted the amount of time they spent in each phase of the painting process. I was able to note their physical distance from the painting through the enlarged or reduced the size of the painted imagery, in the frame, when they moved closer to or farther away from the painting. I wondered whether I should include sections of significant points and ideas from the transcribed texts of the discussions, and whether I should add any background music. I realized the considerable impact such details could have on the general outcomes of my research project. This mode of inquiry accentuated the value of using video footage editing as a research inquiry and systematic analysis mode.

Each edited video was labeled, uploaded to a private YouTube channel, and then saved on my computer and the cloud.

A systematic review of the research process

I made every effort to maintain credibility and transparency, by exploring all of the information generated from the research study from various perspectives. Transcribing and translating conversations added to the multimodal way of looking at the information, akin to triangulation. Words brought ideas and experiences into consciousness, the video honed-in on movements, and imagery formed a conduit to imagination and free thought.

The various modalities complemented, differentiated, and informed one another.

While distilling the results from my sessions with co-researchers, I realized that my attempt not to bias them with my understanding of intimacy led me to avoid asking them, explicitly, to answer the research questions. Instead, I planted the questions in their minds at the beginning of each experimental session, hoping that they would address the questions during the verbal discussions. When specific answers to the research questions were not sufficiently provided, I understood that some change in the research design was required. At least one additional session with co-researchers was required, in which they would specifically address the research questions.

6. *Culminating discussion and review with participant co-researchers*

This phase included two reflective sessions with each co-researcher. In the first session (session number four in sequence), I met with each of the co-researchers to watch their individual edited videos, encouraged their reflection on the video, and discussed the research questions through specific derivatives. The information generated from these discussions was systematically explored and added to the total collection of research materials that was included in the final edited video of the complete research project. During the creation of this final video, which was eight minutes long, I identified elements that were common and different for all the participants, in answering the research questions. Each co-researcher was then invited to a concluding discussion in which they viewed the final edited video, and then reflected and reviewed the research findings.

Final sessions with co-researchers

After the fourth meeting with each co-researcher, I updated my research findings to reflect new information that emerged.

As I found the video footage editing process to be a vitally important resource in my systematic review and meaning making, I created another video to sum-up the research to that point. The summary video was approximately eight minutes long. This inclusive video was comprised of footage from all the participants' processes, as an examination, review, and answers to the updated research questions. After examining and studying the results, co-researchers were invited to a fifth and final individual session, to review and reflect upon the research findings. The sessions were recorded, transcribed, and translated into English. Each session began by watching the inclusive edited video that comprised an interpretation and review of the research project, and was followed by a verbal discussion of the research findings through the following questions:

1. What is your reflection on the inclusive edited video?
2. What do you feel about the research outcomes that were presented?
3. Do you have any reservations about these findings?
4. Do you have any suggestions/thoughts/ideas for future research?
5. What is the value of this research project for you?

These sessions helped to hone and distill the results of the research. After the sessions, I made more changes to the final edited video, *Painting Intimacy — Final Edited Movie,* and updated my research findings.

Results

The participants suggested that the phenomenon of intimacy consists of two operational elements: (1) commitment to the present moment, and (2) looking closely.

Commitment to the present moment, and looking closely

The experimental sessions took place in the private studio space of each co-researcher. While the co-researchers worked, I took care to sit one or two meters away, to minimize distractions during their creative process. This short distance enabled me to become familiar with their artistic space and to see how it was organized. I followed their procedures, rhythms, and movements, and gradually felt closer to them. After the first ten minutes or so, I was completely present in the moment, attentive and focused. I welcomed any thought or question that emerged and wrote it down in my notepad. I paid attention to my breathing, emotions, and any perceptions and thoughts that could inform the research project.

Just as I was committed to the present moment, so were the co-researchers. They had their own ways of setting up their creative space, physically and mentally. During the discussions that followed their painting processes, they all explained how painting required that they be completely present and committed, and that this was possible only if they had gone through the required steps before and during their painting session. Once they were ready, their commitment to the present moment was demonstrated by the qualities that we identified later.

Witnessing their creative processes, I noticed certain changes and transformations taking place in their demeanor, as they painted. I observed differences in their body movements, rhythms, posture, and focus of attention. As time progressed, the participants made fewer and slower movements, and their breathing became steady. They leaned toward their paintings in order to be closer to them. Their painting hand remained in one spot for longer periods of time, and they looked closely at the imagery being created. I experienced similar states in my own response art sessions and during the process of editing the video footage. I became immersed in the creative process as my artwork progressed and developed. I was completely present in the moment. No distractions, physical or mental, interfered with what I did, and I noticed myself looking closely at what was in front of me.

The process of editing footage revealed and strengthened what the co-researchers defined as *intimate moments*. These were signified by a slower rhythm of motion, fewer hand movements, and a steady grip on the painting tools. During such moments, the head-mounted camera movements were much slower, and the proximity of the camera lens to the painting was very close. Such moments were underscored by moments that took place before and after them, showing faster, and rapid handwork on the painted medium, movements toward and away from the painting, with a greater distance between the head-mounted camera and the painting. The participants later described these moments as *non-intimate moments*. Such moments consisted mainly of preparing their studio space and art materials, fidgety gestures, and faster breathing.

I resonated with the co-researchers' perceptions of *intimate moments* and *non-intimate moments* through my own experience of intimacy, as I edited the video footage. I was surprised to find intimacy in this methodological phase of the research project. When I sat in front of my computer screen, looking closely at the photos and streaming visuals, I began to lose track of time and became less aware of my environment. My attention, my body, and my mind were focused entirely on the video footage, and *tempus fugit.* The slower and steadier the images and hand movement on the screen became, the closer I felt to them. Moreover, the I-position viewpoint enabled by the GoPro video camera led me to experience seeing as the other sees, which furthered intimacy. These insights led to the identification of the two qualities: commitment to the present moment and looking closely as necessary components of intimacy.

Features of art-making that further intimate experience

Conversations with co-researchers after each experimental session and after viewing the edited videos, highlighted particular features of their painting processes and materials, as furthering the intimate experience. The empirical facilitators that they mentioned were (1) persistence and continued immersion, (2) being physically close and zooming in, (3) attention to detail, and (4) sensuousness. While I have listed these elements separately for the purpose of presentation and definition, we found them to be interrelated and interdependent components of intimacy.

Persistence and continued immersion

Painting and drawing as creative activities, develop through a process over time. While the participants' subjects, materials, painting style, and techniques differed greatly from one another, some characteristics of their painting processes and the development of their works were similar. Each participant began by getting into the mood of painting. They explained that the transition from their day-to-day tasks to painting required attention, as well as physical and mental preparation.

Eran immerses in painting for four to five hours every morning and ends most days in the same way. He said that during these hours the phone does not ring, everything is quiet, and he can devote himself entirely to the creative process. The time that he devoted to painting drew him closer to himself and enabled him to visit places in himself that he would not have visited otherwise.

All the co-researchers had similar insights. Nir experienced prolonged immersion in painting-as-healing, which could make him physically healthier when he felt ill or alienated. He attributed these features to the repetitive movements of his hand while painting – movements that pulled him toward his center, his core. Ofira lent support to this statement by referring to the movements of her hand and paintbrush as meditative, calm, and intimate.

Being physically close and zooming in

Closeness and zooming in were identified as bearing a direct relation to intimacy. When the co-researchers were asked to define the intimate experience, they used terms such as "being close," "closeness," and "looking closely." The word *close* appeared many times, with variations, across the different methodology stages and information sources.

This was verified when I witnessed co-researchers paint during the sessions. They placed themselves close to the painting that they were working on and to the materials that they used (Image 4). Their painting processes required their direct involvement to develop. A synergy existed between the physical proximity of participants to their painted platforms, materials (referred to as an *other*), and their closeness to their own experiences. Eran used a technical pen with a thin, sharp, point to contour shapes of dried ink on paper. He described this phase within his painting process as intimate because it revealed forms within imagery that he might have overlooked — forms that reminded him of the sea he loved.

Physical closeness to the art materials and the painting was also apparent in Nirit's work. She explained that keeping her body close to the canvas helped her to remain focused on the act of painting and feel closer to the imagery that she was creating. As I edited the video footage, I noticed that the subjects in the frame were enlarged and remained still throughout the long duration of the painting process. The participants' bodies leaned toward their paintings and the movements of their brushes or other painting tools slowed. In the culminating sessions with the co-researchers after they viewed the edited videos, they admitted that the angle and perspective of the shots made the development of their paintings seem tangible. Their experience was intimate and close. They attested to feeling empathy and closeness as they zoomed in on the image that was shown on the screen.

The participants' use of artistic media for bringing back the memory of an *other* also resulted in closeness. Ofira was reminded of her friend by using the color umber brown; Nir's choice of material and technique reminded him of a client who painted in the same way. Nirit said that the subjects of her paintings made her feel close and connected to them. Similarly, in my response to Ofira's first session, I painted a portrait of my stepdaughter and her baby boy and noticed how looking closely at her physical features made me feel closer to her.

Attention to detail

During the culminating sessions with co-researchers, as they viewed the edited videos, they saw their magnified images, due to the close-ups, in such detail that it was almost like seeing them anew. It made Nir pay more attention to details in the painting process and imagery than he did while painting them. Ofira and Nirit, who saw their paintings in their earlier stages, thanks to the video recording, echoed Nir's reaction. Ofira's emotional response to the artwork's unfinished state was like seeing a child's photo album. This analogy felt intimate to her.

All of the participants paid careful attention to detail throughout the painting process. Eran treated the painting materials with respect and appreciation for the way they inform his process. He recalled intimate moments when the imagery revealed small, seemingly insignificant details. The empathy and care he felt for the painting tools, his interest in them and his familiarity with their characteristics, were intimate to him.

During my response art sessions, my method of imitating the co-researchers' painting techniques was similar to Stanislavski's (Benedetti, 1999) "art of experiencing" (p. 202). This helped me gain insight into what they referred to as *intimate* and *non-intimate moments* during their painting processes. My notes following these sessions showed that my attention to the details of their work helped me to think about them during my own painting process and feel intimacy with them.

As the co-researchers and I reflected on imagery, we became aware of elements within the artworks that influenced one another. A line had its own contour, but also framed the elements next to it. Attention to the surrounding space/environment was also evident during the process of editing the video footage. I struggled with the task of choosing photos, looking at one after the other in my search for the ones that reflected the co-researchers' ideas. Each choice highlighted a different momentum within the painting process, and so carried a different quality.

My effort to be accountable for the co-researchers' definitions of intimacy led me to consider various options in great detail, such as the length of time that each photo was shown in the video timeline, the photos in their proximity to one another, the transition between motion and stills, and the addition of subtitles, sound and other details that might inform the research project. Once these elements were combined in the edited video, they felt like siblings within a family, and their permanence, as components of the video established their connection firmly as an intimate community.

Sensuousness

The element of sensuousness was one of the first that the co-researchers identified as furthering an intimate experience. Their descriptions of colors, textures, and smells were consistent throughout our conversations and the concluding discussions. Even when they spoke about an inner voice, they referred to listening as the essential attribute and spoke of how intimacy allowed for the acknowledgment of sensuousness within their painting processes. It was no surprise that all the participants described the painting process as engaging most or all of their senses.

Nir's creative process included touching art materials with his hands, tearing pieces of paper for a collage, placing glue onto the canvas, smearing oil pastels, squeezing the glue tube, and rubbing dried glue off his fingers. During our discussions he explained that the materials' tangible qualities enhanced his experience as he painted, and that touching the art materials helped him to learn their features and discover their creative possibilities.

Eran's painting process also included direct contact with the painting materials. After each painting session, his studio space, clothing, and fingers were covered with blue ink stains. He said that painting was an inseparable part of his identity and his daily life. Similarly, for him, the images that he painted were witnesses of sea life, and the sea was a witness to his painting process: "The sea, my image, the art materials – we are intertwined, intimately involved, and influence one another".

The other participants also said that the sensory qualities of the materials furthered intimate experience. Nirit described a physical sensation she had every time she mixed and stirred color pastes. She explained that this process was intimate because one material touched and influenced the other. Ofira acknowledged that her daily arrival in the studio space, the sensuous smell of oil colors that grew stronger, and her continued immersion in painting invited an experience of intimacy.

All the participants spoke of an embodied perception of detail that was interwoven in the painting process – a perception that required no verbal explanation, which made them feel they belonged and connected to the image they were working on, to their materials, and to their creative space.

Discussion

Intimacy and artmaking ask for a pause in the race of life. I used art-based methodologies that included six interdependent modes of inquiry to explore whether the process of painting, together with witnessing and reflection on the process and imagery, could further our understanding of intimacy.

Operational elements of intimacy

The findings were consistent and affirmative in identifying two operational elements of intimacy: commitment to the present moment and looking closely.

Commitment to the present moment & looking closely

The participants described meditative aspects within their process of painting that can be related to repetitive hand movements and their mindful concentration on the craftsmanship that painting involves. Their views echoed those of Bachelard (1994), who believed that intimacy requires exploration, searching and researching to discover the new in the familiar, and other painters that noted how persistent immersion in painting was meditative and mindful as the writings of many researchers revealed (Kalmanowitz, et al, 2018)

The development of artistic process and product over a period of time required participants in this study to immerse in the task continually and extensively. The effect time had on the participants' experiences of intimacy suggests the temporal nature of intimacy. Similarly, Dissanayake (2015) referred to the aspect of time in both intimacy and artmaking and their capacity to make us feel known by another for a temporary time. Moreover, the process of meaning-making in observation and dialogues (McNiff, 2019), required spending time with imagery as several approaches to art-therapy suggest.

The co-researchers acknowledged a relation between the art materials to the body, the space, and the mind during artmaking. This notion supports art-based researchers, who referred to artmaking as facilitating agents to be in the moment, as an embodied aspect to intimacy (Fried, 2019; Miller, 2012). Other expressive therapists suggested an experience in which the body and mind entwined, bestowing the capacity to enable centering of the self (Dissanayake, 2015; Summer, 2017). This was affirmed by the co-researchers, who indicated that looking closely at their paintings revealed forms within imagery they might have overlooked.

Several other researchers referred to a new aspect of looking during painting, inviting the creator and viewer to see the subject of their familiarity differently (Fish, 2016) by engaging a powerful gaze, intertwined with a deep emotional relationship that was developed towards the imagery (Allen, 2016).

Features of artistic media and processes that further intimacy

In exploring whether certain features of artistic media, processes and reflection through video editing could further intimate experience, four interrelated and interdependent qualities of artistic media were identified: persistence and continued immersion, physical closeness and zooming in, attention to detail, and sensuousness.

Persistence and continued immersion

I found that the creative process was manifold and complex, and that surprises and challenges drew the painters closer to the process and kept them committed. My findings echoed descriptions of artists and educators being pulled by an urge to make art continuously, and their never-ending learning process that informed their self-awareness (Orbach, 2016).

The co-researchers reported that the long periods they spent in painting were necessary for the development of their artworks and that these kept pace with their emotional transformation, by drawing them closer and visiting inner parts, rarely visited. Their words resonate with Schaverien, who proposed that we long for intimacies in art because they reveal places that are normally unacknowledged, unlit, nor seen (2020), and that art could present what we know to exist but are not always aware of (Duckrow Fonda, 2017). Viewing the edited videos, the co-researchers described seeing their images anew, due to the close-ups that magnified and focused on details. This was described to be intimate.

Physical proximity and zooming in

The findings suggest a synergistic integration between physical proximity to the artworks, materials and tools, and our closeness to our own experiences. This echoes Kasulis (2002) who explained that intimate familiarity with *others* occurs when the experiences become second nature, like artists' tools that function as extensions of their hands with familiar qualities. Similarly, the study of Rubesin, Chen, Fried, Lev and Teoli (in press) showed that art-making and close proximity of the painters and viewers to the painting promoted tacit knowledge, contemplation, and deepened their understanding.

Closeness was also achieved by the use of artistic media for evoking the memory of an *other*. A specific hue, painting tool, hand movement, the subjects of the painting, or the technique could bring back the memory of a close person. My findings expand researchers who argued that intimacy involves two or more people (Schaefer & Olson, 1981), in suggesting intimacy to be intra-personal (within the person) as well. My approach was demonstrated by the close proximity of the participants to the painting they worked on and the materials they used.

Attention to detail

The proximity to the paintings during the creative process enabled being attentive to aesthetic elements and qualities of the images; to the lines, hues, forms, and to areas of the paintings that required more care. The observations of McNiff (2018), who spent extensive amount of time in studying the qualities of imagery intimately, were echoed during the discussions with the co-researchers. They indicated that this type of attention increased their interest and curiosity regarding the aesthetic nuances of imagery, materials, and tools.

My prolonged witnessing of the painting process was found to invite intimacy into the creative space in a mode of listening-inward and listening-outward (Lev, 2019). This involved being present in the moment, committed, and attentive to detail. Similarly, interpreting my experience through painting in the response art sessions raised an awareness of details that informed the research questions. This was influenced by becoming close to the material as Havesteen-Franklin and Camarena Altamirano (2015) suggested.

Sensuousness

The co-researchers spoke of how intimacy allowed for the acknowledgment of sensuousness in their painting processes and how it engages most or all of their senses. Their observations support Strawn and Falick, who found that artistic activities performed with the hands, were satisfying (2007). The sensual aspects within intimacy were also observed by Dissanayake, who related the rhythms and sensorimotor engagement within creative activities to inducing primal memories that are instilled in us as humans (2015).

Touching the art materials was also a way for the participants to learn their features and creative possibilities, as Bachelard (1994) noted that intimacy was gained by an inner vision, characterized by a deep familiarity — with one's passion, with light, colors, or form. The participants spoke of an intimate embodied perception of detail that was interwoven in the painting process — a perception that required no verbal explanation, made them feel that they belonged to and were connected to the image they were working on, their materials, and their creative space.

The research findings acknowledge these fundamental elements to be naturally present in creative endeavors and thus, highlight the connection between artmaking and intimacy.

Conclusion

This art-based research suggests that intimacy be included in the general discourse of psychotherapy and no longer regarded as taboo, and that intimacy's healing effect on mental health and well-being for the individual be taken seriously.

Through six methodological phases, participants in this study distinguished between intimate moments and non-intimate moments. The descriptions of colors, textures, and smell were consistent throughout the research in their ability to engage the participants in the creative endeavor for an extended period of time, without draining their energies but instead, rejuvenate them.

The findings also emphasize how video surprisingly furthered intimate experience and how the use of GoPro video camera, the way it was used, enabled seeing experience as others see it, enhancing intimate experience. This discovery could have ramifications for future research in the field.

The research suggests the important role of artmaking in furthering understanding and awareness of intimate experiences and highlights the potential role of expressive therapies in providing the conditions to invite intimacy into our space.

References

Allen, P. (2016) "Art Making as Spiritual Path" (pp. 178-188) in J. A. Rubin (ed.), *Approaches to art therapy: Theory and technique*. Brunner-Routledge.

Antal, A. B. (2013) "Art-based Research for Engaging not-knowing in Organizations" *Journal of Applied Arts & Health,* 4(1), 67-76.

Bachelard, G. ([1969] 1994) *The Poetics of Space* (2nd ed.). Beacon Press.

Blass, R. D. (2017) "Intimacy vs Love: A Tension between New and Traditional Analytic Conceptions of Relatedness" *The IPA 50th Congress: Intimacy*. Buenos Aires, Argentina

Duckrow Fonda, S. (2017) *Filmmaking as Artistic Inquiry: An Examination of Ceramic Art Therapy in a Maximum-security Forensic Psychiatric Facility* [Dissertation, Lesley University]. ProQuest Dissertations & Theses Global.

Fish, B. J. (2016) *Art-based Supervision: Cultivating Therapeutic Insight through Imagery*. Routledge.

Fried, D. (2019) *An Art-Based Study of Adult Perspectives on Attention-Deficit Hyperactivity Disorder*.

Havesteen-Franklin, D., Camarena Altamirano, J. (2015) "Containing the Uncontainable: Responsive Art Making in Art Therapy as a Method to Facilitate Mentallisation" *International Journal of Art Therapy*, 20(2), 54-65.

Intimacy (2012) *English Dictionary – Complete & Unabridged.*

Kabat-Zinn, J., Salzberg, S. (2018) *Lovingkindness: The Revolutionary Art of Happiness*. Shambhala.

Kalmanowitz, D., Marcow Speiser, V., Schwartz, S., Kossak, M. (2018). "Arts-based Disaster Relief: An Overview of Psychosocial Responses and Practices" *Journal of Applied Arts & Health,* 9(2), 149-156.

Leonard, R. C., Knott, L. E., Lee, E. B., Singh, S., Smith, A. H., Kanter, J., Wetterneck, C. T. (2014) "The Development of the Functional Analytic Psychotherapy Intimacy Scale" *The Psychological Record,* 64(4), 647-657.

Lev, M. (2016) *Art as a Mediator for Intimacy* [Pilot Study]. Lesley University.

—. (2020a) "Art as a Mediator for Intimacy: Reflections of an Art-Based Research Study" *Journal of Applied Arts and Health,* 11(3), 1-15.

—. (2020b) "Intimacy through Painting" *Academic Journal of Creative Arts Therapies,* 20(1), 1003-1019.

McNiff, S. (2018) *Using Art Research Learning and Teaching: Multidisciplinary Approaches Across the Arts*. Intellect Books.

—. (2019) "Reflections on What 'Art' Does in Art Therapy Practice and Research" *Art Therapy,* 36(3), 162-165.

Miller, A. (2012) "Inspired by El Duende: One-canvas Process Painting" *Art Therapy Supervision*, 29(4), 166-173.

Schaefer, M. T., Olson, D. H. (1981) "Assessing Intimacy: The Pair Inventory" *Journal of Marital and Family Therapy,* 7(1), 47-60

Schaverien, J. (2020) *The Dying Patient in Psychotherapy: Erotic Transference and Boarding School Syndrome* (2nd ed.). Routledge.

Sinclair, V. G., Dowdy, S. W. (2005) "Development and Validation of the Emotional Intimacy Scale" *Journal of Nursing Measurement,* 13(3), 193-206.

Strawn, S. M., Falick, M. (2007) *Knitting America*. Voyageur Press.
Summer, D., Govani, D., Teoli, L. (2017) *Body Tracing to Dismantle, Confront, and Resist Sources of Power*.
Wieden, J. (2018) *The Impact of Using Intimacy Rituals and Romantic Attachment on Satisfaction among Romantic Couples*. Ann Arbor, CA: Alliant International University.

CHAPTER 14

TEACHING ART THERAPY STUDENTS HOW TO CONDUCT A MULTI-CULTURAL ART BASED RESEARCH

NOGA ARIEL-GALOR

Introduction

In recent years, the question of how to address race and culture in art therapy has been prevalent amongst authors, who found themselves working with patients from different ethnic, cultural, national and religious backgrounds (see for example: Campbell et al., 1999).

However, there have been major shifts in our perception of what constitutes proper cultural-sensitivity in cross-cultural, or multi-cultural therapy. These shifts can be seen as moving from a 'one-person psychology', in which the focus lies on the patient's cultural or ethnic background, and as an attempt to understand the differences between the culture of the majority group and the minority group to which the patient belongs; to a 'two-person psychology' in which the emphasis lies on both therapist and patient, bringing into the therapeutic space not just their personal history, but also the collective history of their large-groups (Volkan, 2001, 2017) and the history between those groups, or the socio-political influences. This shift is parallel to the shift from classical to contemporary psychoanalysis (Aron, 1996). While teaching multi-cultural therapy, therefore, one must teach the therapist both how to observe her patient from a non-biased, non-ethnocentric culturally-relative approach, which seeks to understand her own definitions of etiquette, pathology, relationality, etc; and how to be aware of the different feelings, emotions, and enactments that can be aroused in both therapist and patient, due to the history between their large-groups.

These two approaches, which I will later elaborate on, are very different in nature. The former holds a wish to *know* – to map the differences between cultures, to control our bias, to learn the cultural language through which we can connect. The latter is focused on *not knowing* (Campbell et al., 1999) meaning on raising questions in an attempt to keep a curious and exploratory stance, without jumping to conclusions.

Another form of engaging with cultural issues is related to art therapy in the context of activism and social change. These writers question the role of the art therapist in an unjust society, and how they can contribute to its healing and minimization of differences in representation.

This chapter aims to present the experience of teaching art therapy students how to conduct multi-cultural art-based research. The main rationale and principles will be described, as well as a brief review of the three interconnected pillars of focus to multi-cultural art therapy: cultural sensitivity, socio-political sensitivity, and social action and change. I will discuss some of the potential challenges and rewards of this research topic based on several examples taken from a research seminar group held in The Academic College for Society and the Arts in Israel. The learning process and the structure of the class will be elaborated on, as well as some final conclusions regarding art analysis from a multi-cultural perspective.

Cultural sensitivity: Recognizing our biases and letting go of them

Cross-cultural, or Multi-cultural therapy is something art therapists have been encountering as a regular part of our profession, by working with patients from a varied range of cultural groups. However, across the Western world, art therapists are considered to be predominantly white and middle-class (Kaplan, 2002; Campbell et al., 1999), and therefore the concern was that they are ill-prepared to meet with minority groups of different backgrounds and statuses. As Hocoy (2002) stated: “The history of Western therapeutic traditions is replete with instances in which legitimate cultural expressions are pathologized, marginalized, or misinterpreted” (p. 141). Art therapists wish to depart from this dubious heritage and to assist in cultural expression rather than oppression. However, to do that, they must first recognize and create awareness of how their cultural worldview reflects the privileged, dominant culture, and to become more sensitive to members of minority groups.

Often, when therapists are confronted with issues of multi-culturalism in therapy, they state that “At the end of the day, we are all human beings”, marking that they see the common human traits, rather than the differences.

This "color-blindness", while good-intentioned, can be misleading, and is in danger of shaking the healthy tension between sameness and difference, which is so important in recognizing the other (Benjamin, 2018). Some authors warn us from the danger of declaring oneself "culture blind", meaning that they claim to treat everyone the same regardless of origin, because that alone could lead to wrongful judgments and an unconscious comparison, and holds the danger of unknowingly becoming an agent of cultural assimilation. Thus, some authors rightly emphasize this approach as an ethical danger (Hocoy, 2002).

McNiff (2009) states that cultural differences exist wherever there is a difference, whether it be caused by generational differences, gender, religion, race, people of different sexual preferences, and political values. Therapy must therefore always be approached as a meeting between two cultures, ready to contain the differences.

Subjects such as language, autonomy Vs. dependence, level of acculturation, and certain personality and behavioral traits, are all considered potentially culturally biased (Hocoy, 2002). McNiff (2009) draws from the literature on cross-cultural psychology to define what may apply to art therapists. He emphasizes art therapy research as a tool to understand both sameness and difference of visual imagery between cultures. However, it is important to remember that art interpretation itself is also considered potentially biased. I remember an encounter with a supervisor regarding a patient who was an asylum seeker from Sudan, who said that the house the patient drew – a straw hut, with fine lines depicting the individual straws that constructed it – was an indication of anxiety because instead of drawing the blank square structure we in the Western culture have grown accustomed to, the individual straws made the drawing look blackened. While anxiety in his situation of fleeing the war was not farfetched, that kind of interpretation would have robbed him of the ability to recounter his childhood home in a way that could also express his lost, happy memories and deep longing.

As I have stated in the introduction to this chapter, while understanding our own culture and our biases, as well as learning about the patient's culture is highly important, it shows a very partial picture because it does not take the *emotional* aspect into account when meeting the *Other*: aspects of similarity and difference and how we feel about them – guilt, fear, anxiety, helplessness, sometimes even anger, blame, disgust, and rejection. These are emotions that are also very much influenced by our societal roles, the power structure of society, its patterns of integration and segregation, what we were told about *them* and what they were told about *us,* what encounters we had with other members of their large-group in the past and they had with ours.

Hence, this is a "one-person psychology", based on *knowing* the other and their cultural habits, but the *experience* of meeting the other is so much more complex than that. With this in mind, I introduce the students to the second subject.

Socio-political influences on art therapy

This is another form of addressing the subject of race and culture, which focuses on differences from a point of view that seeks to understand how social, political, and professional reality influences therapeutic relations. While referring to 'The political', I do not mean state politics, which are traditionally left out of the treatment room (at least overtly), but rather to the power relations in society (Avissar, 2016), which permeate the art therapy room and are expressed in the therapeutic relationship and the artwork. The underlying assumption is that our identities are shaped not only by our culture, but also in relation to our place in society regarding other cultures, and in return shape relationships between individuals as well.

Some authors grapple with questions of racial identity, and how it is expressed in art therapy. The literature specific to art therapy is not vast, yet there are important contributions to and from the art therapy field. An especially helpful source is a book titled *Art therapy, race, and culture,* edited by Jean Campbell et al., (2007), which thoroughly explores issues of race from the perspectives of art therapists who belong to both majority and minority groups and their patients. The book places a great emphasis on awareness of social privileges and power as an integral part of the awakening process regarding the role race plays in the therapeutic relationship.

Several authors are members of minority groups who write about their own experience as art therapists who are people of color. Buck (2002) writes about her experiences as an Arab Muslim therapist in post 9/11 United States, and how the bridge between cultures can easily collapse after a national trauma, one she both experienced as an American yet also as it backlashed towards her, as someone who was identified as part of the perpetrating group. An important piece by Gipson (2015) examines the limitations of cultural competency in art therapy education, calling for an immersive engagement with social justice practices, meaning being involved with people who were impacted by systemic violence. As an African-American art therapist, she struggles to help art therapy students to recognize their privileged identities as a step to raising racial awareness. Similarly, Mayor (2012) draws on critical race theory to demonstrate how the therapeutic encounter reproduces, embodies, and recreates cultural and social roles pertaining to race. By engaging with these roles, she adds an ethical component of how to work towards social change.

Cultural competency is gained by the art therapist rigorously and honestly self-examining of their cultural lens, the assumptions and values of their work, but also their discomforts regarding forms of otherness, and facing their prejudice and biases. It is important to recognize that while we consider ourselves non-biased, our patients might see us as such, based on their own experience with "people who look like us." I am reminded of a discussion in a group on cultural and political sensitivity in treatment I held with therapists, in which one of the elder participants, a Jewish Ashkenazi psychiatrist, said that he had never realized before that he was "a white man". While that person was of course previously aware of the color of his skin, he never thought about the way he was potentially being perceived by others, due to his role in society. His "whiteness" was transparent to him, but not necessarily to all of his patients.

Finally, it is at times important to acknowledge that some patients had reached dire places in their lives not because of something inherent in them, but because of limited options society had provided them with, due to their origin group. Here therapists can acknowledge it, yet also instill a sense of agency (Gentile, 2010): it was not their *fault*, but it is their *responsibility* to make a better life for themselves. It is also our responsibility in society as a whole, to make these efforts fruitful and achievable while striving to create equal opportunities and fight injustice. These realizations were what led art therapists to strive for social change.

Social change

Another field in art therapy that has been gaining further attention is that of the art therapist as an activist or a social agent of change. Two books, titled *Art in action: Expressive arts therapy and social change* (Levine & Levine, 2011), and *Art therapy and social action* (Kaplan, 2007) provide many case studies as well as conceptual and practical models. These practices are inextricably related to the understanding of the political forces (power differentials) that rule the world, or as Kapitan put it: "art therapists become social activists when they embrace awareness of the connection between suffering and social imbalance and actively commit to social transformation through advocacy for disenfranchised people" (2015, p. 104). Since art therapists can find their connection to the patient through the unspoken language of art, we are in a better chance to be "out there", in the field, more than verbal therapists, who are more affected by language barriers. And when we are out there, we often come across many forms of oppression, lack of justice, and sometimes hope. By being both artists and healers we are more inclined to observe the injustice of the social order and attempt to change it rather than preserve it (Borowsky et al., 2015). Art therapy gives us the tools to do so.

Thus, these three aspects complement each other – by recognizing cultural differences we become more aware of our own ethnocentricity, replacing an etic point of view with an emic one (Sue & Sue, 2008), making us more tolerant to the other's notions of normalcy and pathology as well as to pathways of reaching them. However, if we neglect to see our differences as social constructs, defining the power relations in society and our roles in them, we are in danger of reenacting the social order in the room, thus awakening our patients' socially induced traumas. These two stances are ethical, because they fully understand the role of the therapist in the life of their patient. But as noted, this realization compels many art therapists to take it even a step further, by becoming agents of social change through art therapy. As Borowsky et al., (2015) noted – once we see it, we want to go blind, but shutting our eyes and doing nothing makes us blind to ourselves.

In the discussed research seminar, I touch upon these three aspects and their manifestation in art therapy. I allow students to research within these possible topics, enabling a wide variety of perceptions for the meaning of "culture" and power relations in treatment. And so, while most students focus on ethnic, cultural or religious differences, some students focus on the different cultures between school teachers and art therapists in the school setting; some on working in mental health clinics with a staff of practitioners from different therapeutic professions and disciplines, and more.

Teaching multi-cultural art-based research in Israel

Israel is a culturally diverse country, with complex relations between the different religious, ethnic, socio-economic and national groups that construct it. These groups are generally left segregated, some by choice and others by chance, and are in many ways enigmatic to one another. Art therapy programs are similarly culturally diverse in nature, attracting students from different groups, with a white, Jewish majority. The personal ties that are formed in these classes are many times novelle and rather emotionally moving to students, who previously had no experience in working together intimately with members of groups which were generally left unknown to them. Furthermore, the art therapy profession itself potentially holds encounters with patients from different cultures, their families and their surroundings. Therefore, it is an essential part of the art therapist's training to familiarize herself with the different complexities that exist in these encounters, complexities she often has no experience in knowing how to think about and contain in a therapeutic and/or academic setting.

However, out of the three main topics I have raised (cultural sensitivity, socio-political sensitivity, and social action and change), talking about socio-political influences in the classroom was the most "explosive", and therefore challenging. The Israeli society as a whole is considered both traumatized and traumatizing (Weinberg, 2017), with arrows pointing both inside – between groups, and outside – towards external enemies. There are various collective traumas and social wounds which were caused by other large-groups, some of their "representative members" sitting in the room right next to each other. In spite of these challenges, I hold in mind that facing them in the classroom is a safe environment for exploration in order to be able to contain the differences later on in the art therapy room. As I will hopefully show in the next examples, maintaining the tension between the personal and professional, between learning from experience and learning from academic knowledge, was highly important in order to create a learning and research environment that could be academically productive as well as personally meaningful and insightful.

Class setting

The research seminar takes place in the Academic college for Society and the Arts (Netanya, Israel), in a culturally diverse group. Its main theme is writing an academic research paper on issues concerning multi-culturalism in art therapy. The students are requested to conduct an art-based mini-research, in which they empirically study participants with both art interventions and a semi-structured in-depth interview. The students are requested to pair-up for the research, and most go through the process in dyads. The first four meetings of the seminar are dedicated to teaching the various subjects I have elaborated on earlier, and the rest are dedicated to accompanying the process through either private or group talks and library work, while strengthening understanding of academic writing and art-based research. The last three or four meetings are dedicated to students' presentations. The class is constructed of experienced therapists, most of whom had been working for several years and came in to complete academic credit points for the purpose of earning an M.A.

Triggers, explosions and hope

As mentioned, while this is an exercise in academic writing and research, it also serves as an opportunity to teach students about multi-culturalism in art therapy, a subject on which they do not know a lot about. However, the setting itself turns out to be challenging, when one considers that these art-therapy groups are often highly multi-cultural themselves! Secular, religious, orthodox Jewish, Muslim and Christian Arab women all sit together in one room, each class member also representing their "large group" (Volkan, 2001; 2017) at that moment. Some of these women might be sitting beside another member whose group might have hurt her own group in one way or another in the past. And yet here we are, together, talking about the complexities of otherness. This is a research group, yet the students wish at times to talk about themselves and the dynamics in the room, and at times wish to disappear from it and just fade away into the background. The temptation to talk about what is happening in the group is great, and yet this is not a therapeutic setting. Therefore, the questions always rise: are we there to learn how to openly talk and experience what it is like to sit together and hold the tension between sameness and difference, or are these materials that we are dealing with here too explosive to contain?

In one group, an older Arab student wearing a hijab was triggered by the conversation. I had just presented the group with a documentary on the experience of men of color in the public sphere. The movie portrayed different Israeli men of Arab, and Jews of Ethiopian or Middle Eastern and North African descent, who openly talked and demonstrated what it is like to be a black man in a white, prejudiced, society. I urged the students to imagine what it is like for these men to encounter a white therapist in the therapy room, after being wounded by the 'white gaze' (The internalized assumption that they need to accommodate to the cultural perceptions of the white person, or else be judged harshly). How the therapist might not consider herself discriminating, but could be perceived as one because of collective wounds. The triggered student wanted to tell the participants that all of it was true, and wished to share what she had gone through every week on the train on her way to college, as a Muslim woman. Yet another student was staring at her accusingly as she talked – that student's brother was killed in a terror attack many years beforehand. Just as the Arab student wished for her classmates to empathize with her everyday struggle of being an openly disliked minority member, of encountering suspicion and too-often hatred, so did the Jewish student wish for the others to see that the suspicion towards her Arab fellow student was justified. For her all Arabs were suspects, potentially dangerous, because maybe if her brother had been more careful, he would have avoided standing next to a terrorist who committed suicide while intentionally taking others with him. What was the class to do at that moment, what was I to do? If we empathized with one, we were in the risk of leaving the other feeling lonely and dropped. Could we justify both their feelings? Should we compare? In an attempt to dismantle the tension, I opted for a third option (Aron & Starr, 2013), to find a vantage point outside of the conflict, and to talk about how painful it is to live in a society that is both hurting and hurtful, and that we must remember that no matter how emotionally triggering it is, the students in this room are not the actual aggressors, and that we share the same values that have allowed us to come together in order to learn how to heal and help others, not to harm them. Yet it wasn't until the next meeting, when I specifically said that this is *not* a therapy group, that the other class members could finally breathe and feel that the room is safe again. Dealing with these matters is so painful, triggering and difficult. How can we talk about it without feeling it and experiencing it ourselves? And especially us, expressive art therapists, who put such an emphasis on experience as a tool for change – should we just dryly discuss this new-found knowledge, detached from how it makes us feel? The delicate tension between therapy, academic class and research group was shaken. I could feel myself turning to the cooling affect of theory, while often times approaching students after class in order to check on them and to acknowledge their struggle. I accepted this fragmented approach, because looking at the whole picture can sometimes be too painful – a picture of oppression, of hurt and loss, rejection, fear and shame. We could touch upon these subjects only vicariously through research, and not directly amongst ourselves. Acknowledging this collusion was an important realization of what this tension could be like in therapy.

Yet I often found that even though speaking about it directly could sometimes be too overwhelming, the research itself became an expressive tool, a way in which students could truly express themselves and their interests, inspired by the early content they had learned. And sometimes presenting their products in front of the other students was their way of speaking out what was previously rendered unspeakable.

One student, an Arab woman with traditional clothing, chose to write a heuristic research paper about her relationship with her Jewish supervisor, during a supervision that took place several years beforehand, but its complexity occupied her thoughts and mind ever since. For the purpose of the research, she revisited her journal at the time, which she had also used as a sketch book, and portrayed her feelings in art. This research was her way of processing what she had experienced then, her feeling of being mute and helpless, her culture judged by her supervisor until she reached a point of feeling torn – if she brought in the material accurately she risked feeling that every hardship was affiliated with her culture; if she kept details hidden, she risked her integrity as a therapist and would not gain insight from her supervision. Combining how she felt and drew with the theory regarding power relations in supervision, and the importance of not being culturally biased, had helped her to better define how small and helpless she felt in that situation, and also to finally express her anger of her supervisor, albeit only in writing and never directly to her, and to feel that she had the class as witnesses who signaled to her that her feelings were just and understandably painful.

And there were also other examples, of classes that contained students who so wanted to learn about the others, who intentionally paired-up with someone who was culturally different from them in order to spend time together, getting to know each other, creating something together. One pair of students – A Jewish and an Arab woman, held an art therapy workshop of Jewish and Arab elementary school girls, who drew on masks together, in order to explore the benefits of holding combined art therapy groups as a pathway to social change. The participants were asked how they imagined meeting the girls from the other national group would feel like before the workshop, and then they were asked what their thoughts were after. All participants described a greater sense of comfort and familiarity following the workshop, and many expressed a wish to visit the other girls in their homes and see how they live differently, or what yummy foods they eat. Being able to share these findings in front of the class while presenting them the research, was a uniting experience for us all. It showed us once again the power of art and the human encounter as a strong unifying force, and the power of research in creating new pathways for thinking and acting.

Some of the research projects led to more continuous ones. A religious woman from the North of the country had expressed a growing curiosity in class regarding a cultural group called Bney Ha'menashe, a tribe of Indian Jews who migrated to Israel, and whose youth had problems assimilating. She decided to contact the municipal authorities and to start an art project with four planned sessions, providing the young members with an opportunity to come together, discuss their culture and express it through art. She showed that the mere intervention had created more confidence in the local authorities, for these adolescents felt seen and heard, and felt more connected to the local youth center. She then continued to work with them, by their own request, and the local authority hired her for that purpose because they recognized the benefits. Thus, something that began as an academic obligation, became a tool for social change and dedication.

Another student chose to work with three generations of women of Moroccan descent – grandmother, mother and daughter, to create cultural empowerment by using clay-work. She asked the Grandmother to mold memories from her homeland, and the next generations created a homage to her work. That student was moved to see how many memories it aroused in the grandmother, how while working she told stories of her homeland that were never told before, and how that affected both her daughter and granddaughter into feeling pride in their Moroccan heritage and a better connection to themselves and the other generations. That student saw these interventions as a way she could be an activist for the empowerment of Mizrahi women, an issue she always felt strongly about, but did not quite know how to fit in. Her research gave her the courage and the pathway to act as both an art therapist and activist.

Conclusions

Watching a research come to life is a beautiful process. The students start off feeling curiosity, which quickly turns into anxiety, and often feel that this project, modest as it may be, is still too much. It is only through carefully taking one step at a time, accompanying them as they go through the troubling stages of finding a research subject, articulating a proposal and then carefully tending to the other segments or chapters, that they slowly begin to see that this process makes a lot of sense. At the end of the course when we sit together and watch the presentations it is a highly moving moment when we come to realize how something which was very much unfathomable just three months prior to that had come into life.

As I hope to have demonstrated, teaching multi-cultural art-based research to art therapy students is both significantly rewarding and challenging. It is highly rewarding because it exposes the students to a new and inciting topic, one which they sometimes felt yet did not know how to articulate; and watching them implement this new-found knowledge and use it as part of their own research is both intellectually interesting and emotionally moving. It is challenging because there is a delicate tension to be preserved between the need to process this subject with the group, and the need to focus on studying and research in light of these highly triggering topics. The degree to which each group will allow this discourse to take place is dynamic, as well as the needed extent and strictness of boundaries.

One final word about observing the art-work as part of this research focus: unlike the way in which we observe our patients' art-work as a signifier for their own intra-psychic and interpersonal processes, in this type of research I encourage the students to observe the art as speaking an internalized societal and cultural voice, and the inter-cultural dynamics as present in the art-work, along with other dimensions of existence. Thus, looking at contrasts, images, colors and shapes, whether abstract or concrete, can tell us several stories at a time. When we practice observing the artwork from different vantage points, we can start seeing how everything is both connected and separate. It is my belief that the cultural and socio-political affect us all as part of our upbringings, and observing their manifestations in patients' artwork should be part of every art therapist's repertoire.

References

Aron, L. (1996) *A Meeting of Minds: Mutuality in Psychoanalysis*. Hillsdale, NJ: Analytic Press.

Aron, L., Starr, K. (2013) *A Psychotherapy for the People: Toward a Progressive Psychoanalysis*. New York: Routledge.

Avissar, N. (2016) *Psychotherapy, Society and Politics: From Theory to Practice*. New York: Palgrave Macmillan.

Benjamin, J. (2018) *Beyond doer and done to: Recognition Theory, Intersubjectivity and the Third*. New York: Routledge.

Borowsky, M. J., Alvarez, J. F., Kellogg, A., Volker, C., Kapitan, L. (2009) "The Art Therapist as Social Activist: Reflections and Visions" *Art Therapy: Journal of the American Art Therapy Association*, 26(3), 107-113.

Buck, H. L. (2002) "Rebuilding the Bridge: An Arab-American Art Therapist Responds to 9/11" *Art Therapy: Journal of the American Art Therapy Association,* 19(4), 164-167.

Campbell, J., Liebmann, M., Brooks, F., Jones, J., Ward, C. (eds.) (1999) *Art Therapy, Race and Culture*. London: Jessica Kingsley Publishing.

Gentile, J. (2010) "Weeds on the Ruins: Agency, Compromise Formation, and the Quest for Intersubjective Truth. *Psychoanalytic Dialogues,* 20(1), 88-109.

Hocoy, D. (2002) "Cross-cultural Issues in Art Therapy" *Art Therapy: Journal of the American Art Therapy Association*, 19(4), 141-145.

Kapitan, L. (2015) "Social Action in Practice: Shifting the Ethnocentric Lens in Cross-Cultural Art Therapy Encounters" *Art Therapy,* 32(3), 104-111.

Kaplan, F. F. (2002) "Cross-cultural Art Therapy: A Now and Future Therapy" *Art Therapy: Journal of the American Art Therapy Association*, 19(4), 138-138.

Kaplan, F. F. (ed.). (2007) *Art Therapy and Social Action.* London: Jessica Kingsley Publishers.

Gipson, L. R. (2015) "Is Cultural Competence Enough? Deepening Social Justice Pedagogy in Art Therapy" *Art Therapy*, 32(3), 142-145.

Levine, S. K., Levine, E. G. (eds.) (2011) *Art in Action: Expressive Art Therapy and Social Change.* London: Jessica Kingsley Publishers.

Mayor, C. (2012) "Playing with Race: A Theoretical Framework and Approach for Creative Arts Therapists" *The arts in Psychotherapy*, 39, 214-219.

McNiff, S. (2009) "Cross-Cultural Psychotherapy and Art" *Art Therapy: Journal of the American Art Therapy Association*, 26(3), 100-106.

Sue, D. W., Sue, D. (2008) *Counseling the Culturally Diverse: Practice and Theory*. Hoboken, NJ: John Wiley & Sons.

Volkan, V. (2001) "Transgenerational Transmissions and Chosen Traumas: An Aspect of Large-group Identity" *Group Analysis,* 34(1), 79-97.

—. (2017) "Large-group Identity and Massive Trauma" in J. L. Alpert., E. R. Goren (eds.). *Psychoanalysis, Trauma and Community: History and Contemporary Reappraisals*. New York: Routledge.

Weinberg, H. (2017) The Social Unconscious of Israeli Jews – Described and Analysed by an Israeli Living in North America" (pp. 129-150) in E. Hopper, H. Weinberg (eds.). *The Social Unconscious in Persons, Groups, and Societies (Volume 3: The Foundation Matrix Extended and Re-configured).* London: Karnac Books.

CHAPTER 15

THEORIZING MUSHINESS FROM THERAPEUTIC PRACTICE TO TEACHING: TWO PERSPECTIVES ON USING LIQUID AND SLIMY MATERIALS IN ART THERAPY

ELANA LAKH AND SHEVY MEDZINI

Introduction

Art therapy operates at various levels and in different areas of the human psyche. It begins with a sensory and motor engagement with materials at the physical level of experience and focuses on its emotional implications. Through planning and implementation of an idea, a mental image is turned into a piece of artwork using materials which can then be viewed to understand its symbolic, personal, and collective meanings. During our years of working as art therapists, we have seen patients go through these transitions in just one therapy session or in multiple sessions that form a process. In teaching art therapy, we formulated our art therapy experience with patients into concepts. In traditional experiential art therapy teaching models that we learned as students and use as teachers, students are given hands-on experience with these concepts in small classes, an experience which is then elaborated in theory classes. One such concept is *mushiness*, which we define as the mental processes that occur while engaging with "mushy" wet, liquid, slimy and soft materials. This concept is basic to the experiences that are formed at the kinesthetic/sensory level (Lusebrink, Martinsone & Dzilna-Silova, 2013). This primal level of working with materials is the foundation for all creative processes, in which the physical qualities of the materials are the focus of experience. These qualities give rise to various sensations during the creative process, and at times to memories and associations with physical experiences.

Our introductory art therapy course begins with this primal level of experience. When preparing for the class, we discovered that each of us experience mushiness in therapy in a different way that derives from our work with patients with various needs. We realized that we needed to distinguish between two kinds of mushiness: *developmental* mushiness and *traumatic* mushiness, which are both discussed in this chapter. Developmental mushiness is characterized by a creative, sensual and developing engagement with the materials, whereas traumatic mushiness has a frozen, forced, and repetitive quality. We describe these two forms of mushiness, and their related mental states in this chapter.

Developmental mushiness

Touch is the primary mode of encountering the world throughout the entire lifespan. The psychoanalyst Thomas Ogden introduced the notion of the "autistic-contiguous position" to characterize this mode of experience as follows: "*a sensory-dominated, pre-symbolic mode of generating experience, which provides a good measure of boundedness of human experience, and the beginning of a sense of the place where one's experience occurs*" (1989, p. 81). This primal mode of sensory experience lays the foundation for the experience of the self. It has a major motor component that corresponds to Piaget's (1969) sensorimotor stage (0-18 months) describing the development of sensory and movement skills as a way to experience the world and interact with the environment.

The first sensorimotor experiences are registered in the psychic layer, termed the Great Round by the Jungian psychoanalyst Erich Neumann (1954). The Great Round, is characterized by unitary reality. According to Neumann, the sensuous and sensory experiences of the primal relationship are registered in their raw form and shape the infant's existential experience, even before the ego exists. These experiences are not evaluated as good or bad, but rather have the potential to be experienced as such by the ego that will develop later on. These early events color the individual's experience in the world in a way that is influenced by the physical sensations of these primal phases. The unitary reality of the Great Round is present in therapy, as well as the observing ego that developed from it. Thus, symbolic representation in therapy can be verbal, stemming from the construction of memory, or emerge from an experience re-lived in the transference, and can be a representation of sensory memory in materials, in a figurative or abstract form.

Example: Hanna, a woman in her forties, is talking about her need for touch. The therapist suggests working with foam. Hanna accepts, touching the foam and playing with it with her hands until the foam is gone. "It feels good", she says, takes off her glasses and puts the foam on her face and on her head. She begins to cry. The therapist hands her a dish of warm water. Hanna puts some foam in the dish and touches it. Her eyes are closed. Throughout the session she plays with the foam in various ways. The therapist, who understands Hanna's primal emotional state, heats some water and wipes Hanna's hands that are covered with foam. Hanna's weeping increases and she does not speak for the rest of the session. In the next session Hanna describes her great relief and her experience of pleasure and comfort after the session. The smell of the foam reminded Hanna of her father who had died a few years previously, whom she missed. The sensory work with foam in the accepting presence of the therapist and the memories it elicited, allowed Hanna to process grief and to enjoy a closer physical connection with her husband.

Engaging with materials begins with the sensuousness and touch of bodily products. During the early stages of life this is an act of discovery at the sensory level. Bodily products are only labelled as "disgusting" or "dirty" after encountering social norms and experiencing reality. Neumann (1973) suggested that early in life, the oral and anal are indistinguishable and are in a continuous cyclic process of eating and secreting. As ego consciousness develops, differentiation begins, accompanied by judgment of good and bad. The result is that whatever is positioned down and behind is perceived as linked to disgust, ugliness, and sin; that is, the smells, secretions, and sex. The pleasure derived from engaging with feces during the anal stage is repressed because of social taboos (Freud, 1938). In Freud's conceptualization, there is an early stage of pleasure, which is short-lived and turns this pleasurable activity into a source of shame and guilt that changes the way individuals relate to their primal sensory experience. Hence, when the art therapist offers mushy materials, she may allow the patient to engage with contents linked with disgust, ugliness and sin on one hand, and contents linked to warmth, softness and pleasure on the other.

The art therapist Felicity Aldridge (1998) referred to the art materials used in therapy as food, and considered the mixtures children make as engaging with food and secretions. Her patients did not only need emotional and symbolic feeding, but also actual, physical feeding. In extreme states of deprivation, the symbolic ability is impaired or does not develop, and it is impossible to use art symbolically (Rabiger, 1990). Thus, the soup of mixed materials or the clay patty might be experienced as real food.

Art therapists offer their patients art materials, which serve as food for the psyche. When therapy deals with the primal phases of psychological development, the appropriate materials may be *pre-material material*; i.e., materials that are not art materials by definition, but can be used for artwork. These are usually liquid or paste materials, such as food (ketchup, mustard, etc…), shaving foam, mud, shampoo, hair conditioner, a water-soaked diaper, an egg, and others. These materials may evoke early memories of smell, touch and sensation. The use of pre-material material or other mushy materials in art therapy allows the patient to connect with primal sensory experiences through the touch on the skin and other senses including smell, hearing and taste. In therapy, the therapist can consider offering these materials based on her understanding of the patient's developmental phase, regardless of chronological age. The art therapist's intervention constitutes a response to what the patients tell her through their actions, and the transference (Moon, 2002). This is an invitation for soft, mushy, limitless and symbiotic action.

Example: Ofra, a 25 year old woman used to choose rough textured bases for her artworks, and to engrave them with a pencil, or stick nails or sharp materials into them. The therapist gently tried to offer her softer and warmer materials, thinking that these materials could elicit an experience of warmth and softness. After a long period of reluctance, Ofra began playing with liquid ink, moving it on a hard surface and adding pre-material materials to it such as ketchup and mud. One day, Ofra brought a hardboiled egg and a raw egg to the session. She was fascinated by the raw egg and used it as art material: she stirred the egg in the same way she had stirred the ink, and later made an egg-like liquid material (she mixed yellow gouache with hair conditioner and glue). As she moved the egg around she said it was like a baby in a cradle. Working with the softness of the fresh egg compared to the stiffness of the hardboiled egg kindled memories of growing up with her difficult mother, as opposed to the soft mother image she missed. Touching the pre-material material allowed Ofra to process emotions relating to the primary relationship with her mother, first in materials and later also in words in a way that corresponds to the cognitive/symbolic level of the ETC model (Lusebrink, Martinsone & Dzilna-Silova, 2013).

Mushiness involves curious exploration of materials. The first stage of engagement with materials, which precedes art-making is what the pioneering art therapist Judith Rubin termed the "manipulation stage" (Rubin, 1978, p. 37-38). In this stage, the child curiously experiments with various materials and discovers sensations, various types of touch, smell, taste, color, and how his or her actions influence them.

We suggest terming this explorative stage "*the mush phase*", a unitary phase which refers to primal developmental states in which there is no differentiation between the infant and its environment, self and object, or between different agencies within the psyche.

In the art therapy studio patients encounter the undifferentiated state through the materials. An experience of sufficient merging will allow the developing psyche to emerge and achieve separateness, the recognition of external reality and an experience of distinct inner and outer worlds. Winnicott thought that in this primal stage the environment needs to support "going on being" (1986), so that the child can gradually accept the reality of separation. Many patients seek therapy due to difficulties with the transition from a state of merging to one of separateness. The "mush stage" in art therapy may allow them to experience this merging.

The art therapist can respond to the client's need for merging at this stage by suggesting finger paints, very wet clay, gouche, ink, and spray bottles with liquid paint, watercolors and similar merging materials. Other options include warm and "snuggly" soft and liquid materials such as play dough in warm water, plaster that gradually warms up, cotton wool and other possibilities. The encounter with these materials may allow for the reconstruction of a soft liquid experience, similar to the physical experience in the womb and the primal mother-infant relationship. Thus, in the mush phase, the patient is in a state of merging with the materials and with the therapist. In this phase, the therapist can create together with the patient: they can work on the same surface, or use liquid and mushy materials together.

The liquid materials, their smell and texture, can make it possible to face unspoken memories and unthought experiences. In her book *Trauma Healing at the Clay Field* (2013, p. 15), the art therapist Cornelia Elbrecht clarifies that touching materials enables access to issues of attachment, developmental delays and traumas etched into the body and the psyche. Elbrecht writes that love, as well as violence, are primarily communicated through touch. She points out that touching material creates memories in the body in a nonverbal mode. Thus touching materials not only enables access to experiences registered in the primal layers of the psyche, but also allows the individual to work with them and create new memory traces.

There is no symbolization in the experiences that take place in these primal developmental psychic areas, nor is symbolization needed. These are formless places of not knowing and not naming that allow the material and the psyche to dwell in a regressive contained state.

Thus, developmental mushiness opens the door to the primal experience of sensory touch, bodily sensations, and dissolving into the material, an experience that sometimes occurs for the first time in therapy. The developmental engagement with these materials has an experiential quality of discovery and play, and needs no conceptualization or symbolization. Words are not important or do not exist, and the experience cannot be explained. At this stage, engagement with the art product is less important, butsometimes the image may take on a symbolic value when reflected upon consciously. The mushy experience itself and the resulting image allow access to unconscious areas of the psyche, and call for a connection between the conscious and unconscious.

Traumatic mushiness

In our work with patients who have experienced trauma, we realized that they produce a different sensory-psychological quality of the mushiness. Traumatic mushiness is not relaxed or pleasant; rather, it usually is frozen, static and does not develop. These ways of touching materials emerge from traumatic experiences occurring during development, and bear the traces of these experiences etched in the body and the psyche. *"Trauma arrests the course of normal development by its repetitive intrusion into the survivor's life"* (Lewis-Herman, 2015, p. 37); hence, a developmental experience of exploration may freeze as a result of trauma. The outcome will affect all realms of the trauma survivor's life, including engagement with materials.

The traumatic state can be the result of life events influencing a cohesive personality, or can be the result of the developmental trauma of an intolerable awareness of separateness from the body of the mother (Tustin, 2013; Alvarez, 2012). Trauma influences individuals in different ways, depending on the developmental phase, the individual's coping mechanisms, their support system, and no less importantly, the traumatic events themselves.

An overwhelming encounter with a sensory experience can color the whole experience in traumatic hues, which can influence the way it is registered in the psyche, as well as in future encounters with materials. The sensory registration linked to the traumatic experience can be expressed in the materials and the way they are used in art therapy; for example, in the way children reconstruct their injuries by "injuring" the clay. Often, in traumatic states, individuals lose control of their body and their bowels. Bodily secretions are then linked to horrible experiences that cause pain, shame and dread. In a situation like this, mushiness is associated with the traumatic experience and can become painful and disgusting, or make the individual avoid touching the materials so as not to experience the difficult emotions arising.

When development takes place in the shadow of the trauma, as for example in children experiencing continuous abuse, the psyche develops around the traumatic experiences and the value attributed to them (Lewis-Herman, 1994). In situations of childhood sexual abuse, the confusion involved with bodily sensations and the awareness of what is being done becomes part of the structure of the psyche and the self-perception of the abused child. Relying on the sensory-motor experiences as the main channel for experiencing the world becomes difficult, since this encounter is very confusing. Confusion and chaos characterize these individuals' engagement with the materials, since they reflect the child's mental state. Materials, especially those reminiscent of the body and relating to it may be both attractive and repelling at the same time, like the bodily sensations during sexual abuse.

Traumatic mushiness has two major aspects: a sensory-motor reconstruction of the sensory and mental experience, and a symbolic representation of the registration of the experience in the psyche. The art therapist Jenny Murphy (1998) described the use of mushy and liquid materials in art therapy by abused children. She reports dirt mixed in containers that are entrusted to the therapist to keep, potions intended to heal or to kill, sensory references to materials and feelings of repulsion and disgust, but also using wet and soft materials with complete enjoyment. Murphy suggests that painting the hands and face allows abused children to express their sense of inner dirtiness openly. Frances O'Brien (2004) claimed that using materials in the shape of bodily fluids and discharges conveys the experience of being dirty and messy inside, and an attempt to find boundaries and distinguish between good and bad feelings. Here, the materials embody the ambivalence experienced toward bodily sensations; namely, disgust and pleasure mixed together, and the secret inner experience of dirtiness, together with the desire to openly reveal it, which is expressed in the manipulation of the materials.

Trauma impairs verbal processing ability and makes it impossible to find meaning in the traumatic experience, which remains at the level of bodily sensations, and is not mediated by human relationships (O'Brien, 2004). The mess and dirt are a pre-symbolic inner representation of the abuse that is projected onto the materials and the therapist, embodying what cannot be said in words. Carol Sagar (1990) raised the question of whether the dual quality of the dirty mixtures produced by abused children in therapy was a way of asking whether the material was good or bad. This reflects the confused feelings experienced by child survivors of sexual abuse towards the perpetrators, including aspects of love, as well as fear, shame and pain.

Example: Orit, a 14 year old survivor of sexual abuse, was busy for weeks mixing colors which always resulted in a brown color reminiscent of feces. Orit was obese, her clothes and hair were always dirty, and she smelled of feces. With time, Orit added paper, dust and dirt she collected in the studio, leftover food, and other things she found to her color mixtures. She put her mixtures into jars, and checked what had happened to them and how much they stank in every session. Apparently, this was Orit's way of telling the therapist about the inner experience of disgust and filth that overwhelmed her, without her being able to understand it. Projecting feelings of disgust into the material was a process of scapegoat transference (Schaverien, 1992) which enabled Orit to get rid of her feelings, while the material, not yet a symbolic image, embodied them. The stench from Orit's jars was intolerable. She nevertheless smiled and asked the therapist if she could bear the smell, and then she challenged: "Would you be willing to put your hand in the jar?" Actually, she was asking whether the therapist would be willing to touch her experience of disgust. If the therapist was willing, maybe she would be too. Orit was sexually abused repeatedly for many years. She did not do well in school, and had little control of her bowels. She felt repulsive and disgusting, and at this stage in therapy she had no way of expressing how she felt other than through the materials which contained her disgust. Later on she was able to express how disgusting she felt by drawing symbolic images.

Trauma freezes the experience and the psyche, and does not allow for movement. Traumatic play repeats the experience again and again without any avenue for change (Terr, 1989; Alvarez, 2012). This petrification is the essence of the difference between the developmental experience of exploration and playfulness and the traumatic experience of stagnant play. In therapy with children and adults who have been traumatized, there is a repetition of the traumatic contents in the material, corresponding to the need of the psyche to tell its story, even if in an unconscious way. In this repetition, materials that have no symbolic representation become available to consciousness and memory (Alvarez, 1992). Orit's repetitive mixtures of disgust were a kind of frozen play in which she created the same thing over and over again. However, inside the sealed jar, the disgusting materials were not stagnant. Even when petrifying influences of the trauma take over the psyche, processes can still occur inside the closed container. Trauma surviving children's curiosity with respect to what is going on inside the closed jar of disgust is a positive sign of movement and life, and an unconscious hope that the powers of change and life are at work within the psyche. Thus exploration of this traumatic mushiness can also be the beginning of a new experience. When using the materials differently during other phases within the therapeutic relationship, mushiness can become a healing experience. This way the material can turn from disgust into the pleasure of the mush phase, and the enmeshment of materials can turn into a pleasant symbiotic experience.

Example: Yair, 8 years old, was referred to therapy after being sexually abused by a friend of the family at the age of six. Yair was over-eating, and suffered from nightmares, bed-wetting, and anxieties. Session after session, Yair would cut clay into pieces, and put them in the therapist's palm. Piles of dry chunks were created, like lumps of stool, which Yair used to leave for the therapist as a "gift" to keep from one session to the next. One day, a leak in the studio got the mountain of clay accidentally wet. This happenstance was a turning point in therapy. Yair started playing with the wet clay. Slowly and gradually, Yair told the story of the sexual abuse in art as well as verbally. His bed-wetting decreased, and he stopped binge eating.

After a while, Yair began to work with clay using warm water. He enjoyed the warm touch and started to form clay containers. He worked with warm play dough and noted how pleasant it felt to the touch. Yair began using watercolors, mostly by dripping and splutters, noting the pleasant experience. Yair was able to shift from the traumatic use of mushy materials to soft and pleasant use of the liquid materials.

Traumatic mushiness tells the story of abuse in two ways. The first is the sensory experience, in which confusing sensations are mixed in a mush that reconstructs the inner experience of disgust and filth together with the physical experience that may be pleasant and painful, and contains conflicting emotions towards the abuser and the traumatic event. This is a non-symbolic level of expressing the physical and mental experience in material that resembles the symbolic equation (Segal, 1957), but is more concrete, since it contains a tangible dimension of real disgust and stench. The process of mixing materials and examining the result indicates the need to tell a story that has no words, as well as to achieve control over the process, which the abused child did not have when the traumatic events took place. The second is the symbolic level, in which the filth and disgust created in materials represent the experience of filth and disgust within the psyche, mediated by the ego. Here the filth and disgust create an embodied image (Schaverien, 1992) that has a life of its own. The symbolic dimension expressed in the life of the artwork allows for the processing of the traumatic experiences embodied in it. Processing (Schaverien, 2000), makes it possible to touch the unbearable contents transferred into the artwork, which serves as a scapegoat. At this point the patient can acknowledge these contents and perhaps even own them and bring them back into the domain of consciousness. After processing, the artwork itself can lose its power, and can be disposed of, since it is not needed any more in its tangible form. Thus, after many months of making mixtures of disgust in jars, after working through the abuse she suffered in other ways, Orit said – "I want to throw this disgusting stuff away, it is not needed anymore".

Discussion

Working with liquid and mushy materials in art therapy involves contact with sensory experiences and the emotional quality accompanying them, and provides an opportunity to touch wordless areas in the psyche in a way that can give form to the emotional nature of the experience. The contact with these materials is like going back to a time when the infant and mother, subject and object, were one, and is thus a return to the emotional qualities of this unity registered in the body and psyche. Similarly, there is no distinction between materials and shapes. The materials mix, one color invades another, dripping and creating the artistic possibility of merging.

Engaging with mushy materials allows for an immediate connection with primal experiences, as well as symbolic expression, observation and the reflection of these areas of the psyche. In this process, internalizations of relationships and occurrences that were held wordlessly in the body and psyche come to life in the here and now of therapy. These internalizations can be important material for working through at different levels of consciousness.

At the sensory level, the mushy engagement can allow parts of the psyche that are in the unitary state to form, with no need for words or interpretations. Thus, mushy engagement can allow stagnant developmental processes to move on in the direction they need to develop. At the Oedipal level (Balint, 1969) of understanding and conscious recollection, observing the experiences arising from engaging with the mushy materials can pave the way to understanding the symbolic meanings within the material and the way to useit, and enable applications to the patient's life.

In this chapter, we described the application of the theoretical concept of mushiness derived from clinical experience to the teaching of art therapy. We defined the engagement with wet, liquid, and slimy materials as mushiness, which is the mental quality of formlessness, liquidity, and merging that touches undifferentiated areas of the psyche. Mushiness is based on touch and sensory experience, and is characterized by the qualities of the sensory experience that existed in the primal object relations that were internalized.

We identified two types of mushiness. Developmental mushiness is linked to a mental experience of oneness that is not yet separated, characterizing the beginnings of life. Developmental mushiness is colored by the object relations that characterized the time of its formation, and is expressed in therapy by transference to the therapist and the materials. The quality of experiencing materials is characterized with creative play and discovery, and the pleasure of engaging with the wet and slimy, even when it is disgusting. Within this engagement, the materials used can be very diverse and include pre-material materials, with their sensory qualities and the associations they give rise to. A therapist who understands the patient's developmental state and is willing to play with unusual materials, can offer various liquid and mushy materials in the studio that enable developmental mushiness. The patient can discover the materials they need, or sometimes the therapist can also suggest them, as a response to the patient's cues (Moon, 2002).

Traumatic mushiness is related to the collapse of the differentiated state into the engulfing mixture in which the distinction between internal and external realms and between self and object has no meaning. The traumatic experience destroys differentiation, sense of meaning, order and logic in the world, leaving a terrifying experience that is meaningless. In this situation, the playful quality of exploring the materials turns into a petrified quality of repeating the stagnant mental experience that is forced to re-occur. Here, the revulsion is not creative, but rather is an expression of the patient's inner sense of disgust, which is a result of bodily experiences during abuse. The disgusting material that patients mix in a state of traumatic mushiness does not symbolize their inner sense of disgust, but rather constitutes a symbolic equation (Segal, 1957) in which the mush embodies the disgust.

The feeling of disgust expressed in the materials is validated by the presence of the therapist who is willing to participate. In so doing, the therapist can enable a movement in the petrified experience, and development toward the symbolization of the sensation, so it can also be consciously referred to.

Here, the materials serve as a container (Symington and Symington, 2002) for the feeling and can also enable the transformation from a symbolic equation of revulsion to a symbolic expression of the feeling of disgust. The materials and the presence of the therapist can enable a shift from the frozen traumatic mushiness to the developmental mushiness which allows playfulness. Then the mush can form into materials and images embodying the emergent differentiation. Here, the variety of materials the therapist can offer is very important, since engagement with mushy materials can bring the patient in touch with the dissociated traumatic experiences, and later on, can pave the way for change in the psychological experience of materials.

Both types of mushiness have a concrete dimension and a symbolic dimension that are fundamental to the tangible essence of art therapy. The mush in the developmental play constitutes a return to the primal unitary mental areas and symbolizes the psychic materials characterizing these areas. The disgusting mixture of the traumatic mush embodies the physical feelings of disgust of the traumatic experience and its implications, and also symbolizes the psychological experience of disgust after the trauma. This way, engaging with the mushy materials can allow the patient to move from a concrete expression of the experience to a symbolic one, and in so doing, promote development and insight.

The concept of mushiness derives from our experiences as art therapists, and was conceptualized during teaching and defined in writing. It became an important part of our students' clinical thinking and professional conceptualization. This concept, like many others in art therapy, stems from our therapeutic experiences in the field, and is returned to the field when our students can use it in their therapeutic work.

References

Aldridge, F. (1998) "Chocolate or Shit Aesthetics and Cultural Poverty in Art Therapy with Children" *Inscape,* 3(1), 2-9.

Alvarez, A. (1992) *Live Company: Psychoanalytic Psychotherapy with Autistic Borderline Deprived and Abused Children*. East Essex and New York: Routledge.

—. (2012) *The Thinking Heart: Three Levels of Psychoanalytic Therapy with Disturbed Children*. East Essex and New York: Routledge.

Balint, M. (1969) *The Basic Fault: Therapeutic Aspects of Regression*. Northwestern University Press.

Elbrecht C. (2013) *Trauma Healing at the Clay Field*. London and Philadelphia: Jessica Kingsley Publishers.

Freud, S. (1938) "Three Contributions to the Theory of Sex" (pp. 553-629) in Freud, S. *The Basic Writings of Sigmund Freud.* A. Brill (trans.). New York: The Modern Library.

Herman, J. L. (2015) *Trauma and Recovery: The Aftermath of Violence – from Domestic Abuse to Political Terror*. Basic Books.

Lusebrink, V. B., Martinsone, K., Dzilna-Silova, I. (2013) "The Expressive Therapies Continuum (ETC): Interdisciplinary Bases of the ECT" *International Journal of Art Therapy*, 18 (2), 75-85.

Moon. K. H. (2002) *Studio Art Therapy*. London and Philadelphia: Jessica Kingsley Publishers.

Murphy, J. (1998) Art Therapy with Sexually Abused Children and Young People" *Inscape,* 3(1), 10-16.

Neumann, E. (1954) *The Origins and History of Consciousness*. R. F. C. Hull (trans.) (pp. 5-38) Princeton University Press: Bollingen Series.

Neumann, E. (1973) *The Child*. R. Manheim (trans.). New York: GP Putnam's Sons.

O'Brien, F. (2004) The Making of Mess in Art Therapy: Attachment, Trauma and the Brain. *Inscape,* 9(1), 2-13.

Ogden, T. H. (1989) *The Primitive Edge of Experience*. New Jersey and London: Jason Aronson Inc.

Piaget, J., Inhelder B. (1969) *The Psychology of the Child*. H. Weaver (trans.). New York: Basic Books.

Rabiger, S. (1990) "Art Therapy as a Container" (pp. 23-38) in Case, C., Dalley, T. (eds.). *Working with Children in Art Therapy.* London and New York: Routledge.

Rubin. J. (1978) *Child Art Therapy: Understanding and Helping cChildren Grow Through Art*. New York: Van Nostrand Reinhold.

Sagar, C. (1990) "Working with Cases of Child Sexual Abuse" (pp. 89-114) in Case, C., Dalley, T. (eds.). *Working with Children in Art Therapy.* London and New York: Routledge.

Segal, H. (1957) "Notes on Symbol Formation" *International Journal of Psychoanalysis*, 38, 391-397.

Schaverien, J. (1992) *The Revealing Image*. London and New York: Routledge.

—. (2000) "The Triangular Relationship and the Aesthetic Countertransference in Analytical Art Psychotherapy" (pp. 55-83) in Gilroy, A., McNeilly, G. (eds.). *The Changing Shape of Art Therapy: New Developments in Theory and Practice*. London and Philadelphia: Jessica Kingsley Publishers.

Symington, J., Symington, N. (2002) *The Clinical Thinking of Wilfred Bion*. London and New York: Routledge.

Terr, L. (1989) "Treating Psychic Trauma in Children: A Preliminary Discussion" *Journal of Traumatic Stress*, 2(1), 3-20.

Tustin, F. (2013) *Autistic States in Children*. London and New York: Routledge.

Winnicott, D. W. (1986) "The Theory of the Parent-Infant Relationship" in Buckley, P. (ed.). *Essential Papers on Object Relations*. New York and London: New York University Press.

CHAPTER 16

SOWING THE SEEDS FOR AN INTEGRATED BRAIN-BODY-MIND HOLISTIC APPROACH IN THE CREATIVE ARTS THERAPEUTIC ARENA

SHARON VAISVASER

Learn how to see. Realize that everything connects to everything else.
(Leonardo da Vinci)

Introduction

Inspiring advances in neuroscience and growing scope of applications, underscore the importance of assimilation and utilization of this knowledge to inform Creative Arts Therapies (CATs) education, training and practice. Neuroscience-informed training can contribute to the development of therapeutic insights and skills, enriching and grounding the work in evidence-based research and recognizing ways in which CATs may shape brain function. Indeed, this multidisciplinary translational approach has received growing interest within CATs modalities in the past decade (Belkofer & Nolan, 2016; Homann, 2010; King et al., 2019; O'Kelly et al., 2016; Payne, 2017; Perryman et al., 2019).

Being trained both as a neuroscientist and a dance/movement therapist, I am deeply interested and invested in the incorporation of neuroscientific insights into the psychotherapeutic toolkit, seeking for a synthesis in which these ideas will be more accessible, natural and useful to CATs educators, students and practitioners. Based on my teaching experience, this chapter will portray ways in which the brain operates, touching upon the clinical relevance and correspondence with mechanisms of CATs, to facilitate their integration into our field of work. Accordingly, when teaching neuroscience in the context of CATs, I find the grounding of the learning process in experiential exercises and the invitation for reflective practices and discussions to be vital.

In the service of interdisciplinary integration, the field of neuroscience will be approached and presented in this chapter from several angles relevant to CATs; these include the embodiment of perception, cognition and emotion; the basic architecture and function of the brain; sensory-motor processing; affectivity and emotion regulation; dynamics of the self and the empathic relationship; transcendent qualities of aesthetic engagement and creativity; finally converging into the neuroplastic moulding of the brain.

Embodiment and grounding of perception, cognition and emotion

Let us first begin with the fundamental recognition that brain processes of representation and meaning creation, at both an emotional and cognitive level, are based on bodily sensory-motor experiences. This view of the brain was, in fact, initially propagated by Sigmund Freud. With training in both neuroanatomy and neurophysiology, Freud tried to link neuronal mechanisms to psychodynamic concepts, in his 'Project for a Scientific Psychology', suggesting an approach to the brain as an intrinsically active and dynamic organ (Freud, 1895). Freud hypothesised that information concerning sensory qualities is dynamically transmitted through the mental apparatus by neural oscillations that would proliferate across 'contact-barriers' (anticipating the synaptic structure and learning and memory processes). The scientific tools of his day were inadequate for such undertakings and Freud's work shifted to exploring psychological models in greater depth, while the recent interdisciplinary field of neuropsychoanalysis fervently explores and anchors Freud's original ideas in contemporary science (Panksepp & Solms, 2012).

Indeed, the remarkable progress in our understanding of the brain has been facilitated by improvements in neuroimaging techniques and methods, predominantly structural and functional magnetic resonance imaging (MRI/fMRI, respectively). fMRI indirectly infers neuronal activity from regional changes in blood oxygenation (hemodynamic response), meaning enhanced blood flow in active brain regions to satisfy energetic demands of the neuronal tissue, offering detailed spatial patterns of whole brain activity. Direct measurement of brain electrical dynamics is recorded mainly through the use of electroencephalography (EEG), offering high temporal resolution. There are possibilities for fusion of imaging modalities, to enhance both spatial and temporal resolution.

As contemporary neuroscience unravels the mystery of the brain, the bidirectional interactive relationship between brain and body is widely expanded, grounded in on-going reciprocity with the environment. An experiential exploration of this idea, while engaging in the arts modalities, might include an invitation to attend to and explore ways of knowing oneself (or consciousness) in the 'here and now', while noting that our brain does not passively process the input from our sense organs, but rather actively and continuously creates and shapes our inner world of representation – perceptions, emotions and cognitions – associating our past experiences with the ongoing one.

Indeed, different brain systems communicate with signals from internal visceral organs (interoceptive), from the neuromuscular system (proprioceptive), and from the surroundings (exteroceptive). The brain is involved in and affected by allostasis, the ongoing processes aimed to maintain homeostasis, thus building and updating internal models of the body in the world. Based on prior experiences, the brain generates predictions of the hidden causes of accumulating incoming sensory signals, from within the body and from the surrounding world. In cases of a mismatch, the discrepancy ('prediction error') moves through the brain's hierarchical system ('bottom-up', from lower to higher level layers of organization) to refine future predictions. These ongoing, multimodal, reciprocal exchanges, termed 'predictive processing', structure our perception, cognition and emotional experiences (Barrett et al., 2016; Friston, 2010).

In accordance, traditional perspectives that view cognition as an isolated module have been challenged. The paradigm shift towards action-oriented cognition recognizes that conceptual representations are grounded in physical experiences associated with them. Indeed, "cognition is not the representation of a pregiven world by a pregiven mind but is rather the enactment of a world and a mind on the basis of a history of the variety of the actions that a being in the world performs" (Varela et al., 1991, p. 9). Higher-level (integrative and abstract) mental representations engage the sensory, motor and affective brain regions in a dynamic way, while interacting with the physical and social environment (Barsalou, 2020; Engel et al., 2013).

These conceptualizations of brain function, further unfolded in this chapter, emphasize the importance of the lived experience in the way we perceive, feel, learn and think about ourselves and about others; This harmonizes with the uniqueness of the arts and the therapeutic potential of the embodied enactive CATs (Koch, 2017; Koch & Fuchs, 2011).

Brain basics – a general outline of the architecture and function of the brain

Delving into the brain's building blocks, we realize its complexity, consisting of about one hundred billion neurons and trillions of supportive cells (glia), approximately the same as the number of stars in our Milky Way galaxy. Neurons are composed of a cell body (soma), dendrites receiving input and a long axon that reaches out to other neurons, propagating the message (nerve impulses). A neuron sends the electrical impulse down its axon, releasing a neurotransmitter at the connection site – the synapse, which then either excites or inhibits the downstream neuron. Individual neurons interact with up to ten thousand other neurons, producing neural assemblies (networks), enabling both segregation (differentiation) and integration of information and functions. Thus, the human brain is investigated in the context of regional neural activity and interregional functional connectivity (temporal correlations between brain regions).

In order to illustrate brain structure and function, educators are encouraged to use a metaphoric approach, such as Siegel's 'hand model' (2002), engaging and giving an experiential-visual example of the relevance of anatomy for coordinated function and neural interconnections (Siegel, 2020). The model uses various parts of the hand to represent major regions, briefly described here and later elaborated on: the brainstem (palm), which is connected to the spinal cord (forearm), communicates with the peripheral nervous system and plays an important role in the regulation of cardiac and respiratory function, consciousness, and the sleep and wake cycle; the limbic region, including the hippocampus and amygdala (the thumb folded over the palm, imagining that you have two), a core region of detection, response and memory of emotional events; and the cerebral cortex or neocortex (fingers encircling the thumb), which contains primary sensory and motor regions and areas of association and integration. The cortex is divided into two hemispheres, with inter-hemispheric connections (for segregation and integration) occurring via a 'white matter' tract (a bundle of fibers/axons), termed the corpus callosum. The frontmost portion (fingertips) is the prefrontal cortex, most evolutionarily and developmentally advanced and generally involved in evaluation, modulation and regulation of emotional stimuli through its connections with subcortical limbic activity.

Is seems valuable for arts therapists to have a general idea of how sensory-motor processing occurs in the brain. Just above the brainstem is the thalamus, an egg shaped area that serves as a gateway and 'relay station' for incoming sensory information, with extensive connections to many brain regions, including the brainstem, limbic area and the cortex above it. Each hemisphere of the cortex is divided into four lobes-frontal, temporal (near the ears, in both sides), parietal (near the center) and occipital (at the back). The cortex is comprised of three primary sensory areas for each modality – auditory (A1), in the temporal lobes; visual (V1), in the occipital lobe; somatosensory (S1), in the parietal lobes; and a primary motor region (M1), in the posterior part of the frontal lobe. Sensations are mapped topographically; for example, the mapping of the body in the somatosensory and motor cortices is constructed in a somatotopic arrangement – in correspondence with specific body areas, with magnified representations of sensitive body parts, visualized as the iconic 'Homunculus' or 'Hermunculus' (little man/woman) (Di Noto et al., 2013).

Primary sensory/motor regions have adjacent association cortical areas, substantially expanded in human, which integrate new inputs with memories of past experiences to process and interpret incoming data and coordinate motor responses. From primary cortices, a ventral pathway is responsible for stimulus recognition and identification (the 'what' stream), while a dorsal pathway is responsible for processing space and motion, locating objects, understanding others' movements (including facial expressions) and guiding our own actions toward objects (the 'where/how' stream).

The crosstalk between sensory and motor regions allows mapping of motor commands onto the sensory consequences of the movement, constructing an internal model of the body in the world. Multisensory integration across modalities is enabled by the response of sensory cortices not only to their own modality but also to other modalities, through their connectedness (Starke et al., 2020; Stein et al., 2020). This may also promote experience-dependent sensory substitution in deprived sensory cortices and favor compensatory plasticity (Xerri & Zennou-Azogui, 2021).

With significant relevance to the multisensory engagement in CATs, brain development, especially in association cortices, is highly dependent on early sensory experiences (Henschke et al., 2018), and heavily influenced, throughout life, by environment and culture and the accumulation of experiences of production and appreciation of art (Nadal & Chatterjee, 2019).

Core players in the emotional orchestra

Psychotherapeutic education would greatly benefit from the investigated domains of affective brain function. While attending to the emotional brain, using creative means of exploration, I begin by challenging the students with the questions "What are emotions?" and "how do you know that you have them?"

The neuroscientific study of emotions is a complex terrain, driven by paradigmatic differences. Introducing CATs students to different neuroscience-based models of emotion might enrich ways in which they can explore self and other's affective repertoire, emotional processing and regulation. We might begin by referring to basic emotions and introducing Panksepp, who coined the term *affective neuroscience* and defined primary emotional brain systems (interconnected regions) for discrete emotional categories, rooted in evolutionary continuities – SEEKING/Exploration, RAGE/Anger, FEAR/Anxiety, LUST, CARE/Nurturing, PANIC/Sadness, and PLAY/Social Joy (Panksepp, 1998). Constructivist (or dimensional) approaches suggest a different viewpoint, conceiving emotions as dynamic social constructions that emerge to make sense of incoming sensory information, experienced and learned based on previous similar experiences, situated and therefore highly variable and shaped by distributed neural functional networks (Barrett, 2017). These affective states are often characterized in terms of valence and arousal dimensions.

Bearing these different perspectives of emotions in mind, we can move on to present core emotion processing regions that have been consistently shown to be engaged during affective experiences. The activation and connections between these key regions play important roles, in mental health and in psychopathology.

The amygdala, an almond-shaped cluster of nuclei, situated in the medial temporal lobe, is a key limbic structure involved in diverse affective states. The amygdala was shown to play a pivotal role in detecting, encoding and triggering responses to potential threats (fear/anxiety), as well as to arousing goal-relevant events, social behaviours like facial expressions, vocal prosody and uncertain or ambiguous external and internal stimuli (Bickart et al., 2014). The amygdala doesn't act alone, its involvement in complex and varied arousing situations relates to the multidimensional responses of its neurons and the multitudes of neural circuits that converge in it, receiving inputs from, and sending outputs to, numerous brain areas (Gothard, 2020). For instance, a region located at the top of the brainstem (midbrain), termed the periaqueductal grey (PAG), is implicated in heightened emotional reactivity and defensive survival functions, through its connectivity with the amygdala, orchestrating behavioural aspects of the defence cascade – fight or flight 'active' responses as well as 'freezing' behaviour.

The hypothalamus (situated underneath the thalamus), closely-connected with limbic and brainstem projections, is a structure that supports the integration between the endocrine (hormonal) and nervous systems, essential for regulation and coordination of biological process such as growth, differentiation, metabolism and reproduction. It regulates many aspects of energy homeostasis and is also a primary stress-integrative brain center. The amygdala is involved in the initiation of the stress response by acting on the hypothalamus (hypothalamic-pituitary-adrenal, HPA-axis), resulting in cortisol release (Phelps & LeDoux, 2005). Cortisol reactively affects memory following an inverted-U shaped function, where moderate cortisol levels enhance hippocampal-based learning processes, while large increases are detrimental (De Kloet et al., 1999). This is why optimal levels of tension or arousal are beneficial and prompt learning and creativity, while extreme, traumatic, or chronic stress leads to diminished cognitive abilities, less coherent memories and psychopathologies, such as anxiety disorders (De Kloet et al., 2005).

The hippocampus, Latin for seahorse named for its shape, is the key region for spatial and contextual information processing and the formation of declarative memory. Its co-activation with the neighbouring amygdala was consistently shown to play a key role in successful encoding and retrieval of emotional episodes (Dahlgren et al., 2020; McGaugh, 2004). During memory encoding, new experiences are associated with established prior information, in a process termed memory consolidation, while long-term memory representations are gradually formed in the neocortex, to be later transmitted back to the hippocampus during retrieval (Frankland & Bontempi, 2005). The hippocampus is fundamental in supporting the associative structure of an event memory and in influencing how the memory is re-experienced at retrieval. Amygdala's contribution leads to the associated implicit subjective emotional experience and to strengthened memory traces (Admon et al., 2018; Vaisvaser et al., 2013). This is why, in addition to the conscious explicit recollection of events that can be verbally articulated, memories include the association and reinstatement of emotions as bodily reactions, such as physiological arousal (McGaugh, 2013). In posttraumatic stress disorder (PTSD), amygdala up-modulation and impaired hippocampal function increases emotional arousal and intrusive imagery, while reducing episodic memory coherence (Bisby et al., 2020). The last section of this chapter refers to the potential for reconsolidation of trauma memories through psychotherapeutic work.

A primal SEEKING urge to engage with the world involves a reward circuit in the brain, where dopamine is released, including the ventral striatum (most specifically a region termed nucleus accumbens, part of the basal ganglia), and the orbital frontal cortex (just above the eyes) (Berridge & Kringelbach, 2015). Decreased activity and connectivity within this reward circuit was related with states of anhedonia and depression (Fan et al., 2021; Forbes et al., 2019), while its amplification may contribute to the onset of hypo/manic symptoms (Damme et al., 2017).

Cortical regions that are implicated in salience detection and emotional processing include the anterior cingulate gyrus, situated above the corpus callosum; and the insula, a folded portion of the cortex responsible for interoceptive awareness, mapping the state of the body in contextually relevant and emotionally significant ways (Craig, 2009).

Functional abnormalities in these aforementioned regions have been identified in a wide array of psychiatric disorders, associated with failure of 'top-down' prefrontal regulation, as further discussed in the next section.

Emotion regulation – the orchestral conductors

Processes of emotion regulation are mediated by higher-level brain regions, also linked with bodily and social experience. To begin to address the concept of emotion regulation, I encourage students to explore it through the art forms, using techniques for grounding, visualizing an imagined or real place where they feel safe, and expressing their experience symbolically. Then I invite them to move into a place of discomfort, so as to again attain physical and mental balance, through their artistic exploration and activate internal resources (imagining an attachment figure), enhancing self-awareness, presence and acceptance.

Emotion regulation broadly refers to the implementation of a conscious or non-conscious modulation of the trajectory of an emotion (Gross, 2015). Emotion dysregulation has emerged as an increasingly important construct for understanding diverse adjustment problems in childhood, adolescence, and adulthood and as a transdiagnostic feature of various mental health outcomes (Beauchaine & Cicchetti, 2019). Based on neuroimaging findings, two broad types of regulation have been distinguished: 'explicit' and 'implicit'. In both, prefrontal cortical regions exert inhibitory control over subcortical limbic regions (e.g. amygdala), reducing anxiety/avoidance (Etkin et al., 2015). Explicit, voluntary emotion regulation, such as the conscious reappraisal, i.e. alteration of self-relevant meaning, is induced mainly by the dorsal and lateral prefrontal cortex (Buhle et al., 2014). Implicit emotion regulation, on the other hand, is modulated by the ventromedial prefrontal cortex (vmPFC), automatically and unconsciously, in the context of safe environments and secure attachments (Etkin et al., 2015). Since amygdala-mPFC connections are bidirectionally shaped, 'bottom-up' processes (from the amygdala to the PFC) may also facilitate regulation.

From a developmental perspective, adolescence is a prolonged transitional period of plastic maturation, related to the slow-developing PFC, demonstrating synaptic reorganization and myelination (the fatty envelope that surrounds axons, crucial for rapid signal propagation), until the third decade of life. Accordingly, this period is associated with intensification of automatic, reactive 'bottom-up' affective processing, reflecting the heightened engagement of subcortical regions (e.g., amygdala), especially in social contexts, and immaturity of 'top-down' regulatory control (Somerville et al., 2010). This signifies adolescence as a period of neural vulnerability to emotion dysregulation, but also a period of more flexible, exploratory style (Crone & Dahl, 2012), with the potential of tapping into the brain's creative capacity in support of the development of self-regulation and formation of identity (Siegel, 2015).

In various affective and trauma-related disorders associated with hyperarousal, emotional dysregulation is caused by insufficient prefrontal modulation of subcortical limbic regions (Admon et al., 2013; Kim et al., 2011). On the contrary, dissociative states and disorders involve overly increased prefrontal activation, resulting in hypoactivation of the amygdala during symptom provocation with concomitant emotional detachment and autonomic blunting (Andrewes & Jenkins, 2019).

Importantly, trajectories of affective regulation draw on the relationship between central and peripheral nervous systems, explained by the Polyvagal Theory, which enlightens our need safe connections in order to regulate intense emotions in a flexible manner (Porges, 2007, 2011). The theory posits that the vagal nerve of the parasympathetic system – the longest cranial nerve, originating in the brainstem and most widely distributed in the body, down-regulating the heart, lungs, and digestive tract – can be divided into two subsystems – ventral (lower) and dorsal (upper). While the dorsal vagal branch sends inhibitory inputs associated with immobilization (freeze/faint), in contrast to active defences mediated by the sympathetic system (fight or flight), the ventral vagal branch induces a calm physiological state, required for social interactions, thus associated with bonding and communicating, producing a 'Social Engagement System'. This ventral nerve branch is covered with myelin and integrates neural regulation of the body with that of the face (expressivity, prosody, and vocalization).

In a process that Porges coined 'neuroception', subconscious reflexive mechanisms in limbic structures continuously pick-up environmental and visceral information, by sensory 'bottom-up' pathways and 'top-down' regulation by the prefrontal cortex, to detect and distinguish features that are either safe and receptive or dangerous and threatening. In safe environments, the 'Social Engagement System' produces more flexible and pro-social behaviours and prevents primitive defensive strategies (fight/flight mobilization or shutdown behaviours mediated by the dorsal vagus). This is reflected in the dynamic balancing of sympathetic/parasympathetic systems that gives rise to variability in heart-rate (HRV) (Porges, 2007). Accordingly, HRV has emerged as a reliable peripheral biomarker of emotion regulation (Mather & Thayer, 2018), as well as respiratory sinus arrhythmia (RSA-HRV in synchrony with respiration; Beauchaine, 2015).

Dysfunctional 'top-down' regulation and autonomic dysregulation in traumatised clients was related to the oscillation between extremes of fight/flight sympathetically-mediated hyperarousal, with accompanying hypervigilance, intrusive imagery and affective over-reactivity and hypoarousal, immobilisation, passivity, emotional numbing and deadness (mediated by the parasympathetic dorsal vagal). Observing these processes in the therapeutic setting forms a first step toward establishing connections and enhancing the ability to modulate raw affects. The therapeutic goal of being present within the 'window of tolerance' of optimal range of arousal, and further expanding it (Ogden et al., 2006; Siegel, 1999), heavily depends on the therapist's own ability to finely attune her/his nervous system, both in preparation for therapy and during moment-to-moment experiential therapeutic work (Geller, 2018).

Receptive attunement to the client's verbal and nonverbal expression, while also staying attuned inwardly, grounded, immersed in the moment, allows the therapist's presence to be experienced, and the client's nervous system to come into alignment, in a bidirectional communication with the therapist's calming presence. Such 'therapeutic presence' promotes 'neuroception' of safety, engaging the 'Social Engagement System' and supporting prefrontal-limbic communication. Creative engagement in a safe atmosphere, enables clients (and therapists) to functionally exercise their neural capacity to regulate behavioural, physiological and emotional state (Porges & Dana, 2018).

Wired to connect – the neuro-symphony of the self and self-other relations

Psychotherapeutic education and practice interweaves intra-subjective aspects related to development of sense of self and self-representations with inter-subjective relatedness and object representations. In this regard, the crosstalk between major functional networks, i.e. interconnected neural assemblies that alter their activity simultaneously, provides a powerful paradigm for characterizing the intra- and inter-subjective experience and the neurobiology of *psychiatric dysfunction* (Menon, 2011; Wig, 2017). These 'large-scale' canonical neural networks relate to the experience of the self, to self-other differentiation and to empathy, supported by the overlap between neural patterns representing the self and others.

The 'salience network', composed mainly of the bilateral anterior insula, anterior cingulate cortex and amygdala, serves to integrate sensory, visceral, and hedonic social signals (Seeley, 2019). This network is crucial for awareness, response and representation of relevant stimuli and imbuing them with emotional weight, supporting both positive and negative affect and showing modality-independent activation (Lindquist et al., 2016).

A different network that supports internal mental exploration is the 'default mode network' (DMN), comprising the cortical midline structures (medial prefrontal cortex and posterior cingulate cortex), also connected with the hippocampus. The DMN was initially revealed as a network consistently activated 'at rest', i.e. during task-free states, undirected by cognitive control. Following extensive research, the DMN is now widely assumed to support self-referential processes, spontaneous introspection, mind-wandering, autobiographical memory, episodic future thinking and mentalizing (Raichle, 2015; Wen et al., 2020).

A third network – the central executive network (CEN, including the dorsal and lateral regions of the prefrontal cortex and the posterior parietal cortex), is engaged in higher-order cognitive and evaluative processes and externally oriented attention. Intriguingly, the salience network was suggested to mediate the interaction and transitions between the intrinsic mentalizing DMN and the extrinsic attention, via CEN, ultimately creating a multidimensional coherent sense of self (Di Plinio et al., 2020; Uddin, 2015). Consequently, abnormal network switching disrupts one's capacity to distinguish between the internal world and external environment. This is why dysregulation of these large-scale networks and their dynamic crosstalk was related, for example, to psychosis (Supekar et al., 2019). The DMN was shown to be active during REM sleep, thus involved in dreaming, yet with reduction in CEN and salience, that might be linked with the lack of reality monitoring, volitional control, and vigilance (Uitermarkt et al., 2020).

Importantly, the interaction and balance between these three networks can be explored with regard to creative processes. Indeed, a cohesive involvement of these networks was shown to be induced in creative processes, across different tasks and domains, such as verbal creativity (divergent thinking) and artistic improvisation (Beaty et al., 2016; Kleinmintz et al., 2019; Shi et al., 2018).

The development of these networks was shown to rely on the nonverbal aspects of social interaction and embodied relational experiences (Atzil et al., 2018), strongly dependent upon on-going, close, and healthy bonds (Long et al., 2020). Indeed, robust literature provides support that "the human brain's primary environment is our matrix of social relationships" (Cozolino, 2014, p. 1). This interpersonal resonance is anchored by neural simulation and synchronisation mechanisms, further described below.

Empathic reflection and mirroring play a key role in the development of the self from infancy and predispose the basis for developing secure attachment. The realisation of a neural mirroring mechanisms, by which an action execution and observation recruit similar neuronal processes, revealed the availability of a direct automatic access to the meaning of others' behavior (Gallese et al., 1996; Rizzolatti et al., 1996). Strikingly, in addition to these action-perception circuits, neuroimaging research has demonstrated that salience regions involved in the subjective experience, like the insula, are also active when these emotions are recognized in others. This mechanism, coined 'embodied simulation' (Gallese, 2003, 2014), emerges through experience sharing, underpinning the capacity to build and maintain attachment, with the involvement of the hormone oxytocin (Feldman, 2017).

In addition to emotional empathy, involving shared embodied representations, neuroscientific evidence point to a separate empathy network for cognitive understanding, involving a theory of mind 'mentalizing' network, largely overlapping the DMN, as well as to the importance of connectivity between these two networks (Abraham et al., 2018; Kanske et al., 2015; Raz et al., 2014; Shamay-Tsoory, 2011). This implies that along with self-referential processes, the DMN is involved in generating and contemplating on thoughts and intentions of others. Consequently, DMN abnormalities were found in multiple psychopathologies (Whitfield-Gabrieli & Ford, 2012).

The interplay between emotional and cognitive components of empathy, established through the crosstalk between these brain networks, seems extremely important to include in therapeutic education. This can be discussed in class by referring to the psychotherapeutic relationship, the movement back and forth between subjective and objective positions and phenomenon such as identification and transference – countertransference (including somatic) transactions.

Another major aspect of our neurophysiology is the capability to synch with others, in the context attachment bonds and in meaningful moments of state-sharing and mutual understanding (Long et al., 2020; Schore & Schore, 2008). Brain-to-brain coupling between people occurs on the basis of transmission of implicit common interpretation (Hasson et al., 2012), affiliated with the development of emotion co-regulation, social understanding and resilience (Feldman, 2020; Hu et al., 2017; Reindl et al., 2018; Wheatley et al., 2012). Moreover, shared artistic experiences were shown induce interpersonal brain synchrony (Babiloni et al., 2012; Jola et al., 2013; Müller et al., 2013; Reddish et al., 2013; Sachs et al., 2020). These insight from the field of social neuroscience empirically ground fundamental CATs ideas in neuropsychological bonding mechanisms.

Brain on art – the aesthetic experience

During (co-)creation processes within the arts modalities, aesthetic engagement emerges, deepens or fluctuates (Samaritter, 2018). The growing field of 'neuroaesthetics' attempts to discover the brain basis of aesthetic experience, wherein aesthetic emotions are savored for their own sake, with subjectively felt intensity and emotional arousal, experienced across a broad range of experiential domains (e.g. body movement, visual artwork, performance, literature, film and music). Aesthetic experiences are integrative in nature, drawing on perception and imagery across multiple senses as well as on memories and associations, thus may also arise in response to imagined objects (Vessel et al., 2019).

Embodied aesthetics, within the field of CATs, was suggested to encompass the active (expression) and the receptive (impression) aspects of the experiences, promoting the experience of body–mind unity (Koch, 2017). Research in the field of neuroaesthetics mostly focuses on perception and individual preference that allow beholders to feel the art in an embodied manner, closely linked to processes of embodied simulation (Gallese, 2017). Recent developments of mobile brain/body imaging technology allow more extensive understandings of brain function also during real-time artistic creation (Cruz-Garza et al., 2019; King, 2018; King & Parada, 2020).

The aesthetic experience emerges from the interaction between distributed neural systems involved in sensory–motor engagement, affective absorption and valuation processes, appraisal and comprehension (meaning) processes (Chatterjee & Vartanian, 2016). Correspondingly, it engages reward and salience circuitry, DMN and higher connectivity between the DMN and both sensorimotor cortices and the salience network (Belfi et al., 2019; Bolwerk et al., 2014; Chatterjee & Vartanian, 2016; Kaimal et al., 2017; Vessel et al., 2013), implementing fundamental aspects of personal involvement, sense of meaning, empathy, imagination, and creativity. The integration of sensory processes with self-reflection was suggested to be related to stress regulation and positive health outcomes (Williams et al., 2018). Importantly, the flexible configuration of neural networks is sensitive to individuals' desires, expectations, goals, mood, context, and the accumulated lifetime of experiences with art (Nadal & Chatterjee, 2019). Moreover, the field of neuroaesthetics teaches us that the arts' potential benefits transcend class, gender, age, race, and culture (Magsamen, 2019).

Neuroplasticity – moulding the brain and fostering therapeutic change

The brain's capacity for change and ways in which CATs might impact the neurobiology of the brain and stimulate neural plasticity is an eminent aspect of neuroscience relevant to psychotherapeutic education and practice. It is well-known that brain development during fetal, neonatal and early infancy periods is critical for establishing the biology of a healthy mind, wherein the interactions with the caregiver(s) play a vital role (Atzil et al., 2018; Curley & Champagne, 2016). Yet, the revolution of neuroplasticity, defined as brain structural and functional reorganization in response to external and internal factors, has taught us that in addition to major early modulations, the brain circuitry continues to be modified throughout the life span (Lepousez et al., 2015). These changes rely on neuroprotective factors (mainly brain-derived neurotrophic factor, BDNF) and include, at micro-level, epigenetic modulations of gene expression, the birth of new neurons (neurogenesis), synapse re-organisation and modified formation and growth of myelin, resulting, at macro-level, in more effective information transfer and improved synchrony between distant regions.

Adverse environments reduce effective brain connectivity, mainly due to impairments in PFC and hippocampus and diminished regulation of core emotional regions, generating negative bias in attention and self-representation (Price & Duman, 2020). Yet, the brain maintains its capacity for neuroplastic change that may allow for subsequent amelioration by positive experiences. What might induce positive neuroplastic changes?

In accordance with the embodied enacted view of brain function, plastic processes were shown to be highly action-dependent and modifiable by experience, suggesting the neuroplasticity-enhancing potential of experiential interventions (Sampaio-Baptista & Johansen-Berg, 2017; Tomassy et al., 2016). Furthermore, creative arts activities were consistently shown to induce significant neural changes, which were related to psychological resilience (Bolwerk et al., 2014; Teixeira-Machado et al., 2019; Zamorano et al., 2019).

Ongoing neuroplasticity has also to do with the possibility to process and update memories. Indeed, Pioneering research has shown that memories are far more malleable than once thought and involve updating processes, both at time of consolidation and at retrieval – in a process of reconsolidation (Phelps & Hofmann, 2019). Retrieved autobiographical memories that involve re-engaged emotional responses can be modulated and updated, potentially changing their impact (Hasson et al., 2015). These processes underline the promise of affective change and reduced emotional consequences that stem from memories of traumatic events, highlighting the potential for clinical avenues (Monfils & Holmes, 2018).

CATs may assist the formulation of a reconsolidated narrative, through processes of creation, observation, reflection, and meaning making, that offer tools for memory processing, also in the implicit realm (Gerge et al., 2019; Hass-Cohen, 2016; Hass-Cohen & Findlay, 2019; Lane et al., 2015). This knowledge could be anchored in experiential learning through artistic exercises involving memory and reminiscence. Using creative means, I guide students to bring to mind events from their past, clarifying that long-term memory is deeply rooted in their sensorium and embodied engagement, as dynamic representations. While reactivating old memories, emotional arousal is induced, reactivated memories are susceptible to modifications, and new facets of the revised memory may be formed.

Recognizing this potential can instill hope that although events of the past cannot be changed, the subjective meaning of the memories associated with them can be changed (Sweatt, 2016). Furthermore, the relational context can help clients' brains overwrite rigid associations learned from earlier dysfunctional relationships and between the trauma memory and intense negative emotions. Through artistic intersubjective experiences one could reconfigure self-narratives, as an interactive agent of transformation.

Summary and final conclusions

Bringing neuroscience perspectives, vocabulary and insights into the CATs arena by teaching these disciplines side by side fosters integration processes in the therapeutic landscape. Recognizing relevant brain mechanisms, psychopathological shifts and ways in which therapy may tap into brain function, could support the acquisition of clinical skills, sparking discussions about development, case formulation, and the therapeutic process. Such interdisciplinary integration processes are supported by the accompanying questions raised, regarding the manner in which the neuroscientific knowledge affects the way students understand their personal and clinical experiences, their clients, themselves, and the therapeutic relationship and processes of change.

The human brain is endowed with generative mechanisms, mapping sensation and action, subserving processing of salient social cues, as well as the ability to develop and change in an experience-based way. It is within a containing relationship and transformative bonds that the client (and therapist) can be challenged, and new avenues for creativity and for personal and social development, can be promoted. The holistic conceptualization of the brain-body-mind coincides with and signifies the emotionally-oriented expressive forms of CATs, encompassing multisensory experiences, agency-driven aesthetic exploration, symbolization and reflective processing. The integrative nature of CATs provides ground for an optimized communication between brain networks that may lead to the constitution of a more coherent sense of self and uniquely shape relational experiences. The inclusion of neuroscience in CATs training, grounded in experiential and reflective modes of teaching and learning, would enable deeper psychic understandings and promote the burgeoning of enriched, multidisciplinary, creative education and practice.

References

Abraham, E., Raz, G., Zagoory-Sharon, O., Feldman, R. (2018) Empathy networks in the parental brain and their long-term effects on children's stress reactivity and behavior adaptation. *Neuropsychologia*, 116, 75-85.

Admon, R., Vaisvaser, S., Erlich, N., Lin, T., Shapira-Lichter, I., Fruchter, E., Gazit, T., Hendler, T. (2018) The role of the amygdala in enhanced remembrance of negative episodes and acquired negativity of related neutral cues. *Biological Psychology*, 139, 17-24.

Admon, Roee, Milad, M. R., Hendler, T. (2013) A causal model of post-traumatic stress disorder: Disentangling predisposed from acquired neural abnormalities. *Trends in Cognitive Sciences*, 17(7), 337-347.

Andrewes, D. G., Jenkins, L. M. (2019) The Role of the Amygdala and the Ventromedial Prefrontal Cortex in Emotional Regulation: Implications for Post-traumatic Stress Disorder. *Neuropsychology Review*, *29(*2), 220-243.

Atzil, S., Gao, W., Fradkin, I., Barrett, L. F. (2018) Growing a social brain. *Nature Human Behaviour*, 2(9), 624-636.

Babiloni, C., Buffo, P., Vecchio, F., Marzano, N., Del Percio, C., Spada, D., Rossi, S., Bruni, I., Rossini, P. M., Perani, D. (2012) Brains "in concert": Frontal oscillatory alpha rhythms and empathy in professional musicians. *NeuroImage*, 60(1), 105-116.

Barrett, L.F. (2017) The theory of constructed emotion: an active inference account of interoception and categorization. *Social Cognitive and Affective Neuroscience*, 12(1), 1-23.

Barrett, Lisa Feldman, Quigley, K. S., Hamilton, P. (2016) An active inference theory of allostasis and interoception in depression. *Philosophical Transactions of the Royal Society B: Biological Sciences*, 371(1708), 20160011.

Barsalou, L. W. (2020) Challenges and Opportunities for Grounding Cognition. *Journal of Cognition*, 3(1), 31.

Beaty, R. E., Benedek, M., Silvia, P. J., Schacter, D. L. (2016) Creative Cognition and Brain Network Dynamics. *Trends in Cognitive Sciences*, 20(2), 87-95.

Beauchaine, T. P. (2015) Respiratory sinus arrhythmia: A transdiagnostic biomarker of emotion dysregulation and psychopathology. *Current Opinion in Psychology*, 3, 43-47.

Beauchaine, T. P., Cicchetti, D. (2019) Emotion dysregulation and emerging psychopathology: A transdiagnostic, transdisciplinary perspective. *Development and Psychopathology*, 31(3), 799-804.

Belfi, A. M., Vessel, E. A., Brielmann, A., Isik, A. I., Chatterjee, A., Leder, H., Pelli, D. G., Starr, G. G. (2019) Dynamics of aesthetic experience are reflected in the default-mode network. *NeuroImage*, 188, 584-597.

Belkofer, C. M., Nolan, E. (2016) Practical applications of neuroscience in art therapy: A holistic approach to treating trauma in children (pp. 157-172.) in *Art Therapy, Trauma, and Neuroscience: Theoretical and Practical Perspectives*. https://doi.org/10.4324/9781315733494

Berridge, K. C., Kringelbach, M. L. (2015) Pleasure Systems in the Brain. *Neuron*, 86(3), 646-664.

Bickart, K. C., Dickerson, B. C., Barrett, L. F. (2014) The amygdala as a hub in brain networks that support social life. *Neuropsychologia*, 63, 235-248.

Bisby, J. A., Burgess, N., Brewin, C. R. (2020) Reduced Memory Coherence for Negative Events and Its Relationship to Posttraumatic Stress Disorder. *Current Directions in Psychological Science*, 29(3), 267-272.

Bolton, T. A. W., Wotruba, D., Buechler, R., Theodoridou, A., Michels, L., Kollias, S., Rössler, W., Heekeren, K., Van De Ville, D. (2020) Triple Network Model Dynamically Revisited: Lower Salience Network State Switching in Pre-psychosis. *Frontiers in Physiology*, 11, 66.

Bolwerk, A., Mack-Andrick, J., Lang, F. R., Dörfler, A., Maihöfner, C. (2014) How art changes your brain: Differential effects of visual art production and cognitive art evaluation on functional brain connectivity. *PLoS ONE*, *9*(7), e101035.

Buhle, J. T., Silvers, J. A., Wage, T. D., Lopez, R., Onyemekwu, C., Kober, H., Webe, J., Ochsner, K. N. (2014) Cognitive reappraisal of emotion: A meta-analysis of human neuroimaging studies. *Cerebral Cortex*, 24(11), 2981-2990.

Chatterjee, A., Vartanian, O. (2016). Neuroscience of aesthetics. *Annals of the New York Academy of Sciences*, 1369(1), 172-194.

Cozolino, L. (2014) *The neuroscience of human relationships: Attachment and the developing social brain* (Second Ed.). W. W. Norton & Company.

Craig, A. D. (2009) How do you feel – now? The anterior insula and human awareness. *Nature Reviews Neuroscience*, 10(1), 9-70.

Crone, E. A., Dahl, R. E. (2012) Understanding adolescence as a period of social-affective engagement and goal flexibility. *Nature Reviews Neuroscience*, 13(9), 636-650.

Cruz-Garza, J. G., Chatufale, G., Robleto, D., Contreras-Vidal, J. L. (2019) Your Brain on Art: A New Paradigm to Study Artistic Creativity Based on the 'Exquisite Corpse' Using Mobile Brain-Body Imaging. In *Brain Art* (pp. 283–308).

Curley, J. P., Champagne, F. A. (2016) Influence of maternal care on the developing brain: Mechanisms, temporal dynamics and sensitive periods. *Frontiers in Neuroendocrinology*, 40, 52-66.

Dahlgren, K., Ferris, C., Hamann, S. (2020) Neural correlates of successful emotional episodic encoding and retrieval: An SDM meta-analysis of neuroimaging studies. *Neuropsychologia*, 143, 107495.

Damme, K. S., Young, C. B., Nusslock, R. (2017) Elevated nucleus accumbens structural connectivity associated with proneness to hypomania: A reward hypersensitivity perspective. *Social Cognitive and Affective Neuroscience*, 12(6), 928-936.

De Kloet, E. R., Joëls, M., Holsboer, F. (2005) Stress and the brain: From adaptation to disease. *Nature Reviews Neuroscience*, 6(6), 463-475.

De Kloet, E. R., Oitzl, M. S., Joëls, M. (1999) Stress and cognition: Are corticosteroids good or bad guys? *Trends in Neurosciences*, 22(10), 422-426.

Di Noto, P. M., Newman, L., Wall, S., Einstein, G. (2013) The hermunculus: What is known about the representation of the female body in the brain? *Cerebral Cortex*, 23(5), 1005-1013.

Di Plinio, S., Perrucci, M. G., Aleman, A., Ebisch, S. J. H. (2020) I am Me: Brain systems integrate and segregate to establish a multidimensional sense of self. *NeuroImage*, 205, 116284.

Engel, A. K., Maye, A., Kurthen, M., König, P. (2013). Where's the action? The pragmatic turn in cognitive science. *Trends in Cognitive Sciences*, 17(5), 202 209.

Etkin, A., Büchel, C., Gross, J. J. (2015) The neural bases of emotion regulation. *Nature Reviews Neuroscience*, 16(11), 693-700.

Fan, J., Liu, W., Xia, J., Li, S., Gao, F., Zhu, J., Han, Y., Zhou, H., Liao, H., Yi, J., Tan, C., Zhu, X. (2021) Childhood trauma is associated with elevated anhedonia and altered core reward circuitry in major depression patients and controls. *Human Brain Mapping*, 42(2), 286-297.

Feldman, R. (2017) The Neurobiology of Human Attachments. *Trends in Cognitive Sciences*, 21(2), 80-99.

Feldman, R. (2020) What is resilience: an affiliative neuroscience approach. *World Psychiatry*, 19(2), 132-150.

Forbes, E. E., Casement, M. D., Forbes, E. E., Casement, M. D. (2019) Reward Disruption in the Development of Depression in *The Oxford Handbook of Positive Emotion and Psychopathology*.

Frankland, P. W., Bontempi, B. (2005) The organization of recent and remote memories. *Nature Reviews Neuroscience*, *6*(2), 119-130.

Freud, S., Freud, S. (1895) Project for a scientific psychology. In *The origins of psycho-analysis: Letters to Wilhelm Fliess, drafts and notes:*

1887-1902.
Friston, K. (2010) The free-energy principle: A unified brain theory? *Nature Reviews Neuroscience*, 11(2), 127-138.
Gallese, V. (2003) The roots of empathy: The shared manifold hypothesis and the neural basis of intersubjectivity. *Psychopathology*, 36(4), 171-180.
Gallese, V. (2014) Bodily selves in relation: Embodied simulation as second-person perspective on intersubjectivity. *Philosophical Transactions of the Royal Society B: Biological Sciences*, *369*(1644), 20130177.
Gallese, V. (2017) Visions of the body. Embodied simulation and aesthetic experience. *Aisthesis (Italy)*. https://doi.org/10.13128/Aisthesis-20902
Gallese, V., Fadiga, L., Fogassi, L., Rizzolatti, G. (1996). Action recognition in the premotor cortex. *Brain*, 119(2), 593-609.
Geller, S. M. (2018) Therapeutic Presence and Polyvagal Theory: Principles and Practices for Cultivating effective Therapeutic relationships (pp. 106-126) In S. Porges, D. Dana (eds.). *Clinical applications of the polyvagal theory*. W.W. Norton & Company Inc.
Gerge, A., Hawes, J., Eklöf, L., Pedersen, I. N. (2019) Proposed Mechanisms of Change in Arts-based Psychotherapies. In *Voices: A World Forum for Music Therapy* (Vol. 19, Issue 2). University of Bergen and NORCE Norwegian Research Centre. https://doi.org/10.15845/voices.v19i2.2564
Gothard, K. M. (2020). Multidimensional processing in the amygdala. *Nature Reviews Neuroscience*, 21(10), 565-575.
Gross, J. J. (2015) Emotion Regulation: Current Status and Future Prospects. *Psychological Inquiry*, 26(1), 1-26.
Hass-Cohen, N. (2016) Secure resiliency: Art therapy relational neuroscience trauma treatment principles and guidelines. In *Art Therapy, Trauma, and Neuroscience: Theoretical and Practical Perspectives*. https://doi.org/10.4324/9781315733494
Hass-Cohen, N., Findlay, J. M. (2019). The art therapy relational neuroscience and memory reconsolidation four drawing protocol. *Arts in Psychotherapy*, *63*, 51-59.
Hasson, U., Chen, J., Honey, C. J. (2015) Hierarchical process memory: Memory as an integral component of information processing. *Trends in Cognitive Sciences*, 19(6), 304-313.
Hasson, U., Ghazanfar, A. A., Galantucci, B., Garrod, S., Keysers, C. (2012) Brain-to-brain coupling: A mechanism for creating and sharing a social world. *Trends in Cognitive Sciences*, 16(2), 114-121.
Henschke, J. U., Oelschlegel, A. M., Angenstein, F., Ohl, F. W., Goldschmidt, J., Kanold, P. O., Budinger, E. (2018) Early sensory

experience influences the development of multisensory thalamocortical and intracortical connections of primary sensory cortices. *Brain Structure and Function*, 223(3), 1165-1190.

Herbec, A., Kauppi, J. P., Jola, C., Tohka, J., Pollick, F. E. (2015) Differences in fMRI intersubject correlation while viewing unedited and edited videos of dance performance. *Cortex*, 71, 341-348.

Homann, K. B. (2010) Embodied Concepts of Neurobiology in Dance/Movement Therapy Practice. *American Journal of Dance Therapy*, 32(2), 80-99.

Hu, Y., Hu, Y., Li, X., Pan, Y., Cheng, X. (2017) Brain-to-brain synchronization across two persons predicts mutual prosociality. *Social Cognitive and Affective Neuroscience*, 12(12), 1835-1844.

Jola, C., McAleer, P. M. A. P., Grosbras, M. H., Love, S. A., Morison, G., Pollick, F. E. (2013) Uni-and multisensory brain areas are synchronised across spectators when watching unedited dance recordings. *I-Perception*, 4(4), 265-284.

Kaimal, G., Ayaz, H., Herres, J., Dieterich-Hartwell, R., Makwana, B., Kaiser, D. H., Nasser, J. A. (2017) Functional near-infrared spectroscopy assessment of reward perception based on visual self-expression: Coloring, doodling, and free drawing. *Arts in Psychotherapy*, *55*, 85-92.

Kanske, P., Böckler, A., Trautwein, F. M., Singer, T. (2015) Dissecting the social brain: Introducing the EmpaToM to reveal distinct neural networks and brain-behavior relations for empathy and Theory of Mind. *NeuroImage*, 122, 6-19.

Kim, M. J., Loucks, R. A., Palmer, A. L., Brown, A. C., Solomon, K. M., Marchante, A. N., Whalen, P. J. (2011) The structural and functional connectivity of the amygdala: From normal emotion to pathological anxiety. *Behavioural Brain Research*, 223(2), 403-410.

King, J. L. (2018) Summary of Twenty-First Century Great Conversations in Art, Neuroscience and Related Therapeutics. *Frontiers in Psychology*, 9, 1428.

King, J. L., Kaimal, G., Konopka, L., Belkofer, C., Strang, C. E. (2019). Practical Applications of Neuroscience-Informed Art Therapy. *Art Therapy*, 36(3), 149-156.

King, J., Parada, F. J. (2020) Using Mobile Brain/body Imaging to Advance Research in Arts, Health & Related Therapeutics. *OSF Preprints*. https://doi.org/https://doi.org/10.31219/osf.io/2avhw

Kleinmintz, O. M., Ivancovsky, T., Shamay-Tsoory, S. G. (2019) The twofold model of creativity: the neural underpinnings of the generation and evaluation of creative ideas. *Current Opinion in Behavioral*

Sciences, 27, 131-138.

Koch, S. C. (2017). Arts and health: Active factors and a theory framework of embodied aesthetics. *Arts in Psychotherapy*, 54, 85-91.

Koch, S. C., Fuchs, T. (2011) Embodied arts therapies. *Arts in Psychotherapy*, 38(4), 276-280.

Lane, R. D., Ryan, L., Nadel, L., Greenberg, L. (2015) Memory reconsolidation, emotional arousal, and the process of change in psychotherapy: New insights from brain science. *Behavioral and Brain Sciences*, 38. https://doi.org/10.1017/S0140525X14000041

Lepousez, G., Nissant, A., Lledo, P. M. (2015). Adult neurogenesis and the future of the rejuvenating brain circuits. *Neuron*, 86(2), 387-401.

Lindquist, K. A., Satpute, A. B., Wager, T. D., Weber, J., Barrett, L. F. (2016) The Brain Basis of Positive and Negative Affect: Evidence from a Meta-Analysis of the Human Neuroimaging Literature. *Cerebral Cortex*, 26(5), 1910-1922.

Long, M., Verbeke, W., Ein-Dor, T., Vrtička, P. (2020) A functional neuro-anatomical model of human attachment (NAMA): Insights from first- and second-person social neuroscience. *Cortex*, 126, 281-321.

Magsamen, S. (2019) Your Brain on Art: The Case for Neuroaesthetics. *Cerebrum: The Dana Forum on Brain Science*.

Mather, M., Thayer, J. F. (2018) How heart rate variability affects emotion regulation brain networks. *Current Opinion in Behavioral Sciences*, 19, 98-104.

McGaugh, J. L. (2004) The amygdala modulates the consolidation of memories of emotionally arousing experiences. *Annual Review of Neuroscience*, 27, 1-28.

McGaugh, J. L. (2013) Making lasting memories: Remembering the significant. *Proceedings of the National Academy of Sciences of the United States of America*, 110, 10402-10407.

Menon, V. (2011) Large-scale brain networks and psychopathology: A unifying triple network model. *Trends in Cognitive Sciences*, 15(10), 483-506.

Monfils, M. H., Holmes, E. A. (2018) Memory boundaries: opening a window inspired by reconsolidation to treat anxiety, trauma-related, and addiction disorders. *The Lancet Psychiatry*, 5(12), 1032-1042.

Müller, V., Sänger, J., Lindenberger, U. (2013). Intra- and Inter-Brain Synchronization during Musical Improvisation on the Guitar. *PLoS ONE*, 8(9), e73852. https://doi.org/10.1371/journal.pone.0073852

Nadal, M., Chatterjee, A. (2019) Neuroaesthetics and art's diversity and universality. *Wiley Interdisciplinary Reviews: Cognitive Science*, 10(3), e1487. https://doi.org/10.1002/wcs.1487

O'Kelly, J., Fachner, J. C., Tervaniemi, M., Nagarajan, S. S. (2016) Editorial: Dialogues in music therapy and music neuroscience: Collaborative understanding driving clinical advances. *Frontiers in Human Neuroscience*, 10, 585. https://doi.org/10.3389/fnhum.2016.00585

Ogden, P., Minton, K., Pain, C. (2006) Trauma and the body: a sensorimotor approach to psychotherapy. In *British Journal of Guidance & Counselling*. Norton. https://doi.org/10.1080/03069880903166509

Panksepp, J. (1998) *Affective neuroscience: the foundations of human and animal emotions*. Oxford University Press.

Panksepp, J., Solms, M. (2012) What is neuropsychoanalysis? Clinically relevant studies of the minded brain. *Trends in Cognitive Sciences*, 16(1), 6-8.

Payne, H. (2017) The Psycho-neurology of Embodiment with Examples from Authentic Movement and Laban Movement Analysis. *American Journal of Dance Therapy*, 39(2), 163-178.

Perryman, K., Blisard, P., Moss, R. (2019) Using Creative Arts in Trauma Therapy: The Neuroscience of Healing. *Journal of Mental Health Counseling*, 41(1), 80-94.

Pessoa, L. (2017) A Network Model of the Emotional Brain. *Trends in Cognitive Sciences*, 21(5), 357-371.

Phelps, E. A., Hofmann, S. G. (2019). Memory editing from science fiction to clinical practice. *Nature*, 572, 43-50.

Phelps, E. A., LeDoux, J. E. (2005) Contributions of the amygdala to emotion processing: From animal models to human behavior. *Neuron*, 48(2), 175-187.

Porges, S. W. (2007) The polyvagal perspective. *Biological Psychology*, 74(2), 116-143.

Porges, S. W. (2011) The polyvagal theory: Neurophysiological foundations of emotions, attachment, communication, and self-regulation. In *The polyvagal theory: Neurophysiological foundations of emotions, attachment, communication, and self-regulation.* WW Norton & Company.

Porges, S. W., Dana, D. (2018) Clinical Applications of The Polyvagal Theory: The Emergency of Polyvagal-Informed Therapies. In *Clinical applications of the polyvagal theory: The emergence of polyvagal-informed therapies*.

Price, R. B., Duman, R. (2020) Neuroplasticity in cognitive and psychological mechanisms of depression: an integrative model. *Molecular Psychiatry*, 25(3), 530-543.

Raichle, M. E. (2015) The Brain's Default Mode Network. *Annual Review of Neuroscience*, 38, 433-447.

Raz, G., Jacob, Y., Gonen, T., Winetraub, Y., Flash, T., Soreq, E., Hendler, T. (2014) Cry for her or cry with her: Context-dependent dissociation of two modes of cinematic empathy reflected in network cohesion dynamics. *Social Cognitive and Affective Neuroscience*, 9(1), 30-38.

Reddish, P., Fischer, R., Bulbulia, J. (2013) Let's Dance Together: Synchrony, Shared Intentionality and Cooperation. *PLoS ONE*, 8(8), e71182. https://doi.org/10.1371/journal.pone.0071182

Reindl, V., Gerloff, C., Scharke, W., Konrad, K. (2018) Brain-to-brain synchrony in parent-child dyads and the relationship with emotion regulation revealed by fNIRS-based hyperscanning. *NeuroImage*, 178, 493-502.

Rizzolatti, G., Fadiga, L., Gallese, V., Fogassi, L. (1996) Premotor cortex and the recognition of motor actions. *Cognitive Brain Research*, 3(2), 131-141.

Sachs, M. E., Habibi, A., Damasio, A., Kaplan, J. T. (2020) Dynamic intersubject neural synchronization reflects affective responses to sad music. *NeuroImage*, 218, 116512.

Samaritter, R. (2018) The aesthetic turn in mental health: Reflections on an explorative study into practices in the arts therapies. *Behavioral Sciences*, 8(4), 41.

Sampaio-Baptista, C., Johansen-Berg, H. (2017) White Matter Plasticity in the Adult Brain. *Neuron*, 96(6), 1239-1251.

Schore, J. R., Schore, A. N. (2008) Modern attachment theory: The central role of affect regulation in development and treatment. *Clinical Social Work Journal*, 36(1), 9-20.

Seeley, W. W. (2019) The Salience Network: A Neural System for Perceiving and Responding to Homeostatic Demands. *The Journal of Neuroscience: The Official Journal of the Society for Neuroscience*, 39(50), 9878-9882.

Seeley, W. W., Menon, V., Schatzberg, A. F., Keller, J., Glover, G. H., Kenna, H., Reiss, A. L., Greicius, M. D. (2007) Dissociable intrinsic connectivity networks for salience processing and executive control. *Journal of Neuroscience*, 27(9), 2349-2356.

Shamay-Tsoory, S. G. (2011) The neural bases for empathy. *Neuroscientist*, 17(1), 18-24.

Shi, L., Sun, J., Xia, Y., Ren, Z., Chen, Q., Wei, D., Yang, W., Qiu, J. (2018) Large-scale brain network connectivity underlying creativity in resting-state and task fMRI: Cooperation between default network and frontal-parietal network. *Biological Psychology*, 135, 102-111.

Siegel, D. J. (1999) *The developing mind: How relationships and the brain interact to shape who we are*. Guilford Press.

Siegel, D. J. (2002) the brain in the palm of your hand. *Psychotherapy Networker*, *26*, 33.

Siegel, D. J. (2015) *Brainstorm: The power and purpose of the teenage brain.* Penguin.

Siegel, D. J. (2020) The Embodied Brain, Awareness, and the Nature of Energy. In *The Developing Mind: How Relationships and the Brain Interact to Shape Who We Are* (third edit). Guilford Press.

Siegel, Daniel J. (2015) Interpersonal Neurobiology as a Lens into the Development of Wellbeing and Reslience. *Children Australia*, 40(2), 160. h

Somerville, L. H., Jones, R. M., Casey, B. J. (2010) A time of change: Behavioral and neural correlates of adolescent sensitivity to appetitive and aversive environmental cues. *Brain and Cognition*, 72(1), 124-133.

Starke, J., Ball, F., Heinze, H. J., Noesselt, T. (2020) The spatio-temporal profile of multisensory integration. *European Journal of Neuroscience*, 51(5), 1210-1223.

Stein, B. E., Stanford, T. R., Rowland, B. A. (2020) Multisensory integration and the society for neuroscience: Then and now. *Journal of Neuroscience*, 40(1), 3-11.

Supekar, K., Cai, W., Krishnadas, R., Palaniyappan, L., Menon, V. (2019) Dysregulated Brain Dynamics in a Triple-Network Saliency Model of Schizophrenia and Its Relation to Psychosis. *Biological Psychiatry*, 85(1), 60-69.

Sweatt, J. D. (2016). Neural plasticity and behavior – sixty years of conceptual advances. *Journal of Neurochemistry*, 139, 179-199.

Teixeira-Machado, L., Arida, R. M., de Jesus Mari, J. (2019) Dance for neuroplasticity: A descriptive systematic review. *Neuroscience and Biobehavioral Reviews*, 96, 232-240.

Tomassy, G. S., Dershowitz, L. B., Arlotta, P. (2016) Diversity Matters: A Revised Guide to Myelination. *Trends in Cell Biology*, 26(2), 135-147.

Uddin, L. Q. (2015). Salience processing and insular cortical function and dysfunction. *Nature Reviews Neuroscience*, 16(1), 55-61.

Uitermarkt, B. D., Bruss, J., Hwang, K., Boes, A. D. (2020) Rapid eye movement sleep patterns of brain activation and deactivation occur within unique functional networks. *Human Brain Mapping*, 41(14), 3984-3992.

Vaisvaser, S., Lin, T., Admon, R., Podlipsky, I., Greenman, Y., Stern, N., Fruchter, E., Wald, I., Pine, D. S., Tarrasch, R., Bar-Haim, Y., Hendler, T. (2013) Neural traces of stress: Cortisol related sustained enhancement of amygdala-hippocampal functional connectivity. *Frontiers in Human Neuroscience*, 7, 313.

Varela, F. J., Thompson, E., Rosch, E., Kabat-Zinn, J. (1991) The embodied mind: Cognitive science and human experience. In *The Embodied Mind: Cognitive Science and Human Experience*.

Vessel, E. A., Isik, A. I., Belfi, A. M., Stahl, J. L., Gabrielle Starr, G. (2019) The default-mode network represents aesthetic appeal that generalizes across visual domains. *Proceedings of the National Academy of Sciences of the United States of America*, 116(38), 19155-19164.

Vessel, E. A., Starr, G. G., Rubin, N. (2013) Art reaches within: Aesthetic experience, the self and the default mode network. *Frontiers in Neuroscience*, 7, 258.

Wen, T., Mitchell, D. J., Duncan, J. (2020) The Functional Convergence and Heterogeneity of Social, Episodic, and Self-Referential Thought in the Default Mode Network. *Cerebral Cortex* (New York: 1991), 30(11), 5915-5929.

Wheatley, T., Kang, O., Parkinson, C., Looser, C. E. (2012) From Mind Perception to Mental Connection: Synchrony as a Mechanism for Social Understanding. *Social and Personality Psychology Compass*, 6(8), 589-606.

Whitfield-Gabrieli, S., Ford, J. M. (2012) Default mode network activity and connectivity in psychopathology. *Annual Review of Clinical Psychology*, *8*, 49-76.

Wig, G. S. (2017). Segregated Systems of Human Brain Networks. *Trends in Cognitive Sciences*, 21(12), 981-996.

Williams, P. G., Johnson, K. T., Curtis, B. J., King, J. B., Anderson, J. S. (2018) Individual differences in aesthetic engagement are reflected in resting-state fMRI connectivity: Implications for stress resilience. *NeuroImage*, 179, 156-165.

Xerri, C., Zennou-Azogui, Y. (2021) Interplay between Primary Cortical Areas and Crossmodal Plasticity. In *Neural Connectivity* [Working Title].

Zamm, A., Debener, S., Bauer, A. K. R., Bleichner, M. G., Demos, A. P., Palmer, C. (2018) Amplitude envelope correlations measure synchronous cortical oscillations in performing musicians. *Annals of the New York Academy of Sciences*, 1423(1), 251-263.

Zamorano, A. M., Montoya, P., Cifre, I., Vuust, P., Riquelme, I., Kleber, B. (2019). Experience-dependent neuroplasticity in trained musicians modulates the effects of chronic pain on insula-based networks – A resting-state fMRI study. *NeuroImage*, *202*, 116103.

CONTRIBUTORS

Ronit Amir, M.A., art therapist for 40 years, a supervisor in private practice. A former lecturer at Haifa University and head of the program of psychotherapy for postgraduate art therapists.
ronit.amiroth@gmail.com

Noga Ariel-Galor, Ph.D., expressive arts therapist and psychoanalytic psychotherapist. Lecture at Ono Academic College, Haifa and Tel Aviv University. Board member of the Israeli Association for Psychoanalytic Psychotherapy and the International Association of Relational Psychoanalysis and Psychotherapy.
ariel.noga@gmail.com

Tsiky Cohen, Ph.D., psychodramatist and psychotherapist in private practice. Senior lecturer at Ono Academic College, and at the Kibbutzim College. A member of The Tel Aviv Institute for Contemporary Psychoanalysis. His research focuses on self-constitution, psychodrama, and psychoanalysis. Author of *On the Brink of the Self: The Phenomenology of Forms of Being and Social Constructs.*
tsiky10@gmail.com

Anat Gilad ,M.A., art therapist, psychotherapist, supervisor, private practice with over 30 years experience. Lecturer at Ono Academic College, Seminar Hakibbutzim College, and the Winnicott Institute of Psychotherapy. Supervisor of staff at the Center for the Treatment of Child Victims of Sexual Assault. Facilitator of workshops in art therapy, especially interested in the connection between Zen Buddhism and art therapy.
anatgil04@gmail.com

Hilla Haelyon, Ph.D., senior lecturer, at the School of Society and the Arts at Ono Academic College. Her research focuses on multiculturalism, gender, education and family.
hilahaelyon@gmail.com

Rachel Hillel-Avraham, Ph.D., Deputy Dean of the Faculty of Humanities and Society, in the School of Education at Ono Academic College. She focuses on multiculturalism, aging, anti-aging medicine and gender, and first generation in Academia.

Debra Kalmanowitz, Ph.D., artist, art therapist and supervisor. Senior lecturer at Ono Academic College. Her work focuses on refugees, social engagement, crisis support, humanitarian aid, resilience and trauma. Co-editor in chief of Creative Arts in Education and Therapy: Eastern and Western Perspectives; Co-author of *The Portable Studio; Art Therapy and Political Violence*: *With art, without illusion* and *Art Therapy in Asia: To the Bone or Wrapped in Silk.*
dkalmanowitz@hotmail.com

Aya Katz, M.A., art therapist and supervisor, private clinic for adolescents and adults. Lecturer at Ono Academic College, and at Ben-Gurion University. Supervising art therapists at the Ministry of Education.
aykapo@gmail.com

Elana Lakh, Ph.D., supervising art therapist and a Jungian analyst, private practice. Senior lecturer at Ono academic college. She specialize in treatment of sexual abuse survivors; studies creation mythologies and her research interests include archetypal aspects of art made in therapy.
elana.lkh@gmail.com

Michal Lev, Ph.D., art therapist, supervisor, and family psychotherapist, private practice. Lecturer at Ono Academic College. She is a social activist, the Israeli representative of International Association for Creative Arts in Education and Therapy (IACAET), and the head of the approval committee of the Expressive Therapies Organization, supporting public legislation for expressive therapies. Her research focuses on intimacy through art, and art-based pedagogy. Author of *Art as a Mediator for Intimacy*; *Painting Intimacy*. Co-Author of *Bridging modalities and playing with identities.*
michlev@gmail.com

Daphna Liber, Ph.D., psychotherapy, psychodrama degrees, with current focus on Clinic in the Digital Age. Private clinic for adolescents and adults. Senior lecturer at Ono Academic College. Head of art therapy programs for a master's degree at the Ono campus.
daphnaliber@gmail.com

Amia Lieblich, Ph.D., Prof. of Psychology, originally from the Hebrew University of Jerusalem. Head of school of society and the arts at Ono Academic College. She has been studying life stories of individuals and communities in Israel and among the international pioneers of qualitative research.
msamia@mail.huji.ac.il

Shevy Medzini, M.A., art therapist and psychotherapist, private practice, supervisor. Lecturer at Ono Academic College. Focuses on treatment of adults and women with infertility problems. She also serves as supervisor to art therapists and social workers.
medzini1@gmail.com

Dalia Merari, Ph.D. Prof. is the Head of the Art Therapy Program at the Academic College for Society and Arts. She holds an M.A. degree in art therapy from Lesley University and a Ph.D. degree in psychotherapy and epidemiology from Tel Aviv University. She is a former chairperson of the Department of Occupational Therapy at Tel Aviv University and a former President of the Israeli Society for Psychosomatic Obstetrics and Gynecology. Her scientific publications are in the areas of psychosomatics, art therapy and psychopathology, and creativity. She is an editorial board member of several professional journals.
daliamerari@yahoo.com

Gili Navoth, M.A., art therapist and supervisor with private practice. Lecturer at Ono Academic College. She has over 25 years of experience in treating children, teenagers and adults.
gili.navoth@gmail.com

Liat Shamri-Zeevi, Ph.D, art therapist, psychotherapist, private practice, supervisor at the Israeli association of creative and expressive therapists. Senior lecturer at Ono Academic College. She founded the Art Based Parental Training model (ABPT).
liatshamri@gmail.com

Janice Shapiro, M.A., artist, art therapist and supervisor, Jungian analyst, senior lecturer at Ono Academic College, teacher in the Israel Institute of Jungian Psychology training program. Israel representative on the international Advisory Board of ARAS Connections. Her private practice includes Jungian oriented experiential workshops on archetypal themes for therapists. She was the head of the art therapy department in the adolescent unit of Eitanim

Psychiatric Hospital for 30 years where she founded the open studio in its present form.
janicesha@gmail.com

Lior Schur, M.A., art therapist, private practice, an artist and curator at Alfred Institute, lecturer and art educator. Specializes in building social programs that combine an educational-therapeutic-artistic perspective. She established a therapeutic department at the Ashdod Museum of Art in Israel. Founder of "Art Animals" - interdisciplinary gallery tours.
liorschur@gmail.com

Yoni Schur, M.A., artist, art therapist and supervisor, private practice. Formerly a senior lecturer at the Academic College of Society and Arts in Israel. He served as Head of Visual Art Therapy Department at the Lesley University extension in Israel for 14 years. Develops models for work practice and diagnosis in the art therapy field. His approach emphasizes the place of the artistic process and the language of art as central and leading in therapy.
yoni.schur@gmail.com

Sharon Vaisvaser, Ph.D., Dance/Movement Therapist, Senior Lecturer and head of DMT program at Ono Academic College. She conducts a private practice and works at the Autism Treatment and Research Center (Association for Children at Risk). She obtained her Ph.D. in neuroscience, focusing on stress, trauma and emotional memory, at Sagol Brain Institute, Tel Aviv Sourasky Medical Center, Tel Aviv University.
ysharonv@gmail.com

Reuma Weinberg, M.A., art therapist and supervisor in private practice in Tel Aviv. She worked as a lecturer at Academic College of Society and The Arts. Former head of the sector of art therapists of the association for children in risk in Ramat Chen.
reuma.weinberg@gmail.com

Hilda Wengrower, Ph.D., Dance/Movement therapist, private practice, and supervision. Senior lecturer at Ono Academic College. Co-head of the DMT section in the Association of Arts Therapies in Israel. Research area: intrinsic health factors of dance in therapy; wellbeing of students in dance movement therapy, migration, arts based research. Book reviews editor of *Body, Movement and Dance in Psychotherapy*. Co-edited *Traditions in Transition in the Arts Therapies*; *The Art and Science of Dance/Movement*

Therapy: Life is Dance; *Dance and creativity within Dance Movement Therapy*.
mshilda@mail.huji.ac.il

Tami Yaguri, Ph.D., holds a degree in philosophy from Tel Aviv University. Senior lecturer at Ono Academic College. A former lecturer in the Philosophy Department, Tel Aviv University; head of the Master of Arts Program in Interdisciplinary Studies at Lesley University Extension in Israel. She is the author of *Human Dialogue with the Absolute*; *Solving the Riddle of Meaning*; *Unraveling Life's Riddle*.
tami.yaguri@gmail.com